REVISED EDITION

THE ULTIMATE
Medical
Mnemonic
COMIC BOOK

DWAYNE A. WILLIAMS

ISAAK N. YAKUBOV

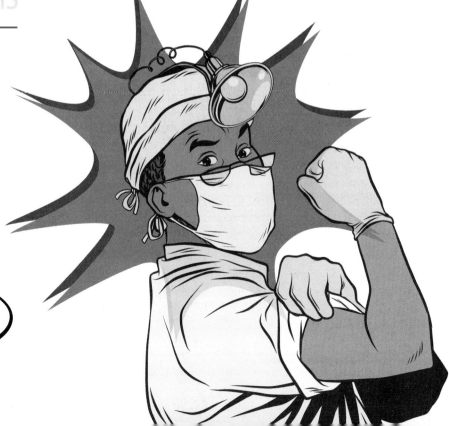

KAPLAN

© 2019 by Dwayne A. Williams and Isaak N. Yakubov

Published by Kaplan Publishing, a division of Kaplan, Inc.
750 Third Avenue
New York, NY 10017

Kaplan Publishing print books are available at special quantity discounts to use for sales promotions, employee premiums, or educational purposes. For more information or to purchase books, please call the Simon & Schuster special sales department at 866-506-1949.

10 9 8 7 6 5 4 3 2 1

ISBN: 978-1-5062-4726-7

Table of Contents

About the Authors v

About the Illustrators vi

How to Use This Book vii

Abbreviations viii

Chapter 1: Cardiovascular 1

Chapter 2: Pulmonary 53

Chapter 3: Gastrointestinal 83

Chapter 4: Musculoskeletal 105

Chapter 5: EENT 139

Chapter 6: Reproductive 159

Chapter 7: Endocrine 185

Chapter 8: Genitourinary 207

Chapter 9: Neurology 227

Chapter 10: Dermatology 257

Chapter 11: Infectious Disease 277

Chapter 12: Hematology 307

Chapter 13: Pharmacology 333

Chapter 14: Procedures 373

Index 393

About the Authors

DWAYNE A. WILLIAMS, PA-C

Dwayne A. Williams has been a practicing physician assistant since 2002 and is the author of the best-selling book, *Pance Prep Pearls*. He currently serves as director of didactic education and as a clinical preceptor for the Long Island University Physician Assistant program. He graduated from the Long Island University program with honors and is a member of the Physician Assistant Honor Society Pi Alpha.

Additionally, Mr. Williams is an adjunct professor for the Weill Cornell Medical College Physician Assistant program (didactic year) and for its PANCE review courses. He frequently teaches physician assistants, residency programs, medical students, and nurse practitioners.

Dedication: This book is dedicated to my PPP warriors and their amazing support; they keep me motivated to work harder. Also, thanks to my family and friends who have been so patient throughout the writing process. God, I thank You for bestowing me with the talents and gifts that You allow me to share with the world. Finally, to my partner, Isaak N. Yakubov, the best is yet to come.

ISAAK N. YAKUBOV, MS, PAS, PA-C

Isaak N. Yakubov has been a practicing physician assistant since 2014, with a specialty in neurosurgery and emergency medicine. He currently serves as a professor at Long Island University's School of Health Professions and at Touro University's Physician Assistant program. He received his master's degree at the Long Island University Physician Assistant program. He is one of the founders of the Flipmed app and is the founder/CEO of LEAA concierge medical service. He teaches board review across the country.

Dedication: I would like to start off by giving thanks G-d for all of the blessings he has bestowed on my family and me. Thank you to Long Island University for transforming me from a student to a medical professional. A huge thank you to my friends, family, and parents; a special thank you to my wife Sharona for being my foundation stone and to Yonah and Caleb. Lastly, I have so much gratitude to my professor and business partner, Akim Dwayne Williams, for being the most amazing, honest, and selfless person I know; you are a true inspiration to the medical community.

About the Illustrators

Ian Baker has been a leading cartoonist, illustrator, and comedy writer in the United Kingdom for over twenty years. His work has been featured in many international publications such as *The Times*, *National Lampoon*, *Reader's Digest*, *Esquire*, and *The Independent on Sunday*. He has illustrated dozens of books including the bestselling *Wit* series as well as writing his own books including *The Codgers' Kama Sutra*, published by Constable and Robinson. His advertising work has included commissions for such corporate giants as Delta Airlines, Thomson Holidays, Merrill Lynch, Shell, Mars Confectionary, JML, Allied Domecq, William Hill, Robinson Healthcare, BBC, and Ryder Haulage. His work in television has included stints as a writer on the comedy series, *Hale & Pace*.

Ngoc (Nicole) Gia Lam has been a physician assistant since 2016. She received her BS from the University of California, Berkeley. She is a Chinese-Vietnamese American and can speak Vietnamese, Cantonese, and Mandarin. Her future goal is to assist underprivileged communities.

Kevin Young is a dancer, artist, entrepeneur, and illustrator dedicated to performance and community outreach for underprivileged youth. He served as a teaching assistant in the area of special education at the Dr. Kenneth B. Clark Academy in New York, and later as director for Cobra Performing Arts, a dynamic drumline and dance team. Most recently, he took on a dance director role with new dance team called Flawless Dance Family in Brooklyn, NY.

Kristen Risom has been a registered physician assistant for over 5 years, currently in the area of orthopedic surgery within a New York City trauma center. She treats patients in both the inpatient and outpatient setting. Earlier in her career she worked as an emergency department technician. She precepts PA students from various programs throughout the New York metropolitan area, and enjoys teaching students new skills and furthering their education.

How to Use This Book

The design of this book is simple:

- Awesome mnemonics to aid in remembering the things you often forget
- Bullet points for last-minute review of significant medical topics
- Useful algorithms and procedures to help ease the life of physicians, PAs, nurses, medical students, and other medical personnel

It is not a traditional textbook but rather a lighthearted, organized approach to mastering many of the conditions you will see in clinical practice.

It is our belief that using multiple sources is the best way to study medicine. Medicine is complex, and it can be taught in various ways. So, laugh at the mnemonics and photos, enjoy the book, and learn in an engaging way!

Note that not all diseases are included here. This book is meant to supplement a traditional/ nontraditional textbook, and should not be used as your sole resource.

Abbreviations

ABE	acute bacterial endocarditis
ABECB	acute bacterial exacerbation of chronic bronchitis
ABI	ankle-brachial index
ACA	anterior cerebral artery
ACE	angiotensin-converting enzyme
ACS	acute coronary syndrome
AFib	atrial fibrillation
AG	aminoglycoside
AGN	acute glomerulonephritis
AI	aortic insufficiency
AIN	acute interstitial nephritis
ALL	acute lymphocytic leukemia
ALS	amyotrophic lateral sclerosis
ANA	antinuclear antibodies
ARB	angiotensin receptor blocker
ARDS	acute respiratory distress syndrome
AR	aortic regurgitation
AS	aortic stenosis
ASA	acetylsalicylic acid (aspirin)
ASD	atrial septal defect
ATN	acute tubular necrosis
AV	atrioventricular
AVM	arteriovenous malformation
AVNRT	AV nodal reentry tachycardia
AVRT	AV reciprocating tachycardia
BAS	balloon atrial septostomy
BB	beta-blocker
BHL	bilateral hilar lymphadenopathy
BNP	B-type natriuretic peptide
BP	blood pressure
BPH	benign prostatic hyperplasia
CABG	coronary artery bypass graft
CAD	coronary artery disease
CAP	community-acquired pneumonia

CBC	complete blood count
CCB	calcium channel blocker
CF	cystic fibrosis
CHD	congestive heart disease
CHF	congestive heart failure
CMV	cytomegalovirus
CLL	chronic lymphocytic leukemia
CML	chronic myelogenous leukemia
CN	cranial nerve
CNS	central nervous system
COA	coarctation of the aorta
CO	coronary output
COPD	chronic obstructive pulmonary disease
CSF	cerebrospinal fluid
DCC	direct current cardioversion
DM	diabetes mellitus
DI	diabetes insipidus
DIC	disseminated intravascular coagulation
DIP	distal interphalangeal
DLCO	diffusing capacity of the lung for carbon monoxide
DTR	deep tendon reflexes
ECF	extracellular fluid
ECG	electrocardiogram
ECRB	extensor carpi radialist brevis
EF	ejection fraction
EGD	esophagogastroduodenoscopy (upper endoscopy)
EM	erythema multiforme
ESR	erythrocyte sedimentation rate
ETOH	ethanol
FQ	fluorinated quinolones
FSGS	focal segmental glomerulosclerosis
FSH	follicle stimulating hormone
FTA-ABS	fluorescent treponemal antibody absorption

GERD	gastroesophageal reflux disease		MAT	multifocal atrial tachycardia
GI	gastrointestinal		MCA	middle cerebral artery
GPA	granulomatosis with polyangiitis (formerly Wegener's)		MEN	multiple endocrine neoplasia
			Mg	potassium
GTT	glucose tolerance test		MI	myocardial infarction
GU	genitourinary		MMA	middle meningeal artery
HAP	hospital-acquired pneumonia		MOA	mechanism of action
HR	heart rate		MR	mitral regurgitation
HIT	heparin-induced thrombocytopenia		MRSA	methicillin-resistant *S. aureus*
HRT	hormone replacement therapy		MRSE	methicillin-resistant *S. epidermidis*
HSV	herpes simplex virus		MS	multiple sclerosis
HTN	hypertension		MTP	metacarpophalangeal
HUS	hemolytic uremic syndrome		MVP	mitral valve prolapse
IBD	inflammatory bowel disease		NSAID	nonsteroidal antinflammatory drugs
ICH	intracerebral hemorrhage		NSR	normal sinus rhythm
ILD	interstitial lung disease		NSTEMI	non-ST elevation MI
IUD	intrauterine device		NVE	native valve endocarditis
IUP	intrauterine pregnancy		OCD	obsessive compulsive disorder
IV	intravenous		OCP	oral contraceptive pill
IVIG IV	immune globulin		ORIF	open reduction and internal fixation
JVD	jugular venous distention		OS	opening snap
JVP	jugular venous pressure		PAS	periodic acid-Schiff stain
LA	left atrium		PCA	posterior cerebral artery
LDH	lactate dehydrogenase		PCI	percutaneous coronary intervention
LDL	low density lipoprotein		PCN	penicillin
LES	lower esophageal sphincter		PCOS	polycystic ovary syndrome
LH	luteinizing hormone		PDA	patent ductus arteriosus
LFT	liver function test		PE	pulmonary embolism
LLQ	left lower quadrant		PEA	pulseless electrical activity
LMWH	low molecular weight heparin		PFTs	pulmonary function tests
LN	lymph nodes		PID	pelvic inflammatory disease
LRS	lactated Ringer's solution		PIP	proximal interphalangeal
LUQ	left upper quadrant		PMS	premenstrual syndrome
LV	left ventricle		PPI	proton pump inhibitor
LVH	left ventricular hypertrophy		PPM	permanent pacemaker
MAC	*Mycobacterium avium* complex		PRN	"pro re nata" (as needed)
MAO	monoamine oxidase		PSVT	paroxysmal supraventricular tachycardia
MAP	multifocal atrial tachycardia		PT	prothrombin time

PTCA	percutaneous transluminal coronary angioplasty
PTH	parathyroid hormone
PTT	partial thromboplastin time
PUD	peptic ulcer disease
RA	rheumatoid arthritis (or right atrium, depending on context)
RAAS	renin-angiotensin-aldosterone system
RBC	red blood cell
RDW	red cell distribution width
RLQ	right lower quadrant
ROM	range of motion
RPGN	rapidly progressive glomerulonephritis
RPR	rapid plasma reagent
RSV	respiratory syncytial virus
RUQ	right upper quadrant
SABA	short-acting beta agonists
SAM	systolic anterior motion
SBE	subacute bacterial endocarditis
SBP	spontaneous bacterial peritonitis
SCC	squamous cell carcinoma
SIRS	systemic inflammatory response syndrome
SJS	Stevens-Johnson syndrome
SLE	systemic lupus erythematosus
SLR	straight leg raise

SNRIs	serotonin and norepinephine reuptake inhibitors
SQ (or SC)	subcutaneous
SSRIs	selective serotonin reuptake inhibitors
STEMI	ST-elevation myocardial infarction
TD	tardive dyskinesia
TEN	toxic epidermal necrolysis
TIBC	total iron binding capacity
TIMI	thrombolysis in myocardial infarction
TM	tympanic membrane
TMP/SMX	trimethoprim/sulfamethoxazole
TOGA	transposition of the great arteries
TPN	total parenteral nutrition
TSH	thyroid-stimulating hormone
TTP	thrombotic thrombocytopenic purpura
UFH	unfractionated heparin
UGT	uridine 5'-diphospho-glucuronosyltransferase
URI	upper respiratory infection
U/S	ultrasound
VDRL	venereal disease research laboratory
vWD	von Willebrand disease
vWF	von Willebrand factor
WAP	wandering atrial pacemaker
WBC	white blood cell

Chapter 1

Cardiovascular

HEART FAILURE

Inability of the heart to pump sufficient blood to meet the metabolic demands of the body at normal filling pressures

Etiology/Pathophysiology

- Initial insult leads to increased afterload, increased preload, decreased contractility

Risk Factors

- Post-myocardial infarction, cardiomyopathies
- Valvular disease
- High output diseases (anemia, Paget's disease of the bone, vitamin B1 deficiency)

Clinical Manifestations/Physical Exam

- Left-sided heart failure: fluid backs up into the lungs
  - Dyspnea (most common symptom), including dyspnea on exertion, orthopnea, paroxysmal nocturnal dyspnea
  - Cheyne-Stokes respiration
  - Pulmonary congestion: tachypnea, rales, chronic cough
  - Pulmonary edema: hypertension (HTN), pink, frothy sputum
  - S3 in systolic failure; S4 in diastolic failure
  - Increased adrenergic activation: dusky, pale skin, diaphoresis, sinus tachycardia, cool extremities (poor perfusion/peripheral arterial vasoconstriction), fatigue, altered mental status
- Right-sided heart failure: fluid backs up into the systemic circulation
  - Peripheral edema in dependent areas (eg, ankles, legs, sacrum)
  - Kussmaul's sign: increased JVD with inspiration
  - GI/hepatic congestion: nausea, vomiting, hepatosplenomegaly
- Systolic heart failure:
  - Decreased EF <55% (reflects decreased force of ventricular contraction)
  - Thin ventricular walls, large ventricular chambers (ventricular dilation)
  - S3 ventricular gallop due to filling of dilated ventricle
- Diastolic heart failure:
  - Normal or increased ejection fraction
  - Thick ventricular walls, smaller ventricular chambers
  - S4 ventricular gallop due to atrial contraction into a stiff ventricle
  - Associated with hypertension, increased age, obesity

Diagnosis

- Echocardiogram (most useful test) measures ventricular function and ejection fraction
- Chest x-ray: cephalization of vascular markings leads to Kerley B lines, butterfly (bat wing) pattern, cardiomegaly, pulmonary edema (if CHF is present)
- Increased BNP may identify CHF as the cause for dyspnea in emergent settings

Management/Prognosis

- Vasodilators: ACE inhibitors, BBs, nitroglycerin, hydralazine (vasodilators decrease afterload)
- Diuretics: hydrochlorothiazides, spironolactone, loop diuretics (diuretics decrease preload)
- Positive inotropes: digoxin, dobutamine, dopamine
- Nesiritide: synthetic B-type natriuretic peptide

In congestive (decompensated) heart failure, manage with **LMNOP**:

- **L**asix (furosemide)
- **M**orphine
- **N**itroglycerin
- **O**xygen
- **P**osition (sit up)/**P**ositive pressure (mechanical ventilation)

> In heart failure, these medications will **BANISH** mortality:
>
> - **B**eta-blockers
> - **A**CEI/ARBs
> - **NI**trates
> - **S**pironolactone
> - **H**ydralazine

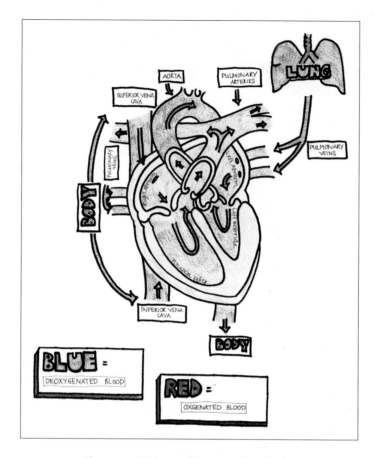

Figure 1.1 Normal Heart Circulation

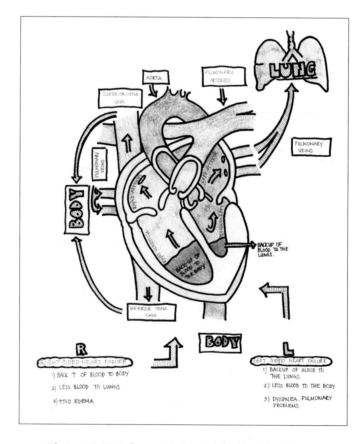

Figure 1.2 Left- vs Right-Sided Heart Failure

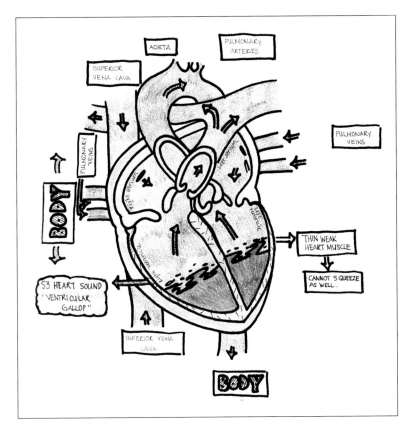

Figure 1.3 Systolic Heart Failure

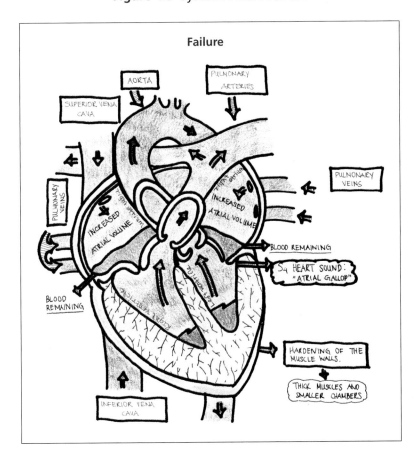

Figure 1.4 Diastolic Heart Failure

ANGINA PECTORIS

Substernal chest pain brought on by exertion (due to decreased supply and increased demand) leading to chest pain

Etiology/Pathophysiology

- Coronary artery disease (most common cause), coronary artery spasm, AS, aortic insufficiency, pulmonary HTN, severe systemic HTN, hypertrophic cardiomyopathy

Risk Factors

- Hypertension, hyperlipidemia, DM

Clinical Manifestations/Physical Exam

- Chest pain: substernal (chest pain, pressure, burning, tightness), poorly localized, nonpleuritic, exertional; radiating to arm, teeth, lower jaw, back, shoulder; duration: usually short in duration (<30 min by definition but typically 1–5 min); relieved with rest or nitrates (predictable pattern); precipitated by exertion/anxiety; Levine's sign: clenched fist over chest
- Associated symptoms: dyspnea, nausea, diaphoresis (sweating), numbness, fatigue
- Physical exam usually normal
- Anginal equivalent: dyspnea, epigastric or shoulder pain (in the absence of chest pain)

Diagnosis

- Primarily a historical diagnosis
- ECG: ST depression is a classic finding; the resting ECG is normal in 50% of patients with angina and may also present with T-wave inversions, nonspecific ST changes, poor R-wave progression, and pseudonormalization of T waves
- Stress test: most useful noninvasive screening tool
  - Myocardial perfusion imaging (stress thallium or technetium): most commonly used in patients with baseline ECG abnormalities; adenosine or dipyridamole are used in the diagnosis
  - Stress echocardiogram (exercise or pharmacologic): increased sensitivity; good to assess left ventricular (LV) function, check for valvular disease, or locate ischemia; dobutamine: positive inotrope/chronotrope
- Coronary angiography: definitive diagnosis; outlines coronary artery anatomy, also defines location/ extent of involvement

Management/Prognosis

- PTCA:
  - Indications: 1- or 2-vessel disease not involving left main coronary artery; ventricular function is normal or near normal
  - Stents: reduces restenosis rates (in 30% of patients); combination of aspirin and clopidogrel is effective in preventing coronary stent thrombosis
- CABG:
  - Indications: left main coronary artery disease, symptomatic 3-vessel disease, left ventricular EF is <40% and critical (>70% stenosis) in all three major coronary arteries
- Medical management: nitroglycerin, BBs, aspirin, CCB

Eating too much fatty <u>SOFT HAM</u> can lead to coronary artery disease.

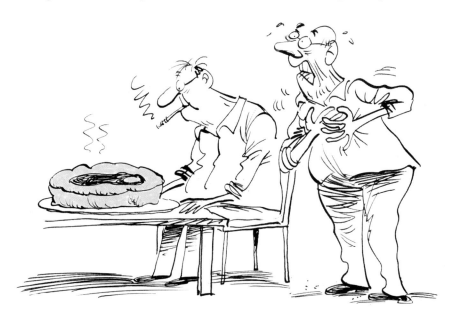

Figure 1.5 Coronary Artery Disease Risk Factors

Fatty (hyperlipidemia)

<u>S</u>moking
<u>O</u>besity
<u>F</u>amily history
<u>T</u>ype 1 & 2 diabetes

<u>H</u>TN
<u>A</u>ge
<u>M</u>ale

ACUTE CORONARY SYNDROME

Spectrum of clinical presentations of acute myocardial ischemia secondary to acute plaque rupture and coronary artery thrombosis (occlusion)

Etiology/Pathophysiology

- Unstable angina: acute myocardial ischemia without evidence of myocardial necrosis; unstable angina is caused by critical stenosis and is a clinical diagnosis (new in onset, increasing symptoms, or symptoms at rest); may not have ECG changes; associated with ST depressions/T-wave inversions, negative troponin/CK-MB
- NSTEMI: acute myocardial ischemia with evidence of myocardial necrosis due to subtotal occlusion: + troponin or CK-MB; ECG: ST depressions and/or TWI
- STEMI: total arterial occlusion (+ troponin or CK-MB, + ST elevations on ECG)

Risk Factors

- Atherosclerosis: most common cause of MI
- Coronary artery vasospasm (2%): cocaine-induced, Prinzmetal variant angina
- Vasculitis: examples include Kawasaki disease, Takayasu arteritis; myocarditis
- Embolism: hypercoagulable states, endocarditis, aortic dissection

Clinical Manifestations/Physical Exam

- Anginal pain: retrosternal "pressure" usually more severe (>30 minutes)
- Sympathetic stimulation: anxiety, diaphoresis, tachycardia, nausea/vomiting, palpitations, dizziness
- Physical exam: usually normal; ± clammy skin, increased or decreased BP, dysrhythmias, CHF; S4 gallop in some patients

Diagnosis

- ECG in ST-elevation MI

Area of Infarction	Q Waves and/or ST Elevations	Artery Involved
Anterior wall	V1 through V4	Left anterior descending (LAD)
Septal	V1 and V2	Proximal LAD
Lateral wall	I, aVL, V5, V6	Circumflex (CFX)
Anterolateral	I, avL, V4, V5, V6	Mid-LAD or CFX
Inferior	II, III, avF	Right coronary artery
Posterior wall	ST depressions V1-V2	RCA, CFX

- Cardiac markers (usually three sets 8 hours apart) (troponin most sensitive and specific).

	Appears	Peaks	Returns to Baseline
CK/CK-MB	4–6 hours	12–24 hours	3–4 days
Troponin I & T	4–8 hours	12–24 hours	7–10 days (most sensitive and specific)
Myoglobin	2–4 hours	4–6 hours	1 day

- Coronary angiography used in the setting of ACS with the goal of revascularization

The LAD will slowly age from 1–4, and when he turns 5–6 he will start to FLEX.

1   2   3   4   5

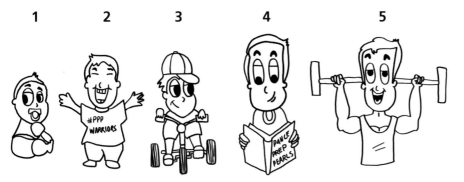

Left **A**nterior **D**escending artery: **V1–V4** Circum**flex** I, aVL V**5** V**6**

Figure 1.6 LAD

Management/Prognosis

- Definitive management: PTCA or CABG
- Medical management: nitroglycerin, BBs, aspirin, CCB if vasospastic disorder is the cause
- Heparin
- TIMI or HEART risk score: used to assess risk of death and ischemic events in patients with unstable angina or NSTEMI ie, to determine benefit of invasive angiography

Historical		TIMI Score Interpretation:
Age ≥65	1	• % risk at 14 days: all cause mortality, new or recurrent MI, or severe recurrent ischemia requiring urgent revascularization
≥3 CAD risk factors (family history, HTN, smoking, increased cholesterol, DM)	1	
Known CAD (stenosis ≥50%)	1	• Score of 0–1 = 4.7% risk
ASA use in past 7 days	1	• Score of 2 = 8.3% risk
Presentation		• Score of 3 = 13.2% risk (≥3 = high risk)
Recent severe angina (<24h)	1	• Score of 4 = 19.9% risk
Increased cardiac markers	1	• Score of 5 = 26.2% risk
ST elevation ≥0.5 mm	1	• Score of 6–7 = ≥40.9% risk

After crashing his **CAR** going **≥65** mph, **TIMI** needed a **CAST** for **3** years!

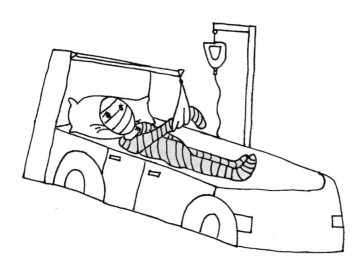

Cardiac marker positivity
Age (>65)
Recent angina (within past 24 hours)

Coronary artery disease history
Aspirin use in past 7 days
ST elevations >0.5 mm

≥3 risk factors for CAD

Figure 1.7 TIMI Risk Scoring

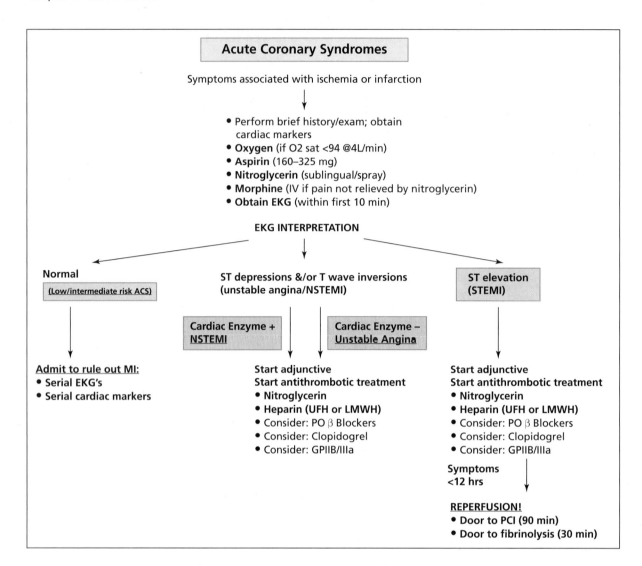

Figure 1.8 Acute Coronary Syndromes

Exceptions For ST Elevation:

- Cocaine-induced MI: O2, ASA, benzodiazepines, heparin, CCB, NTG, NO BBs (cause unopposed alpha vasoconstriction)

- Right ventricular (inferior wall) MI: caution with IV nitrates and morphine use (may cause unsafe drop in preload)

- Viagra use or other erectile meds: no nitrates (drops preload)

Cardiomyopathies are diseases of the heart muscle (myocardium) associated with cardiac dysfunction in the absence of other heart disease.

DILATED CARDIOMYOPATHY

Systolic dysfunction leads to ventricular dilation, "dilated, weak heart"

Etiology/Pathophysiology

- Viral myocarditis (enteroviruses most common), idiopathic, toxic, other: alcohol abuse, cocaine, doxorubicin, vitamin B1 deficiency, pregnancy

Risk Factors

- More common in men than women; ages 20–60

Clinical Manifestations/Physical Exam

- Heart failure: systolic heart failure symptoms

Diagnosis

- Echocardiogram: left ventricular dilation, decreased ejection fraction, regional or global LV hypokinesis
- Chest x-ray: cardiomegaly, pulmonary edema, ± pleural effusion

Management/Prognosis

- Standard heart failure treatment:
  - ACE inhibitors
  - BBs (if not in decompensated CHF)
  - Diuretics: hydrochlorothiazide, loop diuretics, digoxin, sodium restriction
  - Implantable defibrillator if EF is <30–35%
  - Cardiac transplant

The president had an **arrhythmia** when he was about to **VITO** a law that lowered taxes on **alcohol, cocaine, and rubies** in the **REGION** and around the **GLOBE.**

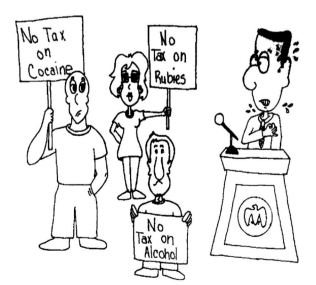

Associated with arrhythmias

Etiologies:
Viral
Idiopathic
Toxic
Other

**Alcohol, cocaine
Doxo**rubic**in

Echo: **shows regional or global hypokinesis**

Figure 1.9 Dilated Cardiomyopathy

RESTRICTIVE CARDIOMYOPATHY

Hallmark is impaired diastolic function with preserved contractility; ventricular rigidity impedes ventricular filling

Etiology/Pathophysiology

- Infiltrative disease: amyloidosis (most common), hemochromatosis, metastatic disease, scleroderma, idiopathic, sarcoidosis

Risk Factors

- History of infiltrative diseases

Clinical Manifestations/Physical Exam

- Right-sided heart failure symptoms more common than left-sided
  ◦ Right-sided failure symptoms: peripheral edema to in dependent areas (eg, ankles, leg, sacrum), Kussmaul's sign (increased jugular venous distention with inspiration), GI/hepatic congestion (nausea, vomiting, hepatosplenomegaly)
  ◦ Left-sided failure symptoms: dyspnea, Cheyne-Stokes respiration, pulmonary congestion (tachypnea, rales, chronic cough), pulmonary edema
- Poorly tolerated arrhythmias

Diagnosis

- Chest x-ray: normal ventricular chamber size, enlarged atria, may have pulmonary congestion
- ECG: low voltage, ± arrhythmias
- Echocardiogram: ventricles nondilated with normal wall thickness; marked dilation of both atria; diastolic dysfunction

Management/Prognosis

- No specific treatment (if hemochromatosis is present, chelation therapy may help; treat symptoms)

AMY, an AMiSH girl, was RESTRICTED from entering the right side of her block because "a tree" that enlarged fell and was too rigid to move.

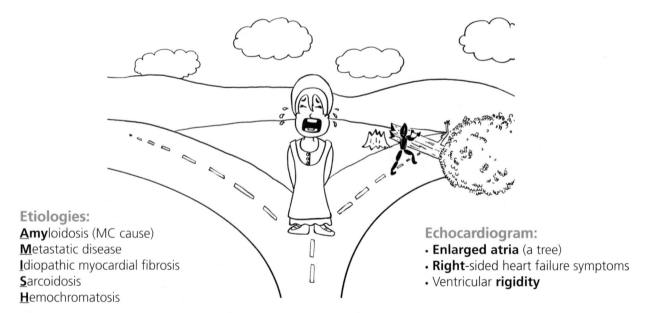

Etiologies:
Amyloidosis (MC cause)
Metastatic disease
Idiopathic myocardial fibrosis
Sarcoidosis
Hemochromatosis

Echocardiogram:
- **Enlarged atria** (a tree)
- **Right**-sided heart failure symptoms
- Ventricular **rigidity**

Figure 1.10 Restrictive Cardiomyopathy

HYPERTROPHIC CARDIOMYOPATHY

Inherited genetic disorder of inappropriate LV and/or RV hypertrophy

Etiology/Pathophysiology

- Subaortic outflow obstruction and narrowed LV outflow tract secondarily to hypertrophied septum, SAM of mitral valve, and papillary muscle displacement
- Diastolic dysfunction: stiff ventricle leads to impaired ventricular filling

Clinical Manifestations/Physical Exam

- Often asymptomatic, first symptom may be sudden cardiac death
    - Dyspnea (90%) most common initial complaint
    - Fatigue
    - Angina pectoris (75%)
    - Syncope (includes presyncope, dizziness) due to inadequate output on exertion
    - Arrhythmias, atrial flutter, ventricular tachycardia, ventricular fibrillation (palpitations, syncope)
    - Sudden cardiac death, especially in (pre)adolescents during extreme exertion; cause is usually ventricular fibrillation
- Harsh systolic crescendo-decrescendo murmur
    - Decreased murmur intensity with increased venous return (eg, squatting, lying down) because increased left ventricular volume preserves outflow
    - Increased murmur intensity with decreased venous return (eg, Valsalva and standing); amyl nitrate

Diagnosis

- Echocardiogram: asymmetrical wall thickness (especially septal) ($\geq$15 mm), SAM of mitral valve
- ECG: left ventricular hypertrophy (LVH), atrial enlargement

Management/Prognosis

- Medical: BB (mainstay), CCB (verapamil), or disopyramide (all are negative inotropes and increase ventricular diastolic filling time); caution with digoxin (increases contractility) and nitrates/diuretics (decrease volume)
- Surgical (myomectomy): resection of the hypertrophied septum (alternative to surgery is alcohol septal ablation)

SAM had a SAD event and DIED from sudden cardiac death from a systole after hitting a thick, stiff wall.

Clinical Manifestations:
Syncope
Angina
Dyspnea.

Di = **di**astolic dysfunction due to **thick, rigid stiff ventricular wall**

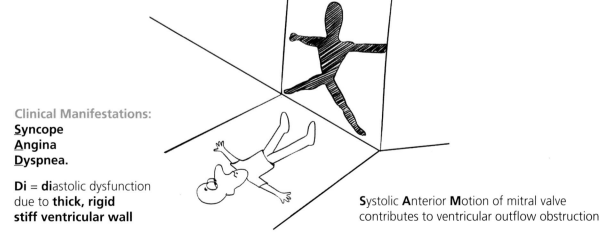

Systolic **A**nterior **M**otion of mitral valve contributes to ventricular outflow obstruction

Figure 1.11 Hypertrophic Cardiomyopathy

MYOCARDITIS

Inflammation of the muscle in the heart; most commonly due to viral infection or post-viral immune cardiac damage

Etiology/Pathophysiology

- Enterovirus and echovirus most common causes
- **Systemic**
- **Toxic**
- **Autoimmune**
- **Medications**
- **Post-infectious**

Clinical Manifestations/Physical Exam

- Viral prodrome: fever, myalgias, malaise over several days leads to heart failure symptoms
- ± concurrent pericarditis: fevers and chest pain, ± friction rub

Diagnosis

- Chest x-ray: cardiomegaly classic (dilated cardiomyopathy); may be normal
- ECG: nonspecific: sinus tachycardia most common, may show pericarditis
- Cardiac enzymes: positive CK-MB and/or troponin
- Echocardiography: ventricular systolic dysfunction
- Other: ESR, CBC, viral cultures and titers (± nasal, mucosal, and/or rectal swabs)
- Endomyocardial biopsy: diagnostic gold standard

Management/Prognosis

- Supportive
- Standard heart failure medications if dysfunction is present

People with myocarditis are **TRAPPED** until they **BUY** a **STAMP** that lets them **ENTER** the country.

Etiologies:
Enterovirus and
Echovirus (most common causes)

Systemic
Toxic
Autoimmune
Medications
Post-infectious

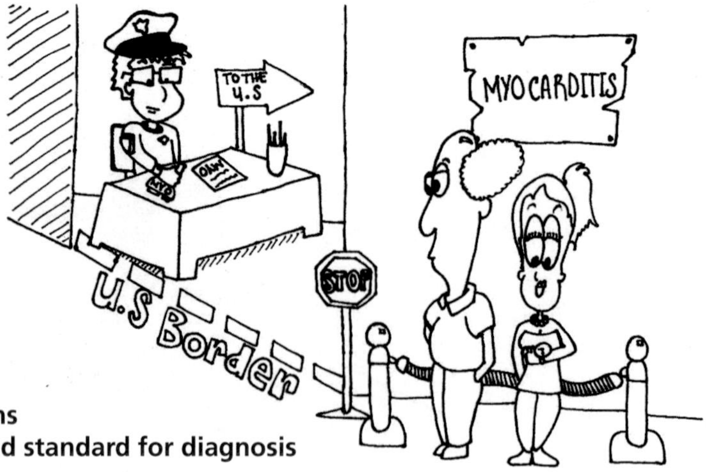

Trap for "Trap-onins": **increased troponins**
Buy for "Buy-opsy": **muscle biopsy is gold standard for diagnosis**

Figure 1.12 Myocarditis

RHEUMATIC FEVER

Acute autoimmune inflammatory multi-systemic illness

Etiology/Pathophysiology

- Molecular mimicry causes a systemic autoimmune reaction
- Preceded by infections with group A β-hemolytic strep (also known as *Streptococcus pyogenes*)

Risk Factors

- Most commonly children ages 5–15

Clinical Manifestations/Physical Exam

- Jones criteria
- Complications: rheumatic disease (valvular): mitral (75–80%), aortic, tricuspid, and pulmonic

Diagnosis

Table 1.1 Jones Criteria for Rheumatic Fever (2 Major or 1 Major + 2 Minor)

Major Criteria	Minor Criteria
"JONES" • **J**oint (polyarthritis) • **O**h my heart (carditis) • **N**odules (subcutaneous) • **E**rythema marginatum • **S**ydenham chorea	Clinical • Fever (38.3–40 C [101–100.4 F]) • Arthralgias Laboratory • Increased acute phase reactants • Increased ESR, C-reactive protein leukocytosis • ECG: prolonged PR interval
Plus supporting evidence of a recent group A streptococcal infection: • Positive throat culture or • Positive rapid antigen detection test and/or • Elevated/increasing streptococcal antibody test (antistreptolysin O)	

Management/Prognosis

- Penicillin G drug of choice (erythromycin if penicillin-allergic)
- Anti-inflammatory: aspirin (2–6 weeks with taper)
- Corticosteroids in severe cases and carditis

Cardiovascular

PERICARDIAL DISEASE

Condition which affects the pericardium, a fibroelastic sac around the heart

Acute Pericarditis

Acute fibrinous inflammation of the pericardium

Etiology/Pathophysiology

- Viral (enterovirus), idiopathic, post-MI (Dressler's syndrome), radiation, autoimmune

Clinical Manifestations/Physical Exam

- Chest pain: pleuritic (sharp and worse with inspiration), persistent and postural (worse when lying down and relieved by sitting/leaning forward); may radiate to trapezius, back, neck, shoulders, arms
- Pericardial friction rub: usually increases when sitting forward

Diagnosis

- ECG: diffuse ST elevations (concave up) especially in most precordial leads; PR depressions (may see opposite changes in aVR); T-wave inversion may be seen in places where previous ST elevations occurred resulting in resolution
- Echocardiogram: used to assess for effusion or tamponade; increase pericardial fluid if effusion present

Management/Prognosis

- Anti-inflammatory drugs: aspirin or other NSAIDS
- Colchicine (second-line management)
- Corticosteroids if severe or refractory

Pericardial Effusion

Fluid build-up in pericardial space

Clinical Manifestations/Physical Exam

- Distant heart sounds because fluid interferes with sound conduction

Diagnosis

- Electrocardiogram: low voltage QRS complex; electrical alternans (alternating QRS amplitudes)

Pericarditis is for **VIP** members only. At resorts, **VIP** members **breathe fresh air** as they **are relieved when they sit up on hammocks and lie down to get rubs from the masseuse.**

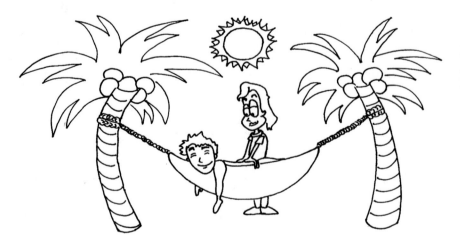

Etiologies:
<u>V</u>iral
<u>I</u>diopathic
<u>P</u>ost MI (Dressler's)
- breathe fresh air =
  pleuritic chest pain worse with inspiration
- sit up on hammocks =
  sitting up relieves the chest pain
- lie down to get rubs =
  lying down reduces the pleural friction rub

Figure 1.13 Acute Pericarditis

Management/Prognosis

- Pericardial effusion: treat underlying cause; ± pericardiocentesis
- Recurrent effusions: ± pericardial window; may need pericardiectomy

Constrictive Pericarditis

Thickened, fibrotic pericardium that impairs diastolic filling of the ventricles

Clinical Manifestations/Physical Exam

- Dyspnea (most common symptom), fatigue, orthopnea; right-sided heart failure signs
- Kussmaul's sign: increased jugular venous distention during inspiration
- Pericardial knock: high-pitched third heart sound

Diagnosis

- Echocardiography: pericardial thickening, ± calcification

Management/Prognosis

- Pericardiectomy definitive treatment

Pericardial Tamponade

Pericardial effusion causing significant pressure on the heart, leading to decreased cardiac output

Clinical Manifestations/Physical Exam

- Beck's triad: distant heart sounds, increased JVP, systemic hypotension
- Pulsus paradoxus (>10 mm Hg decline in systolic BP with inspiration)

Diagnosis

- Echocardiogram: diastolic collapse of cardiac chambers; presence of pericardial effusion

Management/Prognosis

- Pericardiocentesis

BECKy and her **triad** were **DJs** until they died and **COLLAPSED** in their **CHAMBERS** because she failed to put the **needle** to the record, leaving the heart sounds muffled, low pressure in the system, and the neck distended.

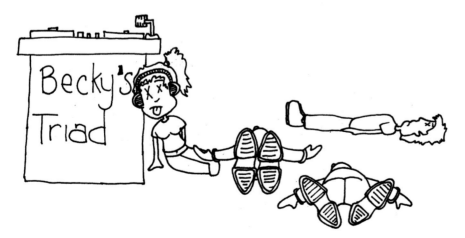

Beck's triad: **D**istant (muffled) heart sound**S**, **J**VD (jugular venous distention), **S**ystemic hypotension
Diagnosis: Echocardiogram will show **collapsed cardiac chambers especially during diastole**
Management: **needle decompression**

Figure 1.14 Pericardial Tamponade

VALVULAR DISEASE

Damaged valve structure that impairs valvular mechanics

Timing of Murmurs

- **Diastolic murmurs—PaRTS** of the **ARMS REST**:
    - Pulmonic Regurgitation
    - Tricuspid Stenosis
    - Aortic Regurgitation
    - Mitral Stenosis best heard in diastole (when the heart rests)
- **Systolic murmurs—MR. AS TRaPS** in Systole:
    - Mitral Regurgitation
    - Aortic Stenosis
    - Tricuspid Regurgitation, Pulmonic Stenosis

Murmur Accentuation

- **Mitral murmurs**
    - MR & MS best heard with patient lying on left side
    - MR & MS mitral must lie down on their left side in order to hear each other
- Inspiration increases murmurs on the right side
    - **Inspiring** people is the **right** thing to do!
- Expiration increases murmurs on left side
    - People who **Expire** are **left** to rest in peace
- **Handgrip**
    - Handgrip **increases** murmurs of **MS, MR,** and **AR**
    - After lying on their left side **MR & MS AR** had a strong handgrip
    - Handgrip **decreases** murmurs of **MVP, hypertrophic cardiomyopathy,** and **AS**
- **Increased venous return**: squatting/lying down increases the sound of both left- and right-sided murmurs (exception is hypertrophic cardiomyopathy and the click of MVP)
- **Decreased venous return**: standing/Valsalva maneuver decreases the sound of both left- and right-sided murmurs (exception is hypertrophic cardiomyopathy and the click of MVP)

When the **MVP** with **hypertrophied** arms **squatted,** the sound of the crowd got **lower** in anticipation.

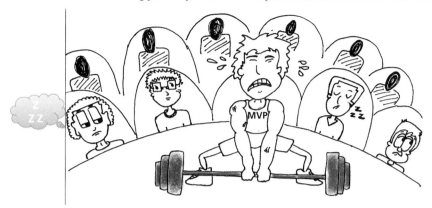

Part 1 of the Valvular Disease Golden Rule: an increase in venous return increases the intensity of ALL murmurs EXCEPT hypertrophic cardiomyopathy and the click of mitral valve prolapse.

Squatting and going into a supine position increases venous return to the heart. With INCREASED VENOUS RETURN, hypertrophic cardiomyopathy murmurs **decrease in intensity** and the **ejection click of MVP occurs later** (and leads to shorter murmur duration IF mitral regurgitation is present with the ejection click–the click can be heard without MR).

Figure 1.15 Increased Venous Return

When the **MVP** with **hypertrophied** arms **stood up,** the sound of the crowd got **louder.**

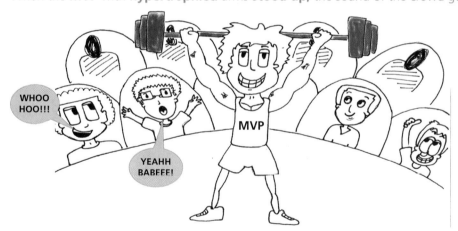

Part 2 of the Valvular Disease Golden Rule: a decrease in venous return decreases the intensity of ALL murmurs EXCEPT hypertrophic cardiomyopathy and the click of mitral valve prolapse!

Valsalva and standing decrease venous return to the heart. With DECREASED VENOUS RETURN, hypertrophic cardiomyopathy murmurs **are intensified** and the **ejection click of MVP occurs earlier** (and leads to longer murmur duration IF mitral regurgitation is present with the ejection click–the click can be heard without MR).

Figure 1.16 Decreased Venous Return

AORTIC STENOSIS

Obstruction of LV outflow of blood across the aortic valve

Etiology/Pathophysiology

- Stenosis leads to left ventricular outflow obstruction (fixed cardiac output), increased afterload (pressure overload), LVH, LV failure

Risk Factors

- Degenerative heart disease: calcifications (atherosclerotic disease), age ≥ 70
- Congenital heart disease: (eg, bicuspid aortic valve), age ≤ 70
- Rheumatic heart disease

Clinical Manifestations/Physical Exam

- **A**ortic **S**tenosis **C**omplications in order of worsening severity:
  - **A**ngina (5-year mean survival)
  - **S**yncope (exertional, 3-year mean survival)
  - **C**ongestive heart failure (2-year mean survival)
- Systolic "ejection" crescendo-decrescendo murmur at right upper sternal border; radiates to carotid (neck); signs of severity: late peaking murmur, paradoxically split S2
- Signs of LVH: LV heave and loud S4
- Pulsus parvus et tardus: small, delayed carotid pulse

Diagnosis

- Echocardiogram: small aortic orifice during systole, LVH, thickened/calcified aortic valve
- ECG: left ventricular hypertrophy; nonspecific changes (LAE, LBBB, $\pm$ AFib, ischemic changes)

Management/Prognosis

- Surgery: aortic valve replacement only effective treatment
- Percutaneous balloon aortic valvotomy (BAV)
- Intra-aortic balloon pump
- Medical therapy: no medical treatment truly effective
  - Mild AS: no exercise restriction
  - Severe AS: avoid physical exertion, venodilators (eg, nitrates), and negative inotropes (CCB, BBs)

AORTIC REGURGITATION/AORTIC INSUFFICIENCY

Backflow of blood across the aortic valve

Etiology/Pathophysiology

- Incomplete aortic valve closure during diastole leads to regurgitation of blood from aorta to LV, LV volume overload, LV dilation, CHF

Risk Factors

- Valve disease: rheumatic heart disease, endocarditis, bicuspid aortic valve
- Aortic root disease/dilation: HTN, Marfan syndrome, syphilis, rheumatoid arthritis, lupus, aortic dissection, ankylosing spondylitis

Clinical Manifestations/Physical Exam

- Acute: pulmonary edema, ± hypotension
- Chronic: clinically silent while LV dilates, leads to LV decompensation, CHF
- Diastolic decrescendo, blowing murmur maximal at left upper sternal border (high pitch); Austin Flint murmur (mid-late diastolic rumble at apex secondary to retrograde regurgitant jet competing with antegrade flow from LA into the ventricle)
- Bounding pulses: secondary to increase stroke volume
  - Pulsus bisferiens: seen with AR + AS together or severe AR; double pulse carotid upstroke
- Wide pulse pressure; laterally displaced point of maximal impulse

Table 1.2 Classic Signs of Widened Pulse Pressure in AR/AI (seen only with chronic AR/AI)

Sign	Description
Corrigan's pulse (water hammer)	Rapid swelling of wrist and fall of radial pulse accentuated with wrist elevation
Hill's sign	Popliteal artery systolic pressure > brachial artery by 60 mm Hg (most sensitive)
Duroziez's sign	Gradual pressure over femoral artery leads to systolic and diastolic bruits
Traube sign (pistol shot)	Double sound heard at femoral artery with partial compression of femoral artery
de Musset's sign	Head bobbing with each heartbeat (low sensitivity)
Müller's sign	Visible systolic pulsations of the uvula
Quincke's pulse	Visible fingernail bed pulsations with light compression of fingernail bed

Diagnosis

- Echocardiogram: regurgitant jet seen with Doppler flow

Management/Prognosis

- Surgical therapy: acute or symptomatic AR; asymptomatic AR with LV decompensation (EF is <55%)
- Medical therapy: afterload reduction with vasodilators (ACE inhibitors, ARBs, nifedipine, hydralazine)

MITRAL STENOSIS

Narrowed mitral valve which blocks blood flow from LA to LV

Etiology/Pathophysiology

- Obstruction of left ventricular inflow leads to increased left atrial pressure/volume overload, pulmonary congestion, pulmonary HTN, CHF

Risk Factors

- Rheumatic heart disease most common cause
- Congenital, left atrial myxoma, thrombus, valvulitis (SLE, amyloidosis)

Clinical Manifestations/Physical Exam

- Slow progression until symptoms occurs, then rapid progression
  - Pulmonary symptoms: dyspnea (most common symptom), pulmonary edema, hemoptysis, cough, frequent bronchitis, and pulmonary HTN
  - AFib: embolic events (especially CVA)
  - Right-sided heart failure: prolonged pulmonary HTN
  - Mitral facies: ruddy (flushed) cheeks with facial pallor
  - Signs of left atrial enlargement: dysphagia (esophageal compression), laryngeal nerve compression, and hoarseness
- Prominent (loud) S1 due to delayed forceful closure of mitral valve
- Opening snap (OS): high-pitched early diastolic sound of the opening of stenotic valve; severity of MS: shorter S2–OS interval and prolonged diastolic murmur
- Early-mid diastolic rumble at apex (low pitched) especially in the left lateral decubitus position

Diagnosis

- Echocardiogram: narrowed mitral valve
- ECG: left atrial enlargement (LAE/P mitrale); ± AFib or right ventricular hypertrophy (pulmonary HTN)
- Chest x-ray: nonspecific, left atrial enlargement (straightening of the left heart border)

Management/Prognosis

- Surgical management:
  - Balloon valvuloplasty: best for younger patients (valve is not calcified)
  - Mitral valve repair/replacement: symptomatic MS, pulmonary HTN; mechanical better than porcine
- Medical management does not alter natural history:
  - Loop diuretics and sodium restriction (if congestion)
  - BBs; digoxin (if AFib)

MITRAL REGURGITATION

Improper valve closure that results in backflow of blood into LA

Etiology/Pathophysiology

- Retrograde blood flows from the LV into the LA (but the refluxed blood in LA returns to LV during diastole)
- Leads to LV volume overload: left atrial dilation as blood backflows to lungs (increased LA/pulmonary pressures) and decreased CO due to diminished effective forward flow

Risk Factors

- Leaflet abnormalities: MVP (most common cause), rheumatic heart disease, endocarditis, valvulitis, annulus dilation, Marfan syndrome
- Papillary muscle dysfunction: ischemia/infarction, cardiomyopathy
- Ruptured chordae tendineae: collagen vascular disease, dilated cardiomyopathy, MVP

Clinical Manifestations/Physical Exam

- Acute: pulmonary edema, hypotension, dyspnea, fatigue
- Chronic: AFib, CHF, pulmonary HTN, hemoptysis

Diagnosis

- Echocardiogram: regurgitant jet, hyperdynamic LV (an EF of <60 results in LV impairment)
- ECG: nonspecific: LAE (left atrial enlargement - P mitrale), LVH, ± AFib
- Chest x-ray: nonspecific: cardiomegaly, ± pulmonary congestion
- Blowing holosystolic (pansystolic) murmur at apex with radiation to axilla (high pitched)
- Widely split S2, laterally displaced PMI, ± thrill

Management/Prognosis

- Surgical repair preferred over replacement:
  - Acute or symptomatic MR; asymptomatic MR with LV decompensation/dilation (EF <55–60%)
  - Intra-aortic balloon pump for stabilization/bridge to surgery
- Medical: indicated if patient not operative candidate
  - ± vasodilators to decreased afterload (ACE inhibitors, hydralazine/nitrates)
  - ± diuretics to decreased preload (decreased amount of mitral regurgitation)
  - ± digoxin (AFib or need for positive inotropy)

MITRAL VALVE PROLAPSE

Myxomatous degeneration of the mitral valve apparatus

Risk Factors

- Connective tissue diseases (eg, Marfan syndrome, Ehlers-Danlos syndrome)
- Most commonly affects young women

Clinical Manifestations/Physical Exam

- Most are asymptomatic
- Autonomic dysfunction: anxiety, atypical chest pain, panic attacks; arrhythmias causing palpitations, syncope, dizziness, fatigue
- Symptoms associated with MR progression: fatigue, dyspnea, paroxysmal nocturnal dyspnea, congestive heart failure
- Stroke, endocarditis
- Possible narrow anteroposterior diameter, low body weight, hypotension, scoliosis, pectus excavatum
- Midsystolic click best heard at apex ±mid-late systolic murmur; any maneuver that makes the left ventricle smaller (Valsalva, standing), results in an earlier click and longer murmur duration (secondary to increased prolapse of abnormal valve with normal valve)

Diagnosis

- Echocardiogram: shows posterior bulging leaflets (with tissue redundancy)

Management/Prognosis

- Reassurance (most cases have a good prognosis)
- ± BBs for symptomatic autonomic dysfunction

CONGENITAL HEART DISEASE

Structural heart defects present at birth

- Cyanotic Lesions:
  - Right-to-left shunt
  - Occurs when right heart pressures are greater than left heart pressures. Blood passes from right side of the heart (without getting oxygenated) to the left side, causing cyanosis. Associated with hypoxia that is resistant to O_2 therapy (the blood doesn't go to the lungs)
  - Cyanotic babies are totally (**TTLE**) blue!
  - TOGA: **T**etralogy of Fallot, **L**ate VSD, **E**isenmenger syndrome
- Non-Cyanotic Lesions:
  - Left-to-right shunt
  - Oxygenated blood from the left side mixes with deoxygenated blood from the right side
  - Non-cyanotic babies make PAs **PACE** from Left to right
  - **P**DA, **A**SD, **C**oarctation (can be both), **E**arly VSD

Cyanotic babies are totally (TTLE) blue!

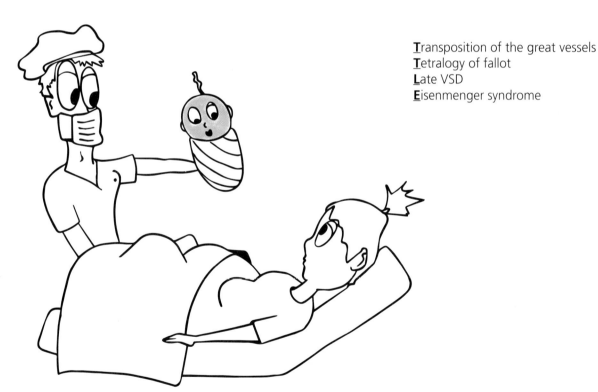

Transposition of the great vessels
Tetralogy of fallot
Late VSD
Eisenmenger syndrome

Figure 1.17 Cyanotic Congenital Heart Conditions

ATRIAL SEPTAL DEFECT

Blood flow from left to right atrium

Etiology/Pathophysiology

- Left-to-right shunting (depending on size)
- Most common type of congenital heart disease (especially ostium secundum)
- Usually asymptomatic until middle age

Clinical Manifestations/Physical Exam

- Symptoms usually minimal in childhood (may present with failure to thrive); adults: exertion, fatigue, clubbing, cyanosis
- "Widely fixed split S2" (does not vary with breathing); loud S1; ± RV lift
- Systolic ejection murmur heard over the pulmonic area

COARCTATION OF THE AORTA

Narrowed aorta that leads to increased afterload and cardiomegaly

Clinical Manifestations/Physical Exam

- Usually asymptomatic
- Bilateral claudication, headache, HTN, fatigue
- Bicuspid aortic valve (70%)
- Increased BP in upper extremities > lower extremities
- Absent/weak/delayed femoral pulses
- Systolic murmur that radiates to the chest/back
- HTN in upper extremities (secondary HTN)

Diagnosis

- Angiogram
- Chest x-ray: rib-notching, "figure 3 sign" on enlarged aortic knob

Management/Prognosis

- Surgical, prostaglandin E1 (maintains a patent ductus arteriosus, reducing symptoms)

PATENT DUCTUS ARTERIOSUS

Failure of DA closure that results in blood flow from descending aorta to pulmonary artery

Etiology/Pathophysiology

- Left-to-right shunt

Risk Factors

- Most commonly affects women, preterm infants

Clinical Manifestations/Physical Exam

- Continuous machinery murmur over pulmonic region, wide pulse pressure, bounding pulses

Management/Prognosis

- Ibuprofen in preterm infants (PGE2 maintains patency of the duct); surgical repair

VENTRICULAR SEPTAL DEFECT

Blood that flows from left to right ventricle

Etiology/Pathophysiology

- Usually congenital but may be acquired (eg, post-myocardial infarction)

Clinical Manifestations/Physical Exam

- Loud, harsh, high-pitched holosystolic murmur at the left sternal border
- Initially, there is a left-to-right shunt; over time, $\pm$ increased blood on the right side leads to pulmonary HTN until the right-sided pressure is greater than the left-sided pressure resulting in a right-to-left shunt (Eisenmenger syndrome phenomenon)

TETRALOGY OF FALLOT

Cardiac anomaly marked by four structural heart defects

Etiology/Pathophysiology

- Right-to-left shunt due to
  - Right ventricular outflow obstruction
  - RVH
  - VSD
  - Overriding aorta

Clinical Manifestations/Physical Exam

- Blue baby syndrome is most common congenital cyanotic heart disease
- "Tet-spells" in children during feeding or crying; older kids squat to relieve symptoms

Diagnosis

- Chest x-ray: boot-shaped heart

TRANSPOSITION OF THE GREAT ARTERIES

Most common cyanotic heart disease diagnosed in the neonatal period

Etiology/Pathophysiology

- 8% of all CHD
- Two parallel non-connected circulations; without mixing of the circulations, there is profound hypoxia (patent ductus arteriosus helps to reduce cyanosis by increased mixing)

Clinical Manifestations/Physical Exam

- Cyanosis is not affected by exertion (crying or feeding) or use of supplemental oxygen; CHF, acidosis, and tachypnea >60 bpm
- If large VSD present or patent ductus arteriosus, there is less cyanosis

Diagnosis

- Echocardiogram: primary means of diagnosis
- Chest x-ray: classic triad
  - "Egg on a string" or "egg on a side" appearance (due to great arteries forming a narrowed pedicle when transposed)
  - Mildly increased pulmonary vascular congestion (despite hypoxemia)
  - Mild cardiomegaly
- Catheterization (angiogram)

Management/Prognosis

- Surgical repair: arterial switch operation is the treatment of choice
- Temporary intercirculatory mixing:
  - Prostaglandin E1 analog (alprostadil) maintains PDA patency
  - Balloon atrial septostomy (BAS): promotes intercirculatory mixing

INFECTIVE ENDOCARDITIS

Infection of endocardial surface of the heart (including but not limited to heart valves)

Etiology/Pathophysiology

- Native valve endocarditis (NVE): Mitral > Aortic > Tricuspid > Pulmonic
  - Acute bacterial endocarditis (ABE): typically, normal valves with virulent organisms (eg, *Staph. aureus*, GBS). Usually aggressive course of illness (days to weeks)
  - Subacute bacterial endocarditis (SBE): typically, abnormal valves (structural valvular disease) with low virulence organisms (eg, *Strep. viridans*) with slow progression (weeks to months)
- Prosthetic valve endocarditis (PVE):
  - Early: (<60 days) *Staph. epidermis* & *Staph. aureus*, gram negatives
  - Late: (>60 days) resembles the pathogens causing native valve disease
- IVDA endocarditis: 50% tricuspid valve involvement! *Staph. Aureus* (most common organism) (especially MRSA), *Pseudomonas, Candida albicans*
- Nosocomial endocarditis: predominantly staphylococci and enterococci. Often related to IV catheters and surgical procedures
- "HACEK" organisms:
  - *Haemophilus, Actinobacillus, Cardiobacterium, Eikenella, Kingella*; associated with large vegetations that may embolize

Clinical Manifestations/Physical Exam

- **"JP ROSS JR"**:
  - **J**aneway lesions
  - **P**etechiae
  - **R**oth spots
  - **O**sler nodes/Ouch (Osler nodes are painful)
  - **S**eptic emboli
  - **S**plinter hemorrhages
- DUKE criteria = 2 major, 1 major plus 3 minor, or 5 minor:
  - Major criteria: **DUKE** = **D**iagnose **U**nder two positive **K**ultures (blood) and positive **E**chocardiogram
  - **JR** = minor criteria = 5 manifestations of JP ROSS ± fever

Diagnosis

Table 1.3 Duke Criteria

Major	Minor
• + blood culture • Endocardial involvement: ○ + echocardiogram: (vegetation, perforated valve, abscess) ○ Clearly established, new (aortic or mitral regurgitation)	• Predisposing condition abnormal valves, IVDA, indwelling catheters • Fever (>38°C [100.4°F]) • Vascular phenomena: Janeway lesions, septic arterial or pulmonary emboli, mycotic aneurysms, intracranial hemorrhages • Immune phenomena ○ Osler's nodes, Roth spots ○ + Rheumatoid factor ○ Acute glomerulonephritis • + culture not meeting major criteria • + echocardiogram not meeting major criteria (eg, worsening murmur)

Management/Prognosis

- Penicillin G and gentamicin or ceftriaxone for 4–6 weeks
- Vancomycin and gentamicin (if MRSA infection is suspected or if penicillin-allergic)
- Good oral hygiene to reduce bacteremia

Table 1.4 Endocarditis Prophylaxis

Cardiac conditions	• Prosthetic (artificial) heart valves • Heart repairs using prosthetic material (not including stents) • Prior history of endocarditis • Congenital heart disease
Procedures	• Dental: involving manipulation of gums, roots of the teeth, oral mucosa perforation • Respiratory: surgery on respiratory mucosa, rigid bronchoscopy • Procedures involving infected skin/musculoskeletal tissues (including abscess incision and drainage)
Regimens	Amoxicillin 2 g 30–60 minutes before procedure (clindamycin 600 mg if penicillin-allergic)

Prophylaxis no longer routinely recommended for GI/GU procedures or for most types of valvular heart disease (including MVP)

CIRCULATORY SHOCK

Inadequate organ perfusion and tissue oxygenation to meet the body's oxygenation requirements

Etiology/Pathophysiology

- **Hypovolemic shock**: loss of blood or fluid volume: decreased CO, decreased PCWP, increased SVR
- **Cardiogenic shock**: primary myocardial dysfunction leads to the heart being unable to maintain cardiac output: decreased CO, increased PCWP, increased SVR
- **Obstructive shock**: extrinsic or intrinsic obstruction to circulation (eg, PE, pericardial tamponade): decreased CO, increased PCWP, increased SVR
- **Distributive shock**: excess vasodilation and altered distribution of blood flow—neurogenic, anaphylactic, septic, endocrine, and septic shock (increased CO, increased or decreased PCWP, decreased SVR)
- SIRS (systemic inflammatory response syndrome) **must have >2 of the following** criteria:
  - Temperature >38°C (100.4°F) or <36°C (96.8°F)
  - Pulse >90 bpm
  - RR >20 bpm or PaCO2 <32 mm Hg
  - WBC count >12,000 or <4,000
- Sepsis: SIRS and focus of infection; often associated with increased lactate (>4 mmol/L)
- Severe sepsis: SIRS and MSOF (multi-system organ failure)
- Septic shock: sepsis and refractory hypotension after fluid administration (SBP <90 mm Hg, MAP <65 mm Hg or drop in SBP 40 mm Hg from baseline)

Risk Factors

- Often associated with hypotension (but not always); a patient may be in shock without hypotension or may have hypotension without shock
- Shock is determined by low SVR or low cardiac output (CO = HR × stroke volume (a function of preload, contractility, and afterload)

Management/Prognosis

The ABCDEs

- **A**irway: may need intubation
- **B**reathing: mechanical ventilation and sedation decreases work of breathing (reducing the oxygen demand of tachypnea)
- **C**irculation: isotonic crystalloids (normal saline, lactated Ringer's); often given multiple liters and titrated to CVP 8–12 mm Hg or urine output 0.5 ml/kg/hr (30 ml/hr) or improved heart rate
- **D**elivery of oxygen: monitor lactate levels
- **E**ndpoint of resuscitation: urine output 0.5 ml/kg/hr, CVP 8–12 mm Hg, MAP 65–90 mm Hg, central venous oxygen concentration >70%

Patients with SIRS criteria will start going downhill (get sepsis) and if they are wearing a hat, it will be FLAT.

Fever >38°C (100.4°F) or
    T <36°C (96.8°F)
Leukocytosis/penia WBC >12,000 or <4,000
    or 10% bands
Accelerated respiratory rate >20 bpm
    or PaCO2 <32 mm Hg
Tachycardia: pulse >90 bpm

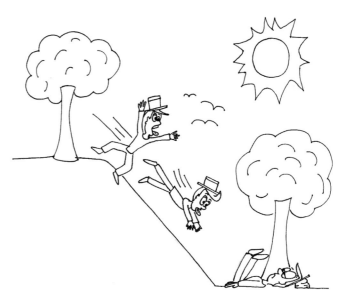

Figure 1.18 SIRS Criteria

HYPERTENSION

Elevated arterial BP

Etiology/Pathophysiology

- Primary (essential; 95%): idiopathic
- Secondary (5%): HTN due to an underlying, identifiable, and often correctable cause (eg, renovascular, endocrine, ETOH)

Clinical Manifestations/Physical Exam

Blood pressure should be based on an average of ≥2 careful readings on ≥2 days. Adults being treated with hypertensive medication are designated as "having hypertension."

	JNC7	ACC/AHA 2017
SBP <120 and DBP <80	Normal BP	Normal BP
SBP 120–129 and DBP <80	Prehypertension	Elevated BP
SBP 130–139 or DBP 80–90	Prehypertension	Stage 1 hypertension
SBP 140–159 or DBP 90–99	Stage 1 hypertension	Stage 2 hypertension
SBP ≥160 or DBP ≥100	Stage 2 hypertension	Stage 2 hypertension

Management/Prognosis

- Goal <140/90 mm Hg
- Lifestyle modifications: weight loss, diet, exercise
- Diuretics: hydrochlorothiazides, loop diuretics, potassium-sparing diuretics
- Vasodilators: ACE inhibitors, angiotensin receptor blockers, CCBs, BBs, alpha-1 blockers
- **Eighth Joint National Committee (JNC 8) guidelines have established important new changes:**
  - BP goal in those age <60 and with chronic kidney disease (after diet/exercise): 140/90 mm Hg
  - BP goal in those age ≥60: 150/90 mm Hg
  - For uncomplicated HTN in non-African-American patients, initial drug should be any one of the following: thiazide-type diuretic, ACE inhibitor, ARB, or CCB

HARASSING others is the MC UN**SAFE** side effect of smoking **CUSH,** drinking **ALCOHOL,** and eating **COCO P**uffs.

Hyper**A**ldosteronism, **R**enal
Artery **S**tenosis (most common)

Sleep **A**pnea
Fibromuscular dysplasia
ETOH (**Alcohol**)

Cushing's syndrome

COX-2 inhibitors
COarctation of aorta
Pheochromocytoma

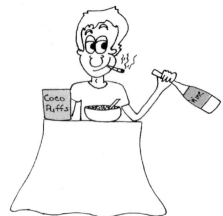

Figure 1.19 Causes of Secondary Hypertension

PERIPHERAL ARTERIAL DISEASE

Atherosclerotic disease of the lower extremities

Clinical Manifestations/Physical Exam

- Intermittent claudication (most common presentation); reproducible pain/discomfort in lower extremity brought on by exercise/walking and relieved with rest; may occur at rest if severe
- Acute arterial embolism: usually caused by sudden occlusion: **6 Ps** (paresthesias, pain, pallor, pulselessness, paralysis, poikilothermia)
- Gangrene
  - Wet gangrene: ulcers lead to malodorous, copious, purulent, infected, blackened regions
  - Dry gangrene: mummification of digits of foot
- Decreased/absent pulses; ±bruits (>50% occlusion); decreased capillary refill, cool skin
- Atrophic skin changes (muscle atrophy, thin/shiny skin, hair loss, thickened nails, cool limbs)
- Pale color on elevation, dusky red with dependency (dependent rubor), cyanosis; if ulcers present, usually involves toes or points of trauma (eg, lateral malleolar ulcers)

Diagnosis

- Ankle-brachial index: most useful screening tool (normal 1–1.2); positive PAD if <0.90 (0.50 severe)
- Arteriography: gold standard
- Duplex B-mode U/S: noninvasive (used for visualizing stenosis)
- Hand-held Doppler may be used to help assess distal blood flow

Management/Prognosis

- Medical: cilostazol mainstay of treatment, aspirin, clopidogrel: ADP inhibitor, pentoxifylline
- Revascularization: percutaneous transluminal angioplasty, bypass graft (eg, fem-pop), endarterectomy
- Supportive: foot care; exercise: fixed distance walking
- Amputation: if severe/gangrene
- Acute arterial occlusion: heparin for embolism; thrombolytics if thrombus; embolectomy

After a **Painful .9** mile walk, **ABI** placed a gauze **PAD** on a **PLUM**-shaped **RASH** she noticed on the **Later** side of her ankle.

Worse with walking
Ankle Brachial Index > .9 = PAD
Pallor/**P**ulseless **L**eg **U**lcers **M**ottled skin
Rubor **A**strophy **S**hiny skin **H**air-loss
Ulcers on LATERAL Malleolus

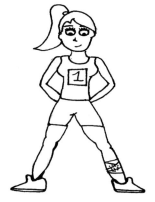

Figure 1.20 Management of Peripheral Arterial Disease

ECG CHEAT SHEET

- **Step 1: Determine rhythm**, regular or irregular? Use rhythm strip (regular is <0.12 sec difference) and note abnormalities eg, dropped QRS, PVC, PAC
- **Step 2: Determine rate**
  - Regular rhythm? 300-150-100-75-60-50 method **or** 1500/number of small squares
  - Irregular rhythm? Number of R waves in a 6-second strip ×10
- **Step 3: Determine QRS axis**

	Normal	**LAD**	**RAD**	If LAD, check lead II; if positive, this indicates a normal axis
Lead I	+	+	−	If predominantly negative, this indicates LAD
AvF	+	−	+	

- **Step 4: Evaluate P waves/PR interval**
  - Look in lead II and V1 for P-wave morphology
    - Sinus? (upright in I, II, avF; negative in avR, each P followed by QRS)
    - PR interval normal? [0.12–.20 sec (or 3–5 boxes)] or is it prolonged/shortened?

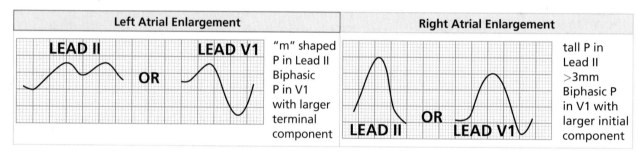

Left Atrial Enlargement — "m" shaped P in Lead II Biphasic P in V1 with larger terminal component

Right Atrial Enlargement — tall P in Lead II >3mm Biphasic P in V1 with larger initial component

- **Step 5: Evaluate QRS complex**
  - Narrow or wide? (normal <0.12 seconds); bundle branch blocks?

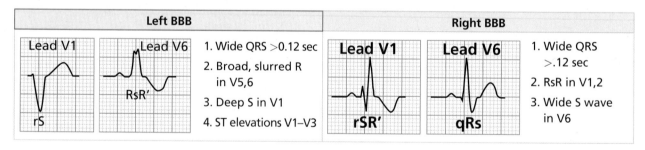

Left BBB
1. Wide QRS >0.12 sec
2. Broad, slurred R in V5,6
3. Deep S in V1
4. ST elevations V1–V3

Right BBB
1. Wide QRS >.12 sec
2. RsR in V1,2
3. Wide S wave in V6

- Ventricular hypertrophy
  - RVH: look at V1: R>S in V1 or R >7 mm in height in V1
  - LVH: S in V1 + R in V5 >35 mm (men); 30 mm (women)
  - Cornell criteria: R in avL + S in V3 >24 (men); >20 (women)
- Pathological Q waves? (Q wave >1 box tall or wide)
- Step 6: Evaluate ST segment
  - ST depression or elevation (>1 mm in height)?
- Step 7: Evaluate T waves
  - Any T-wave inversions (TWI); T wave flattening?

NORMAL SINUS RHYTHM

Impulse originates in the SA node

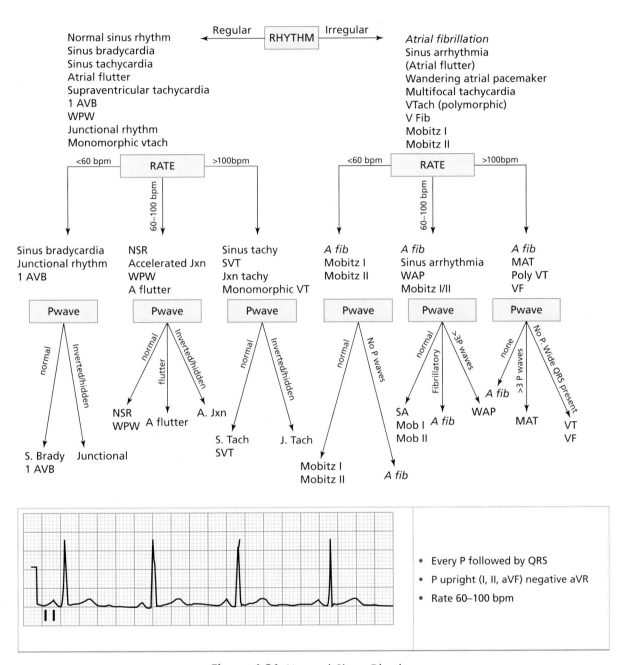

Figure 1.21 Normal Sinus Rhythm

- Every P followed by QRS
- P upright (I, II, aVF) negative aVR
- Rate 60–100 bpm

SINUS TACHYCARDIA

Same as normal sinus rhythm except rate >100 bpm

Risk Factors

- Physiologic: exercise, emotional stress, young children/infants
- Pathologic: fever, infection, hemorrhage, hypoglycemia, anxiety, pain, thyrotoxicosis, hypoxemia, hypovolemia, shock, sympathomimetics (eg, decongestants, cocaine)

Clinical Manifestations/Physical Exam

- Gradual onset and termination

Diagnosis

- ECG:

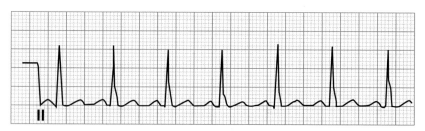

Figure 1.22 Sinus Tachycardia

Management/Prognosis

- None usually; treat underlying cause

SINUS BRADYCARDIA

Same as normal sinus rhythm except rate is <60 bpm

Risk Factors

- Physiologic: young athletes, vasovagal reaction, increased intracranial pressure, nausea/vomiting
- Pathologic: BBs, CCBs, digoxin, carotid massage, SA node ischemia (inferior wall myocardial infarction), gram-negative sepsis, hypothyroidism

Diagnosis

- ECG:

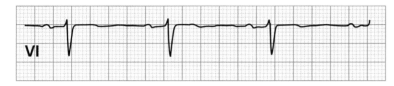

Figure 1.23 Sinus Bradycardia

Management/Prognosis

- No treatment needed if asymptomatic
- Atropine first-line treatment in symptomatic bradycardia
- Epinephrine, transcutaneous pacing
- Permanent pacemaker (PPM) (definitive treatment)

SINUS ARRHYTHMIA

Same as normal sinus rhythm except rhythm is irregular and increases with inspiration

Etiology/Pathophysiology

- Normal variant (especially with slower heart rates)

Diagnosis

- ECG:

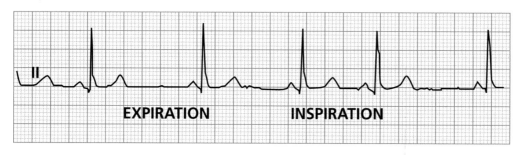

Figure 1.24 Sinus Arrhythmia

SICK SINUS SYNDROME (TACHY-BRADY)

Combination of sinus arrest with alternating paroxysms of atrial tachyarrhythmia and bradyarrhythmia

Risk Factors

- Caused by sinoatrial node disease, corrective cardiac surgery

Diagnosis

- ECG:

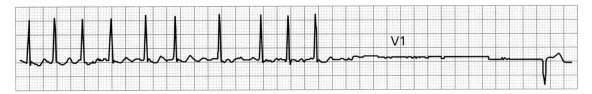

Figure 1.25 Sick Sinus Syndrome

Management/Prognosis

- ± PPM if symptomatic (dual chamber pacing usually preferred over ventricular pacing)
- If ventricular bradycardia alternating with ventricular tachycardia, use permanent pacemaker (with automatic implantable cardioverter defibrillator

MOBY the 2nd got SICK from his SINUSES for the 3rd time, so his BLOCK to receive a PPM was lifted.

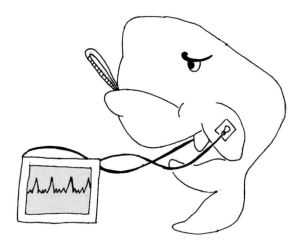

- **Mobitz type 2**

- **Sick sinus syndrome**

- **3rd degree heart block**

Figure 1.26 Candidates for Permanent Pacemakers

ATRIOVENTRICULAR BLOCKS

Interruption of normal impulse from SA node to AV node via AV node and PR interval; helps mostly in determining AV conduction blocks

First Degree AV Block

- Constant, prolonged PR interval (>0.20 sec)
- ECG: every P wave followed by QRS (all impulses conducted from atria to ventricle)
- Management/Prognosis: none, observation

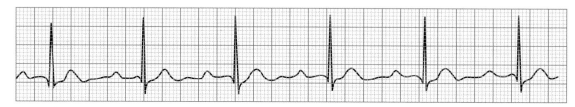

Second Degree AV Block

- Intermittent nonconducted impulses ("dropped QRS")
- **Mobitz I: Wenckebach**
    - Progressive PR interval lengthening leads to dropped QRS
    - ECG: intermittently non-conducted P waves with progressive PR interval lengthening
    - Management/Prognosis: atropine, epinephrine, ± pacemaker if symptomatic

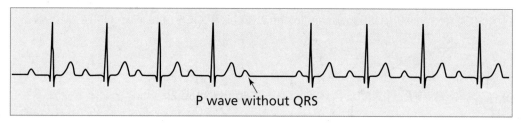

P wave without QRS

- **Mobitz II**
    - Constant/prolonged PR interval leads to dropped QRS
    - ECG: intermittently non-conducted P waves with constant PR intervals
    - Management/Prognosis: permanent pacemaker (high progression to third)

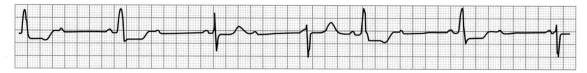

Third Degree AV Block

- AV dissociation with P waves unrelated to QRS
- ECG: all Ps NOT followed by QRS leads to decreased cardiac output
- Management/Prognosis: Permanent pacemaker definitive; temporary pacing

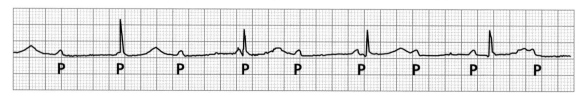

ATRIAL FLUTTER/ATRIAL FIBRILLATION

Irregular rhythms in atria

Atrial Flutter

- ECG: flutter ("saw tooth") waves (no Ps) at 250–350 bpm
- Rate is usually regular

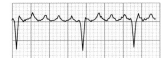

Atrial Fibrillation

- ECG: No P waves (fibrillatory waves at 350–600 bpm)
- Irregularly irregular rhythm

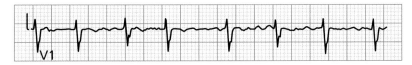

Management/Prognosis

- Vagal, CCB, or BB
- Direct current cardioversion if unstable; DCC also performed after 3–4 weeks of anticoagulation or TEE showing no atrial thrombi
- ± Digoxin
- Prevention of stroke: warfarin or aspirin as prophylaxis against thromboembolism based on CHADS2 score; the atrial quivering causes clots in atria that can embolize to lung/brain

CHADS2 Criteria	Points	Recommended Therapy
Congestive heart failure	1	High risk: ≥2 warfarin (INR 2–3)
Hypertension	1	
Age ≥75	1	Moderate: 1 warfarin or aspirin
DM	1	
S$_2$: stroke, TIA, thrombus	2	Low: 0 none or aspirin

WANDERING ATRIAL PACEMAKER AND MULTIFOCAL ATRIAL TACHYCARDIA

Cardiac arrhythmias due to nodes misfiring electrical impulses

Etiology/Pathophysiology

- Atrial arrhythmia that occurs when $\geq$3 ectopic atrial foci discharge in a random fashion

Clinical Manifestations/Physical Exam

- MAT associated with severe COPD

Diagnosis

- ECG:
    - WAP: heart rate <100 bpm and $\geq$3 P wave morphologies
    - MAT: heart rate >100 bpm

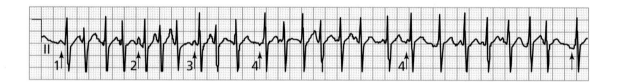

PAROXYSMAL SUPRAVENTRICULAR TACHYCARDIA

Condition that causes episodes of rapid heart rate that begin and end suddenly

Etiology/Pathophysiology

Most commonly preceded by a premature atrial contraction; rhythm originates above the ventricle (supraventricular)

- AVNRT (most common) two pathways both within AV node (slow and fast)
- AVRT: one pathway within the AV node and a second accessory pathway outside the AV node (eg, WPW and LGL)

Clinical Manifestations/Physical Exam

- Orthodromic AVNRT (95%): impulse goes forward (antegrade) down normal AV node pathway and returns retrograde to atria via accessory pathway in circles, perpetuating the rhythm
- Antidromic AVNRT (5%): impulse goes forward (antegrade) through accessory pathway and returns to atria retrograde via normal pathway; this preexcitation leads to a wide QRS (loss of normal impulse delay of AV node)

Diagnosis

- Orthodromic AVNRT
  - ECG: narrow complex tachycardia

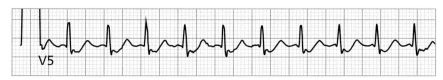

- Antidromic AVNRT
  - ECG: wide complex tachycardia (mimics ventricular tachycardia)

Management/Prognosis

- Orthodromic AVNRT:
  - Vagal maneuvers, adenosine, BBs, CCBs, DCC, especially if unstable
  - Radiofrequency catheter ablation is the definitive treatment for PSVT (destroys pathway in both AVRT and AVNRT)
- Antidromic AVNRT
  - Procainamide or amiodarone
  - Avoid AV-nodal blocking agents (BBs, CCBs) in antidromic AVNRT because AV inhibition by these agents may cause preferential conduction through the fast pathway

WOLFF-PARKINSON-WHITE

Aberrant electrical pathway resulting in tachycardia

Etiology/Pathophysiology

- Accessory pathway (Kent bundle) "pre-excites ventricle"; leads to slurred, wide QRS
- WPW is a type of AVRT

Clinical Manifestations/Physical Exam

- Patients prone to tachyarrhythmias

Diagnosis

- ECG delta wave (slurred QRS upstroke, wide QRS >0.12 seconds) and short PR interval

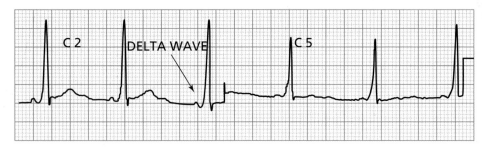

Management/Prognosis

- Vagal maneuvers
- Antiarrhythmics (eg, procainamide, amiodarone)
- Radiofrequency ablation definitive

ATRIOVENTRICULAR JUNCTIONAL DYSRHYTHMIAS

Abnormal cardiac rhythms generated from the area around the AV junction node (the dominant pacemaker of the heart)

Risk Factors

- Most common rhythm seen with digitalis toxicity

Clinical Manifestations/Physical Exam

- Junctional rhythm: heart rate is usually 40–60 bpm (intrinsic rate of AV junction)
- Accelerated junctional: HR 60–100 bpm
- Junctional tachycardia: HR >100 bpm

Diagnosis

- ECG: regular rhythm; P waves inverted if present or not seen; usually narrow QRS (± wide)

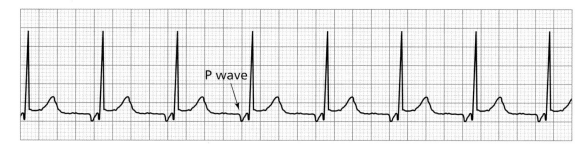

VENTRICULAR DYSRHYTHMIAS

Abnormal heart rhythms that are frequently unstable and unpredictable; stroke volume and coronary flow are compromised; potentially lethal

Premature Ventricular Complex

- Premature beat originating from ventricle
- Etiology: premature beat results in wide, bizarre QRS occurring earlier than expected; usually the T wave is in opposite direction of the R; associated with compensatory pause thus overall rhythm unchanged
- Diagnosis: unifocal (1 morphology); multifocal (>1 morphology); couplet (2 in a row); bigeminy (every other beat is a PVC)
- Management: recall that most ventricular arrhythmias start as a premature ventricular complex

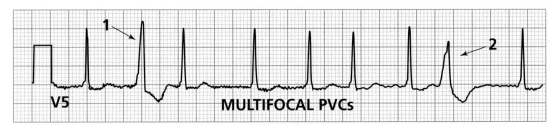

V5   MULTIFOCAL PVCs

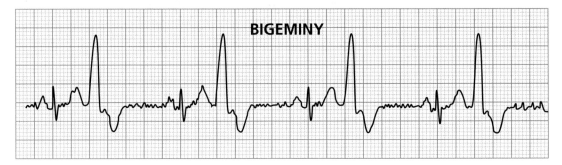

BIGEMINY

Ventricular Fibrillation

- ECG

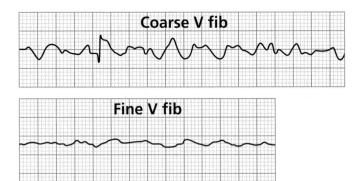

Coarse V fib

Fine V fib

- Management/prognosis: unsynchronized cardioversion (defibrillation) and CPR

Ventricular Tachycardia

- ≥3 consecutive PVCs at rate >100 bpm
- Clinical manifestations: patient hemodynamically stable or unstable? sustained or non-sustained?
  - ◦ Sustained: duration ≥30 seconds
  - ◦ Ventricular tachycardia: prolonged QT interval often cause
  - ◦ Torsades de pointes: most common due to hypomagnesemia, hypokalemia

Diagnosis

- ECG:

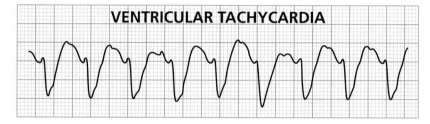

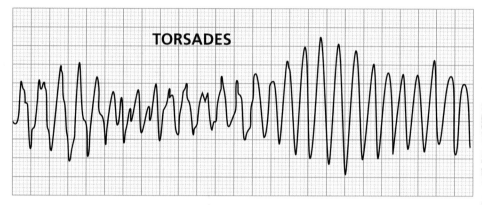

Management/Prognosis

Stable sustained VT	Antiarrhythmics (amiodarone, lidocaine, procainamide)
Unstable VT with a pulse	Synchronized cardioversion (direct current)
VT (no pulse)	Unsynchronized cardioversion (defibrillation) + CPR (treat as ventricular fibrillation)
Torsades de pointes	IV magnesium

Pulseless Electrical Activity

- Clinical manifestations: organized rhythm seen on monitor but patient has no palpable pulse (electrical activity is not coupled with mechanical contraction)
- Management: CPR, epinephrine, check for "shockable" rhythm every 2 minutes

Asystole Rhythm

- Ventricular standstill
- ECG:
- Management: (same as PEA) CPR, epinephrine, check for "shockable" rhythm every 2 minutes

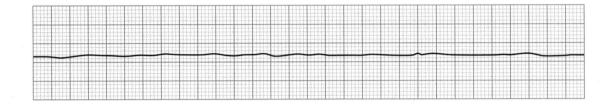

Chapter 2

Pulmonary

LUNG DISEASE

Obstructive Lung Disease

People with obstructive lung disease cannot sing the ABCCCs.

Asthma
Bronchiectasis
COPD
Cystic fibrosis
Coal workers' lung

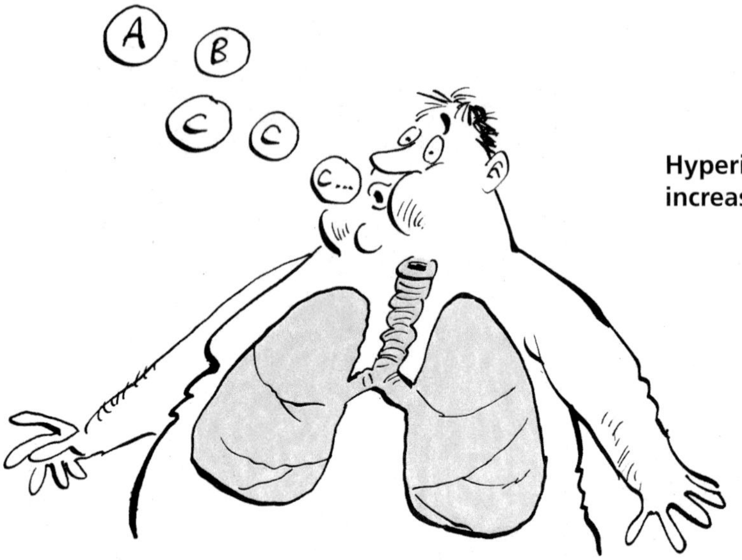

Hyperinflated lungs: increased lung volumes

Figure 2.1 Obstructive Lung Disease

Restrictive Lung Disease

People with restrictive lung disease cannot SIPP from a straw.

Sarcoidosis
Idiopathic
Pulm fibrosis
Pneumoconiosis

Decreased lung volumes

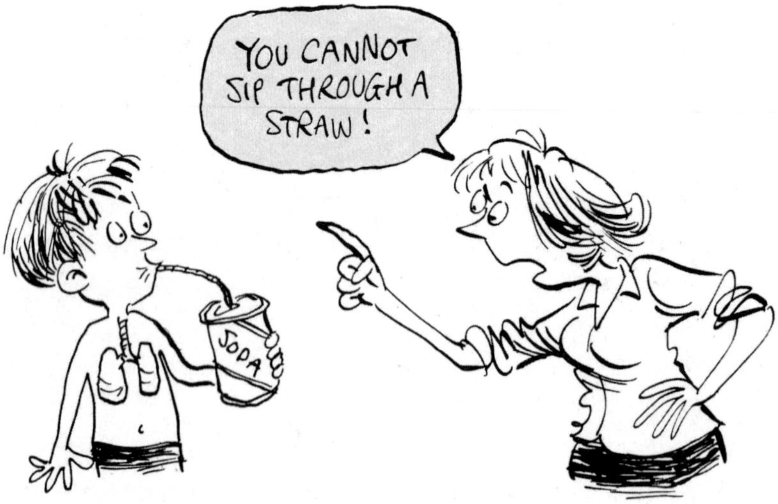

Figure 2.2 Restrictive Lung Disease

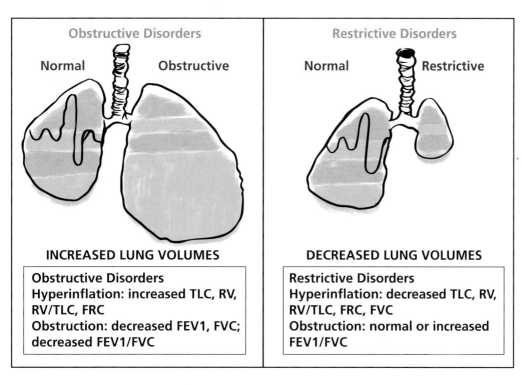

Figure 2.3 Obstructive vs. Restrictive Lung Disease

ASTHMA

Reversible hyperirritability of the tracheobronchial tree resulting in bronchoconstriction and inflammation (airway obstruction)

Risk Factors

- Extrinsic (allergic) asthma: triggers associated with allergies include animal dander, pollen, mold, dust; associated with increased IgE
- Intrinsic (non-allergic) asthma: triggers of asthma not associated with allergies include anxiety, stress, exercise, cold air, dry air, hyperventilation, viruses
- Environmental: smoke and air pollution

Clinical Manifestations/Physical Exam

- Dyspnea, cough (especially at night), wheezing, chest tightness
- Physical exam: prolonged wheezing (especially expiratory), decreased breath sounds, tachypnea, tachycardia, and use of accessory muscles
- Samter's triad: asthma, nasal polyps, and ASA/NSAID allergy

Diagnosis

Table 2.1 Classification of Asthma Severity

	Intermittent	Persistent		
		Mild	**Moderate**	**Severe**
Symptoms	≤2x/day ≤2/week	>days/week (not daily)	Daily	Throughout the day
Short-acting beta 2 agonist (SAB2A) use for symptoms	≤2x/day ≤2/week	>days/week (not >1x/day)	Daily	Several times a day
Nighttime awakenings	≤2/month	3–4x/month	>1x/week (not nightly)	Often (7x/week)
Interference with normal activity	None	Minor limitation	Some limitation	Extremely limited
Lung function	• Normal FEV1 between attacks • FEV1 >80% predicted	• FEV1 ≥80% predicted • FEV1/FVC normal	• FEV1 60–80% predicted • FEV1/FVC reduced 5%	• FEV1 <60% predicted • FEV1/FVC reduced >5%
Management	• Inhaled SABA PRN	• Inhaled SABA PRN + • Low dose ICS	• Low ICS + LABA or • Increase ICS (medium) or • Add LTRA	• High dose ICS + LABA ± omalizumab (anti-IgE)
Requiring PO steroids	0–1/year	≥2/year		

Management/Prognosis

- Acute exacerbations
  - **Short-acting beta 2 agonists (SABA):** first-line therapy in acute asthma exacerbation (eg, albuterol, levalbuterol). Cause dilation of the peripheral airways (fastest and most effective initial treatment). Usually 3 treatments are administered in the first hour. Side effects include beta-1 cross reactivity (tachycardia, arrhythmias, muscle tremors, CNS stimulation) and hypokalemia.
  - **Short-acting antimuscarinic (anticholinergic) agents** may be added to SABA therapy (eg, ipratropium). They work on the central airways. Side effects include increased thirst, dry mouth, blurred vision, urinary retention, dysphagia, worsening of glaucoma, worsening of benign prostatic hypertrophy.
  - **Systemic glucocorticoids** are recommended in all but the mildest cases of acute asthma exacerbation (eg, prednisone, methylprednisolone, prednisolone). Reduces the inflammatory component of asthma. Onset of action ~6 hours. Side effects include immunosuppression, catabolic effects, hyperglycemia, fluid retention, osteoporosis, growth delays.
  - **IV magnesium sulfate:** added in life-threatening exacerbations, severe symptoms, or persistent symptoms even after bronchodilator therapy. Dilates the bronchial airways.
- Long-term (chronic control) maintenance
  - **Inhaled corticosteroids:** initial long-term treatment of choice. Reduces inflammation. Side effects include oropharyngeal candidiasis (usage of a spacer and rinsing the oral cavity after use reduces incidence).
  - **Long-acting beta-2 agonists (LABA):** bronchodilator that may be added to inhaled corticosteroids (not used as monotherapy or in acute exacerbations). Examples include salmeterol and formoterol.
  - **Mast cell modifiers:** may be an adjunct to albuterol as prophylaxis of asthma induced by cold air or exercise. Minimal side effects (eg, throat irritation). Used as prophylaxis only. Effective prophylaxis may take several weeks. Examples include cromolyn and nedocromil.
  - **Leukotriene receptor antagonists:** blocks leukotriene-mediated neutrophil migration, capillary permeability, smooth muscle contraction via leukotriene cysLT1 receptor inhibition. Zileuton does so via 5-lipoxygenase inhibition. Useful in asthmatic with allergic rhinitis, aspirin-induced asthma and exercise-induced asthma (prophylaxis only). Side effects include increased LFTs, headache, gastrointestinal symptoms, myalgias. Zileuton associated with behavioral disturbances.
  - **Omalizumab:** anti IgE antibody that inhibits Ig-E mediated inflammation. Used in severe asthma not controlled with other medications.

Asthmatics gotta PAC their PILS before they get on a SHIP or it will CAPSIZE.

Clues to Asthma Severity
Psychiatric d/o
Albuterol (how often they need to use it)
Comorbid illnesses

Prolonged attack
Inconsistent with their meds
Low **S**ocioeconomic status

Steroid usage
Hospital admissions
ICU admissions previously for asthma
Previous intubations due to asthma

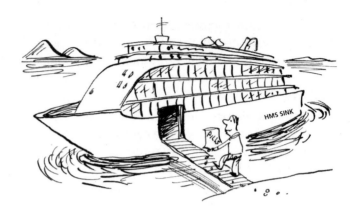

Status Asthmaticus
Cyanosis
AMS = altered mental status
Pulsus paradoxus
Silent chest (ominous sign)
Inability to speak in full sentences
Zzz = fatigue/somnolent
Expiratory flow rate <40% predicted

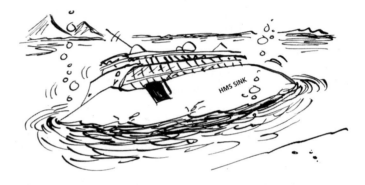

Figure 2.4 Clues to Asthma Severity

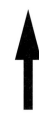

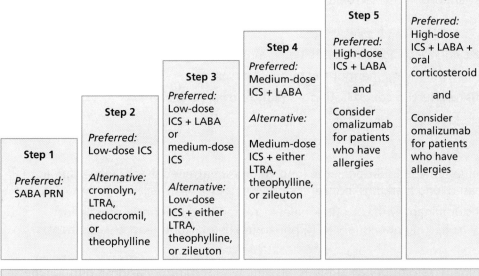

Intermittent asthma	Persistent asthma: daily medication Consult with asthma specialist if Step 4 care or higher is required. Consider consultation at Step 3.

Step 1

Preferred:
SABA PRN

Step 2

Preferred:
Low-dose ICS

Alternative:
cromolyn, LTRA, nedocromil, or theophylline

Step 3

Preferred:
Low-dose ICS + LABA or medium-dose ICS

Alternative:
Low-dose ICS + either LTRA, theophylline, or zileuton

Step 4

Preferred:
Medium-dose ICS + LABA

Alternative:
Medium-dose ICS + either LTRA, theophylline, or zileuton

Step 5

Preferred:
High-dose ICS + LABA

and

Consider omalizumab for patients who have allergies

Step 6

Preferred:
High-dose ICS + LABA + oral corticosteroid

and

Consider omalizumab for patients who have allergies

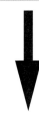

Step up if needed

(first, check adherence, environmental control, and comorbid conditions)

Assess control

Step down if possible

(and asthma is well controlled for at least 3 months)

Each step: patient education, environmental control, and management of comorbidities:
Steps 2-4: consider subcutaneous allergen immunotherapy for patients who have allergic asthma.

Quick-relief medication for all patients

- SABA as needed for symptoms. Intensity of treatment depends on severity of symptoms; up to 3 treatments at 20-minute intervals as needed. Short course of oral systemic corticosteroids may be needed.
- Use of SABA >2 days a week for symptom relief (not prevention of EIB) generally indicates inadequate control and the need to step up treatment.

Figure 2.5 Stepwise Approach to Asthma Therapy

Pulmonary

CHRONIC OBSTRUCTIVE PULMONARY DISEASE

Inflammatory lung disease causing airflow obstruction

Risk Factors

- Smoking is the most important risk factor, α-1 antitrypsin deficiency

Clinical Manifestations/Physical Exam

- Patients often have evidence of both, with one being more predominant in many cases
  - Emphysema: permanent enlargement of the terminal airspaces
  - Chronic bronchitis: productive cough lasting >3 months over ≥2 years

Diagnosis

- Chest x-ray:
  - Emphysema dominant: hyperinflation: large lung volumes, flattened diaphragms, dark lung fields with decreased lung markings, bullae
  - Chronic bronchitis dominant with cor pulmonale: increased lung markings, prominent pulmonary artery (reflecting pulmonary HTN, horizontal heart, right heart enlargement)
- ABG:
  - Emphysema dominant: respiratory alkalosis at baseline with respiratory acidosis during illnesses
  - Chronic bronchitis dominant: acute or chronic respiratory acidosis in patients with chronic bronchitis
- PFTs: decreased FEV1/FVC ratio <70%; normal or decreased FVC; normal or increased TLC; decreased DLCO in emphysema

Management/Prognosis

- **COPD Stops** with Me
  - **C**orticosteroids
  - **O**xygen (if signs of cor pulmonale, O2 sat <88%, PaO2 <55 mm Hg)
  - **P**revention of exacerbations (antibiotics, vaccinations, pulmonary rehabilitation)
  - **D**ilators (bronchodilators)
  - **Stop** smoking (smoking cessation)

Emphysema-Dominant COPD

Pink puffers breathe RAPID and FAST.

Respiratory **A**lkalosis (from hyperventilation)
Pursed lip breathing
Increased AP diameter (on physical exam and CXR)
Dyspnea on exertion/Decreased lung markings on CXR

Flattened diaphragms on CXR
Alpha-1 antitrypsin deficiency (acquired or genetic)
Spaces/**S**pots (bullae on CXR)
Tachypneic (hyperventilation)

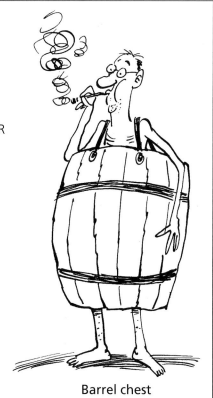

Barrel chest

Figure 2.6 Emphysema-dominant COPD

Chronic Bronchitis Dominant COPD

Blue bloaters exhale air SLOW as CRAP.

Severe V/Q mismatch
Low oxygen (hypoxic)
Obese
Wheezing

Cor pulmonale (right heart enlargement/failure)
Rales/rhonchi
Acidosis (respiratory)
Productive cough (≥3 mos x ≥2 yrs)

Obese & Cyanotic

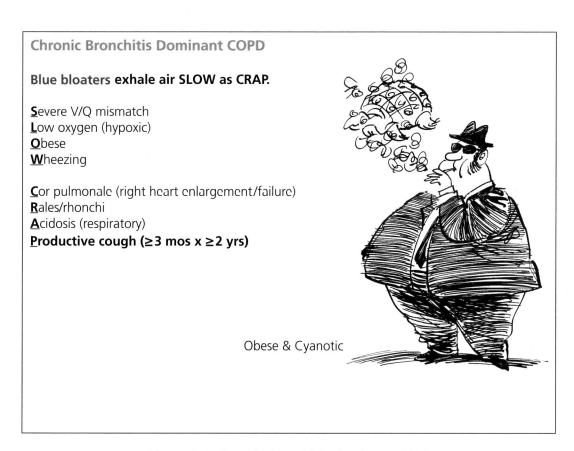

Figure 2.7 Chronic Bronchitis-dominant COPD

BRONCHIECTASIS

Permanent enlargement of the medium-sized bronchi, leading to airway obstruction

Etiology/Pathophysiology

- Recurrent lung infections (eg, *Haemophilus influenzae*, tuberculosis, *Pseudomonas*)
- 50% of cases due to cystic fibrosis
- Alpha-1 antitrypsin deficiency, local obstruction (eg, foreign body), autoimmune disease

Clinical Manifestations/Physical Exam

- Daily chronic cough with mucopurulent sputum, hemoptysis
- Physical exam: persistent crackles, wheezing, rhonchi

Diagnosis

- Chest x-ray: nonspecific abnormal findings, bronchial wall thickening with "tram track lines" is the only specific finding
- CT scan (high resolution): airway dilation, lack of tapering of bronchi, bronchial wall thickening (tram track), consolidation
- Pulmonary function: obstructive pattern decreased FEV1/FVC ratio <70%

Management/Prognosis

- Antibiotics are the cornerstone of treatment, chest therapy, surgery

He Flew and left TRAM tracks on the MAP.

H. Flu most common organism in general but *Pseudomonas* if due to CF

Diagnosis:
CT scan: tram track appearance due to thickened bronchial walls

Problematic Pathogens:
MAC
Aspergillus
Pseudomonas

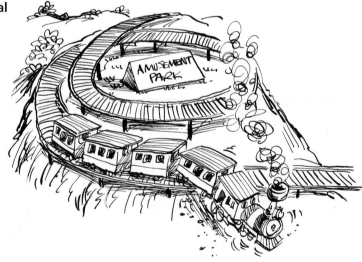

Figure 2.8 Bronchiectasis

CYSTIC FIBROSIS

Autosomal recessive disorder due to defect in the cystic fibrosis transmembrane receptor; result is protein buildup causing thick mucus and secretions in lungs, pancreas, liver, and intestines

Risk Factors

- Most commonly Caucasians

Clinical Manifestations/Physical Exam

- Respiratory: recurrent lung infections (especially *Pseudomonas* & *S. aureus*), productive cough, dyspnea, chest pain, wheezing, chronic sinusitis
- GI: meconium ileus at birth, later failure to thrive, chronic diarrhea, pancreatic insufficiency, malabsorption
- Systemic: infertility, heat exhaustion

Diagnosis

- Sweat chloride test: >60 mEq/L
- Genetic testing

Management/Prognosis

- Airway clearance treatment, pancreatic enzyme replacement, vitamin A, D, E, K replacement, lung transplantation

OLD PIE will lead to a BIG MI.

Obstructive Lung Disease
Pancreatic Insufficiency, Elevated chloride in sweat diagnostic
Bronchiectasis, Infertility, Growth delays
Meconium Ileus (most common initial presentation)

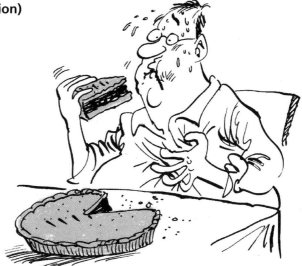

Figure 2.9 Cystic Fibrosis

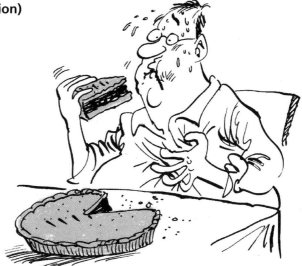

SARCOIDOSIS

Exaggerated T-cell response leading to granuloma formation

Risk Factors

- Most commonly African Americans, Northern Europeans, women ages 20–40

Clinical Manifestations/Physical Exam

- 50% asymptomatic (found incidentally on chest x-ray)
- Pulmonary: cough, dyspnea, chest pain; lymphadenopathy
- Skin: erythema nodosum, lupus pernio, maculopapular rash; parotid enlargement
- Visual: uveitis, conjunctivitis
- Cardiomyopathy
- Joint involvement
- Neurologic involvement

Diagnosis

- Chest x-ray: BHL (stage I); BHL + ILD (stage II); ILD only (stage III); fibrosis (stage IV)
- Labs: increased serum ACE levels, hypercalcemia, hypercalciuria
- PFTs often show a restrictive pattern
- Biopsy: noncaseating granulomas classic

Management/Prognosis

- Observation if asymptomatic or mild; corticosteroids if more severe

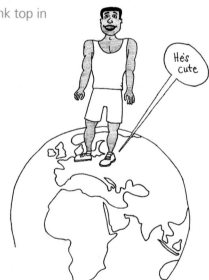

When a muscular **African American** on **steroids** wears a **HANES** tank top in **Northern Europe**, young women **CALL** him **CUTE**.

Hilar lymphadenopathy (classic chest x-ray finding)
ACE levels (elevated)
Noncaseating granulomas (classic biopsy finding)
Erythema nodosum
Steroids (treatment of choice)

Calcium (elevated in urine, blood)
Lung most commonly involved

Cutaneous anergy, **E**osinophilia

Figure 2.10 Sarcoidosis

PNEUMOCONIOSIS

Chronic lung disease due to inhalation of mineral dust

Silicosis

- Small nodules seen primarily in upper lobes due to quartz exposure
- Mining of granite/quartz, slate, pottery, sandblasting
- Chest x-ray: eggshell calcifications (classic sign)

Coal Worker's Lung

- Only pneumoconiosis associated with hyperinflation and obstruction
- Black lung appearance on gross examination
- Most commonly in upper lobes ("head" of the lung)

Berylliosis

- Beryllium is pneumoconiosis associated with inhalation of beryllium dust/fumes; often alloyed with nickel, aluminum, and copper, so people working in those industries are at increased exposure
- Aerospace, ceramics, computer, automotive, tool and dye manufacturing, electronics and jewelry making
- Berylliosis causes an increased risk of lung, stomach, and colon cancers
- Chest x-ray: normal in 50% of cases; abnormal findings include hilar lymphadenopathy, increased interstitial lung markings
- Positive beryllium lymphocyte proliferation test and noncaseating granulomas on biopsy

---

Extubation Criteria: ECSTUBATE

To identify patients who can begin weaning off mechanical ventilation:

- **E**dema of larynx should be ruled out with Cuff leak
- **C**ough strength: patient should be able to cough when prompted to
- **S**tate of consciousness: Glasgow coma score should be >8
- **T**rial of CPAP: patients should undergo trial of CPAP before extubation
- **U**nstable patients must be hemodynamically stable
- **B**reathing: able to initiate inspiratory effort
- **A**irway protection: ability to guard against aspiration during spontaneous breathing
- **T**reatment of cause of respiratory failure
- **E**levated pH >7.25 is necessary for extubating patients

Dyspnea on exertion due to silicosis will make you drop your Eggs, quarters, and pottery onto the granite floor, leaving Eggshells everywhere.

Dyspnea on exertion (most common symptom)

Risk Factors:
mining of granite/quartz, slate, pottery making, sandblasting

Chest x-ray:
Eggshell calcifications seen, small nodules in upper lobes

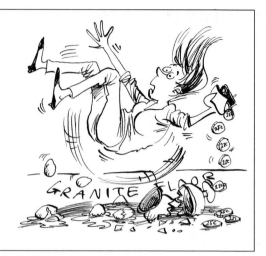

Figure 2.11 Silicosis

Coal workers must wear a **BLACK CAP** on their **INFLATED HEADS** in the mines.

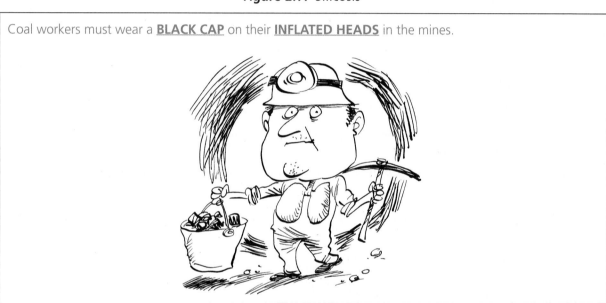

Figure 2.12 Coal Worker's Lung

Picking **BERRIES** in an open **SPACE** using **ELECTRONIC TOOLS** without **FLUORESCENT LIGHTS** on can permanently **DYE** your clothing!

Beryllium used in:
• **Electronics**
• **Fluorescent light bulbs**
• **Tool and dye manufacturing**
• **Aerospace products**
• **Ceramics**

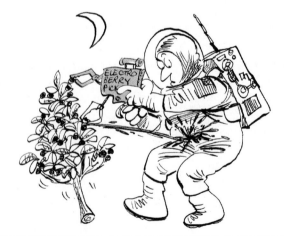

Figure 2.13 Berylliosis

BRONCHOGENIC CARCINOMA

Most common sites of metastasis: brain, bone, liver, lymph nodes, adrenal glands

Small-Cell Carcinoma (15%)

- Increased association with smoking
- Classically located centrally
- SVC syndrome: dilated neck veins, facial plethora (redness), prominent chest veins; due to tumor compressing the superior vena cava
- SIADH: hyponatremia (ectopic ADH production)
- Cushing's syndrome: tumors produce ectopic ACTH
- Eaton Lambert syndrome: tumor cells cause immune system to attack the body; antibodies "eat" presynaptic calcium channels, resulting in less acetylcholine release and weakness that improves with continued usage of the muscles
- Small-cell lung carcinoma: chemotherapy with or without radiotherapy

Non-Small Cell Carcinoma

- **BALS** are not small cells: **B**ronchoalveolar, **A**denocarcinoma, **L**arge cell, **S**quamous cell
- Bronchoalveolar carcinoma has the best prognosis
- Adenocarcinoma: most common type of lung cancer (in smokers, nonsmokers, and women); 40%; typically peripheral
- Large cell (anaplastic): (5%) worst prognosis
- Squamous cell (20%)
    - Pancoast syndrome: tumors in the apex of the lung causing Horner's syndrome: ptosis, miosis, and anhidrosis
    - **SHAC** loves to play Ball: **S**houlder pain, **H**orner's syndrome, **A**trophy of hand/arm muscles, **C**ervical cranial sympathetic compression
- Non-small cell lung carcinoma: surgery usually first-line treatment (often associated with local spread)

You can get **squamous cell lung cancer** if you **smoke** in the **center** of **red** square in Russia. (Russia used to be known as CCCP)

Centrally located lesions

Cavitary lesions

Calcium elevations

Pancoast syndrome

Hemoptysis = red

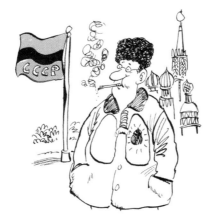

Figure 2.14 Squamous Cell Lung Carcinoma

PULMONARY EMBOLISM

Thrombus in the pulmonary artery or its branches

Etiology/Pathophysiology

- Virchow's Triad: **SHE** has a DVT: **S**tasis, **H**ypercoagulability, **E**ndothelial damage

Risk Factors

- 95% of cases arise from lower extremity/pelvic DVTs

Clinical Manifestations/Physical Exam

- Dyspnea most common symptom, tachypnea most common sign
- Also presents with pleuritic chest pain, tachycardia, ± hemoptysis, cough

Diagnosis

- Well's criteria for DVT: **TAPP** the **CUBES** into **A** well (add 1 point for each)
  - **T**enderness along deep veins, **A**ctive cancer, **P**aralysis, paresis or recent immobilization of lower extremities, **P**revious DVT
  - **C**ollateral superficial vein swelling (non-varicose in symptomatic leg), **U**nilateral calf swelling (≥3 cm), **B**edridden recently (≥3 days or major surgery requiring regional or general anesthetic in past 12 weeks), **E**dema (unilateral, pitting), **S**welling of entire leg
- Subtract 2 points for **A**lternative diagnosis to DVT as likely or more likely
- Score <2 is considered low risk for DVT

Management/Prognosis

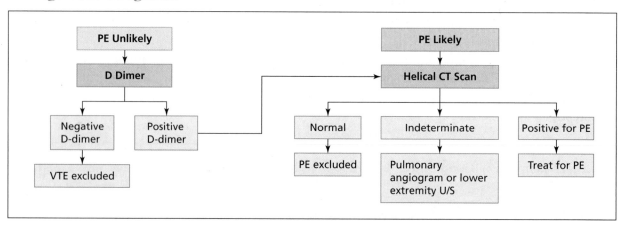

Figure 2.15 Pulmonary Embolism Workup

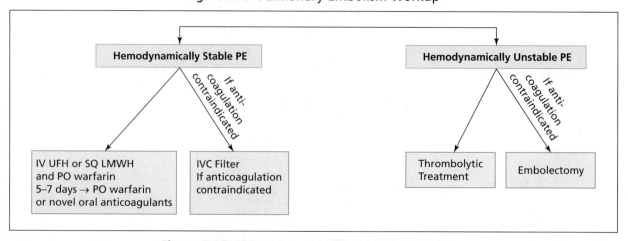

Figure 2.16 Management of Pulmonary Embolism

PLEURAL EFFUSION

Build up of excessive fluid around the lungs

Etiology/Pathophysiology

- Transudate
  - Circulatory system fluid due to increased hydrostatic and/or decreased oncotic pressures (not by inflammation); CHF (most common cause >90%); nephrotic syndrome, cirrhosis (right side), atelectasis
  - Taking Lasix for CHF transudative effusions will make you run **N P.E** over 175 **CC**s
  - **N**ephrotic syndrome **P**ulmonary **E**mbolism (often exudate but may be transudate), **CH**F, **C**irrhosis
- Exudate: any fluid that filters from circulatory system into areas of inflammation (increased plasma proteins, WBCs, platelets, ± RBCs) due to infection, malignancy, PE, pericarditis, uremia

Clinical Manifestations/Physical Exam

- Asymptomatic, dyspnea (most common), chest pain (pleuritic); cough
- Physical exam: dullness to percussion, decreased fremitus, decreased breath sounds; ± audible pleural friction rub

Diagnosis

- Chest x-ray: positive menisci (blunting) of costophrenic angles ± loculations; lateral decubitus films great to evaluate effusions
- Light criteria are exclusive to exudates
  - Pleural fluid protein:serum protein >0.5
  - Pleural fluid LDH:serum LDH >0.6
  - Pleural fluid LDH >2/3 upper limit of normal LDH

Management/Prognosis

- Treat underlying condition
- Thoracentesis: diagnostic or therapeutic:
  - Empyema drainage indications: pleural fluid pH <7.2, glucose <40 mg/dL, positive Gram stain
- Chronic or recurrent effusions: pleurodesis with talc or bleomycin (obliterates pleural space) or long-term drainage catheter

PNEUMOTHORAX

Air within the pleural space

Etiology/Pathophysiology

Positive pleural pressure causes collapse of the lung (especially during expiration)

Risk Factors

- Spontaneous: (atraumatic and idiopathic) ruptured bleb
  - Primary: no underlying pulmonary disease; mainly tall, thin men ages 20–40 (especially smokers, family history)
  - Secondary: underlying pulmonary disease without trauma (eg, asthma, COPD)
- Traumatic: iatrogenic (eg, CPR, thoracentesis, PEEP ventilation, subclavian lines), trauma (eg, car accidents, etc.)
- Tension: positive air pressure pushes lungs, trachea, and heart to contralateral side; immediately life threatening

Clinical Manifestations/Physical Exam

- Symptomatic: chest pain (usually pleuritic), dyspnea
- Physical exam findings: If large, decreased fremitus and breath sounds and increased hyperresonance (tympany), unequal respiratory expansion, tachycardia, tachypnea, wheezing, crackles
- Physical Exam in Tension PTX: pulsus paradoxus, hypotension, JVD, respiratory distress

Diagnosis

- Chest x-ray, expiratory view
  - Linear shadow of visceral pleura with lack of lung markings in periphery, $\pm$ companion lines (radiopaque lines following the 1st/2nd ribs), deep sulcus sign
  - Tension PTX: mediastinal shift to the contralateral side

Management/Prognosis

- Observation: if small (<20%) often closes spontaneously
  - Oxygen increases air resorption 3–4 times faster than 1.25% qd
- Chest tube placement: if large pneumothorax
- Needle aspiration if tension pneumothorax; done at second intercostal space at midclavicular line leads to chest tube placement
- Avoid high altitudes, smoking, unpressurized aircraft, scuba diving

TUBERCULOSIS

Lung infection caused by infection with *Mycobacterium tuberculosis* leading to granuloma formation

Risk Factors

- Primary rapidly progressive TB: most commonly in children and immunosuppressed patients
- Secondary (reactivation) TB: reactivation of latent infection in people with waning immunity (eg, elderly, patients on chronic steroids, HIV, malignancy, immunosuppressants)

Clinical Manifestations/Physical Exam

- Active infection: (infectious) active infection occurs if immune system is overwhelmed/suppressed leading to cavitary lesions that erode into larger airways; expelled through talking, coughing, sneezing
- Latent infection: TB contained in granuloma (occurs in 90% of patients with intact immune systems) and becomes dormant (noninfectious); positive PPD but have normal chest x-ray and no symptoms

Management/Prognosis

- Primary progressive or reactive infection:
  - RIPE(S)—initial 4-drug therapy (total treatment duration for active is 6 months): rifampin, isoniazid, pyrazinamide, ethambutol (or streptomycin)
- Latent TB infection:
  - Isoniazid/INH (+ pyridoxine) over a period of 9 months
- Side effects of anti-tuberculosis medications:
  - Isoniazid (**INH**): **I**nhibitor of cytochrome P450, **N**europathy (prevented by giving pyridoxine/vitamin B6), **H**epatoxicity
  - Rifampin (**RIF**): **R**ed-orange colored secretions, **I**nactivity of platelets (thrombocytopenia), **F**lu-like symptoms
  - Pyrazinamide (**PZA**): **P**hotosensitive rashes, **Z**aps the liver (hepatitis), **A**rthritis
  - Ethambutol: E = **E**yes (optic neuritis)
  - Streptomycin (Ami**NO**glycoside): **N**ephrotoxic **O**totoxic

PNEUMONIA

Infection that inflames the air sacs (alveoli) of the lungs; may affect one lung or both

Etiology/Pathophysiology

- Community-acquired pneumonia (CAP):
  - Typical pneumonia: if doctors misdiagnose pneumonia, patients sue for large amounts of **KASH**: *Klebsiella*, *S. Aureus*, *Strep pneumoniae* (most common cause), *Haemophilus influenzae*
- Atypical pneumonia: *Mycoplasma pneumoniae* (most common cause of walking pneumonia), *Legionella pneumophila*, *Chlamydophila pneumoniae*, viral pneumonias
- Hospital-acquired pneumonia includes *Pseudomonas*, *Klebsiella*, *Enterobacter*, *Serratia*, *Acinetobacter*, and *S. Aureus* (MRSA)

Management/Prognosis

Clinical Scenario	Empiric Treatment Guidelines
Community-acquired (outpatient)	Macrolide or doxycycline (FQ if co-morbid conditions/recent antibiotic use)
Community-acquired (inpatient)	β-lactam + macrolide (or doxycycline) or broad spectrum FQ
Community-acquired (in ICU)	β-lactam + macrolide or β-lactam + broad spectrum FQ If β-lactam allergy, use FQ ± aztreonam (or clindamycin + aztreonam)
Hospital-acquired	Anti-pseudomonal β-lactam & anti-pseudomonal AG or FQ • If legionella suspected, add macrolide or FQ • If MRSA suspected, add vancomycin • If *Pneumocystis* pneumonia suspected, add TMP-SMX ± steroids *If documented β-lactam allergy: FQ ± clindamycin (aztreonam, AG)
Aspiration	FQ + clindamycin
Route of therapy	Inpatients should initially be treated with IV antibiotics; change to PO when clinically responding, eg, 7–10 days (minimum of 5 days)

To treat the pneumonia, you must RACE and AIM at the PC.

Beta-lactams:
Rocephin (Ceftriaxone)
Ampicillin sulbactam
Cefotaxime
Ertapenem

Antipseudomonal:
Imipenem
Meropenem

Piperacillin-tazobactam
Cefepime

Macrolides:
Azithromycin
Clarithromycin
Erythromycin

Aminoglycosides:
Tobramycin
Amikacin
Gentamicin

Respiratory fluoroquinolones: levofloxacin, moxifloxacin, gemifloxacin

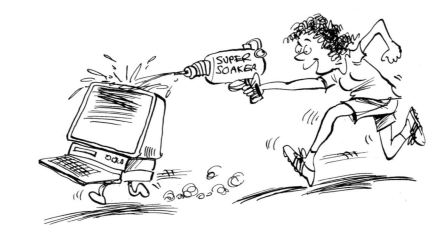

Figure 2.17 Treatment of Pneumonia

Pulmonary

ACUTE EPIGLOTTITIS (SUPRAGLOTTITIS)

Inflammation of epiglottis

Etiology/Pathophysiology

- Haemophilus influenza type B (HiB) most common but reduced incidence due to vaccination
- May be caused by *Streptococcus pneumoniae*, *Staphylococcus aureus*, GABHS

Risk Factors

- Most commonly children age 3 months to 6 years

Clinical Manifestations/Physical Exam

- Three **D**s (**d**ysphagia, **d**rooling, **d**istress), fevers, odynophagia, inspiratory stridor, dyspnea, hoarseness, tripoding (sitting leaned forward with elbow on lap)

Diagnosis

- Laryngoscopy: definitive diagnosis (provides direct visualization but may provoke spasm); cherry-red epiglottis; if high suspicion, don't attempt to visualize epiglottis with tongue depressor
- Lateral cervical x-rays: thumbprint sign (enlarged epiglottis seen)

Management/Prognosis

- Support and maintain airway: place child in a comfortable position and keep calm; do tracheal intubation to protect airway if necessary
- Antibiotics: second/third generation cephalosporins ($\pm$ add penicillin, ampicillin, or anti-staphylococcus coverage)

PERTUSSIS (WHOOPING COUGH)

Pertussis (whooping cough): infection secondary to *Bordetella pertussis* (gram-negative coccobacillus)

Clinical Manifestations/Physical Exam

- Catarrhal phase: URI symptoms last 1–2 weeks and lead to paroxysmal phase
- Paroxysmal phase: severe paroxysmal coughing fits (with inspiratory whooping sound after cough fit); post-coughing emesis leads to convalescent phase
- Convalescent phase: resolving of the cough and the emesis (although the coughing stage may last for up to 6 weeks; coughing fits may occur spontaneously or provoked by laughing, yawning, etc.)

Diagnosis

- Nasopharyngeal swab (done in first 3 weeks of symptom onset)

Management/Prognosis

- Supportive: antibiotics have no effect on duration of illness, only decrease contagiousness of affected patient
- Macrolides; bactrim if allergic to macrolides
- Complications: pneumonia, encephalopathy, otitis media

Pulmonary

LARYNGOTRACHEOBRONCHITIS (CROUP)

Inflammation secondary to acute upper airway infection (larynx, subglottis, trachea)

Etiology/Pathophysiology

- Infection leads to subglottic larynx/trachea swelling leads to stridor, "barking" cough, hoarseness
- Parainfluenza virus most common cause, adenovirus etc.; rarely seen due to diphtheria (because of widespread vaccination)

Risk Factors

- Common (affects ~15% of children in childhood); most commonly age 6 months to 6 years

Clinical Manifestations/Physical Exam

- "Seal-like barking" cough, ± URI symptoms either preceding or concurrent, fever
- Stridor: both inspiratory and expiratory (worsened by crying and agitating child)
- Hoarseness (due to laryngitis)
- Dyspnea (especially worse at night)

Diagnosis

- Usually a clinical diagnosis
- Cervical x-ray (frontal): steeple sign (subglottic narrowing of trachea) in 50% of cases

Management/Prognosis

- Cool air mist is a mainstay
- Supplemental O_2 in patients with O_2 sats <92%
- Corticosteroids, eg, dexamethasone IM; nebulized epinephrine if severe

If a child is not treated with **steroids** for __CROUP__, they will em__BARK__ to fall down a __STEEP__ and __NARROW__ cliff without a __PARA__chute, __SEAL__ing their doom!

- **"Seal-like" barking cough**

- **Steeple sign** on plain x-ray
  (represent narrowing of the trachea)

- **Parainfluenza virus** MC cause

- **Corticosteroids** reduce tracheal narrowing

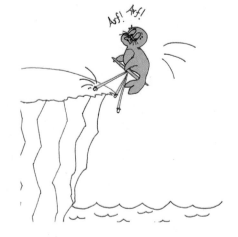

Figure 2.18 Laryngotracheobronchitis (Croup)

RESPIRATORY DISTRESS SYNDROME

Severe lung condition in which oxygenation of the lungs is reduced

Acute Respiratory Distress Syndrome

Life-threatening hypoxemic respiratory failure (organ failure from prolonged hypoxemia)

Etiology/Pathophysiology

- Inflammatory lung injury leads to diffuse alveolar damage, increased permeability of alveolar-capillary barrier, pulmonary edema, and alveolar fluid influx

Risk Factors

- Most commonly affects critically ill patients

Clinical Manifestations/Physical Exam

- Acute dyspnea and hypoxemia with multi-organ failure if severe
- Severe refractory hypoxemia (hallmark); not responsive to 100% O_2 (PaO_2/FIO_2 ratio <200 mm Hg)
- Diffuse bilateral pulmonary infiltrates on chest x-ray

Diagnosis

- ABG: PaO_2/FIO_2 ratio <200 mm Hg not responsive to 100% O_2
- Chest x-ray: diffuse bilateral infiltrates lead to white-out pattern (resembles CHF on chest x-ray)
- Cardiac catheterization of pulmonary artery (Swan-Ganz): pulmonary capillary wedge pressure <18 mm Hg

Management/Prognosis

- Noninvasive or mechanical ventilation CPAP with full face mask, PEEP
- Nonspecific treatment for **ARDS** (treat underlying disease):
  - **A**bsence of cardiogenic pulmonary edema
  - **R**efractory hypoxemia (PaO2/FIO2 ratio <200 mmHg)
  - **D**iffuse bilateral pulmonary infiltrates
  - **S**wan-Ganz (pulmonary capillary wedge pressure <18 mmHg)

Infant Respiratory Distress Syndrome

Disease of premature infants secondary to insufficiency of surfactant production and lung structural immaturity

Clinical Manifestations/Physical Exam

- Usually presents shortly postpartum: tachypnea, tachycardia, chest wall retractions, expiratory grunting, nasal flaring, and cyanosis

Diagnosis

- Chest x-ray: bilateral diffuse reticular ground-glass opacities, air bronchograms, poor expansion, domed diaphragms
- Histopathology: waxy appearing layers lining the collapsed alveoli, may show airway distention

Management/Prognosis

- CPAP, IV fluids, exogenous surfactant
- Prevention: steroids given to mature lungs if premature delivery expected (between 24–36 weeks)

INFLUENZA

Contagious, viral respiratory condition of the nose, throat, and lungs

Etiology/Pathophysiology

- Influenza A associated with more severe outbreaks compared to B
- Transmitted primarily via airborne respiratory secretions (eg, sneezing, coughing, talking, breathing); contaminated objects
- Children are important vectors for the disease (the highest rates of infection are seen among children but those age ≥65 are at highest risk for complications)

Risk Factors

- Age ≥65; pregnancy; immunocompromised status

Clinical Manifestations

- Abrupt onset of a wide range of symptoms: headache, fever, chills, malaise, URI symptoms, pharyngitis, pneumonia
- Myalgias most commonly involve the legs and lumbosacral areas

Diagnosis

- Rapid influenza nasal swab
- Viral culture

Management

- Supportive management (acetaminophen, salicylates, rest) for those with **mild disease but otherwise healthy**
- Antivirals for those that are **hospitalized or have high risk of complications** (age ≥65, cardiovascular disease [except isolated hypertension], pulmonary disease, immunosuppression [malignancy, DM, HIV infection, post-transplant], chronic liver disease and hemoglobinopathies [sickle cell, thalassemia]
- Neuraminidase inhibitors: oseltamivir best if initiated within 48 hrs of symptom onset
  - Work against both A and B
  - Side effects include skin reactions, nausea/vomiting, and transient neuropsychiatric events
  - Alternatives include peramivir and zanamivir (egg allergy contraindicated with zanamivir)
- Amantanes: amantadine and rimantadine are effective against influenza A only (high level of resistance), so not recommended for treatment or prophylaxis against influenza A
- **Chemoprophylaxis**
  - In cases of outbreak and exposure in high-risk groups, oseltamivir can be used for high-risk patients age ≥1
  - During influenza outbreak in long-term facilities, all residents should receive chemoprophylaxis regardless of immunization status; for the general population, only those who did not receive the annual influenza vaccine should be given chemoprophylaxis

Influenza Vaccine

Indications

- **Inactivated vaccine:** annual vaccination for all individuals age ≥ 6 months (including pregnancy); high dose vaccination for individuals age >65
- **Live attenuated** (intranasal) **vaccine:** can be used for annual vaccination for all individuals age 2–49

Contraindications/Cautions/Side Effects

- **Contraindications** (to both types): anaphylaxis to influenza vaccine; Guillain-Barre within 6 wks after a previous influenza vaccination; high fever; infants age <6 mos
- Although allergy to protein egg used to be a contraindication, **patients with egg allergy of any severity (including anaphylaxis) can safely receive the egg-based inactivated influenza vaccine** in a medical setting
- **Live attenuated vaccine only:** immunocompromised status (including HIV); pregnancy; age ≥ 50; having taken influenza antiviral medication within last 48 hrs; close contacts/caregivers of severely immunocompromised patients who require a protected environment
- **Side effects:** injection site reaction, fever, myalgia, irritability; nasal spray may cause upper or lower respiratory tract symptoms; allergic reaction and anaphylaxis rare

ACUTE BRONCHIOLITIS

Lower respiratory tract infection of the bronchioles

Etiology/Pathophysiology

- Respiratory syncytial virus (RSV) 85%
- Parainfluenza, adenovirus, rhinovirus, influenza, echovirus, *Mycoplasma pneumoniae*, *Chlamydia trachomatis*
- Critical airway narrowing/obstruction: mucous plugging secondary to necrosis of respiratory epithelium and destruction of ciliated epithelial cells

Risk Factors

- Most commonly children age 2 months to 2 years; highest incidence in November–February

Clinical Manifestations/Physical Exam

- History: initially fever and URI symptoms, 1–2 days leads to respiratory distress
- Physical: tachypnea (>50–60 breaths/minute), wheezing, nasal flaring, cyanosis, retractions, ± rales, tachycardia, prolonged expiration (decreased/absent breath sounds, cyanosis, altered mental status if severe)

Diagnosis

- Pulse oximetry: single best predictor of disease in children
- Chest x-ray: ± hyperinflation, segmental atelectasis, peribronchial thickening, consolidation, pneumonia
- RSV testing: nasal swabs done with monoclonal antibody testing

Management/Prognosis

- Supportive: fluids, supplemental oxygen, acetaminophen/ibuprofen for fever (steroids and antibiotics not usually helpful); ± beta 2 agonist (no clinical proven benefit of outcome); ± racemic epinephrine
- Prevention (high-risk patients): palivizumab (prophylaxis in high risk infants [anti-RSV antibody given 55% reduction of RSV hospitalization])

INFANTS that are **WHEEZING** due to bronchiolitis don't need to **RSVP** in order to get **SUPPORT** at the hospital.

- **Infants** age 2 mos–2 yrs

- **Wheezing** (respiratory symptoms)

- **RSV** (most common cause) **R**espiratory **S**yncytial **V**irus

- **P**arainfluenza can cause bronchiolitis as well

- **Supportive** mainstay treatment

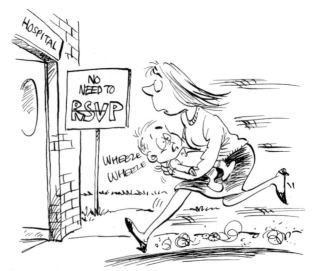

Figure 2.19 Acute Bronchiolitis

ACID-BASE DISORDERS

Blood pH changes due to impairment in the kidneys, lungs, or buffer systems which increase or decrease the level of acids and bases in the body

Metabolic Acidosis

High anion gap

- The acid dissociates into H^+ and an unmeasured anion (Ua); the H^+ is buffered by HCO_3^- and the unmeasured anion accumulates, creating the AG: $HUa + NaHCO_3 \rightarrow NaUa + H_2CO_3 \rightarrow CO_2 + H_2O$

Normal gap (hyperchloremic)

- Loss of HCO_3^- followed by reabsorption of Cl^- resulting in elevated blood Cl^- levels, so there is no change in AG but there is an accumulation of Cl^- concentration
- In other cases (diarrhea, type II RTA), there is loss of $NaHCO_3$ and the kidney tries to preserve volume by retaining NaCl: $HCl + NaHCO_3 \rightarrow NaCl + H_2CO_3 \rightarrow CO_2 + H_2O$

Anion Gap Metabolic Acidosis	Non-Gap Metabolic Acidosis
"MUDPILERS"	"HARDUPS"
Methanol	Hyperalimentation
Uremia	Acetazolamide
DKA/alcoholic KA	Renal tubular acidosis
Paraldehyde	Diarrhea
Isoniazid	Uretero-pelvic shunt
Lactic acidosis	Post-hypocapnia
ETOH/ethylene glycol	Spironolactone
Rhabdo/renal failure	
Salicylates	
Too much acid or too little bicarbonate	Too much acid or too little bicarbonate

Metabolic Alkalosis

- Increased HCO_3^- (serum) with increased pH requires generating and maintenance factors (because able to excrete large amounts of HCO_3^-)
- Loss of H^+ from GI tract/kidneys: vomiting/NG suction (loss of gastric HCl maintained by ECF volume depletion, chronic diarrhea (maintained by ECF volume depletion), loop diuretics
- Exogenous alkali: contraction alkalosis: diuresis leads to excretion of HCO_3^- and poor fluid leads to ECF volume "contracts" around fixed HCO_3^- leads to increased HCO_3^-
- Post hypercapnia: rapid correction of respiratory hypercapnia (ex mechanical ventilation) leads to transient excess HCO_3^-

Pulmonary

Respiratory Acidosis

- Anything that decreases respiration
- Acute respiratory failure: CNS depression (opiates, sedatives, trauma), chest wall disorders, cardiopulmonary arrest, pneumonia
- Chronic respiratory failure: COPD, obesity, neuromuscular disorders (myasthenia gravis, Guillain Barré syndrome, poliomyelitis, ALS)

Respiratory Alkalosis

- Anything that increases respiration

Etiology/Pathophysiology

- Hyperventilation: CNS disorders, pain, anxiety, salicylates, progesterone, pregnancy, hepatic failure, stimulation of pulmonary receptors (pneumonia, asthma)

Acute Respiratory Acidosis	Metabolic Alkalosis	Respiratory Alkalosis
Anything that causes hypoventilation: • CNS depression (drugs/CVA) • Airway obstruction • Pneumonia edema • Hemo/pneumothorax • Myopathy	"CLEVER PD" Contraction Licorice* Endo (Conn's, Cushing, Bartter's) Vomiting Excess alkali* Refeeding alkalosis* Post-hypercapnia Diuretics* * Associated with increased UCI-	"CHAMPS" Anything that causes hyperventilation, i.e.: CNS disease Hypoxia Anxiety Mech ventilators Progesterone Salicylates/sepsis
Anything that decreases respiration	Little acid or too much bicarbonate	Anything that causes hyperventilation

---

Three-Step Approach to Acid Base Disorders

Step 1: Identify the most apparent disorder. (ideal 7.40)

- If pH >7.45, alkalosis
- If pH <7.35, acidosis
- If pH is not within normal limits (especially if not 7.40 exactly), check HCO_3^- and PCO_2; if they are abnormal, there may be full compensation of an underlying acid-base disorder

Step 2: Look at PCO_2. Is it normal low or high? (ideal 40)

- If it corresponds with pH, leads to a disorder that is respiratory in nature; meaning, in primary respiratory disorders, PCO_2 & pH go in opposite directions
- If PCO_2 is going in same direction as pH, leads to a partial respiratory compensation

Step 3: Look at HCO_3^-. Is it normal low or high?

- If HCO_3^- corresponds with pH, primary disorder is metabolic in nature; meaning in primary metabolic, pH and HCO_3^- go in the same direction
- If HCO_3^- is in opposite direction of pH, partial metabolic compensation

> **Normal ranges:**
>
> Na: 135–145
>
> Cl: 105
>
> HCO_3 -: 22–26
>
> PCO_2: 38–42
>
> AGNa (Cl + HCO_3): 10–12
>
> pH: 7.35–7.45
>
> PO_2: 80–100

Chapter 3

Gastrointestinal

ESOPHAGITIS

Inflammatory condition affecting the esophagus

Etiology/Pathophysiology

- GERD most common cause
- Infections in immunocompromised: *Candida albicans*; CMV; HSV
- Radiation therapy, ingestion of medications or corrosive agents

Risk Factors

- Pregnancy, smoking, obesity, alcohol, chocolate, spicy foods
- Medications: NSAIDs, BB, CCB, nitroglycerin, bisphosphonates

Clinical Manifestations/Physical Exam

- Odynophagia, dysphagia, retrosternal chest pain

Diagnosis

- Upper endoscopy (EGD):
    - *Candida*: linear yellow-white plaques
    - CMV: **M**ega (large), shallow ulcers on EGD
    - HSV: **S**mall deep ulcers on EGD
- Double-contrast esophagram

Management/Prognosis

- Treat underlying cause
- *Candida* esophagitis: fluconazole oral treatment of choice
- CMV: ganciclovir
- HSV: acyclovir, valacyclovir

PLUMMER-VINSON SYNDROME

Dysphagia, esophageal webs, iron deficiency anemia

Risk Factors

- Most commonly Caucasian women ages 30–60

Clinical Manifestations/Physical Exam

- Atrophic glossitis, angular cheilitis, koilonychia, splenomegaly may also be present

The female PLUMMBER using an iron tool SAID EW when she saw spider webs near the SIDE of the SINK.

Splenomegaly
Atrophic glossitis
Inflammation of angles of mouth (cheilitis)
Dysphagia

Esophageal
Webs

Plummer-Vinson Triad
Serum **I**ron decreased (anemia)
Dysphagia
Esophageal webs

Iron Deficiency
Stores (Ferritin) decreased
Increased **I**ron binding capacity (TIBC)
Non-food substances (pica)
Koilonychia (spooning of nails)

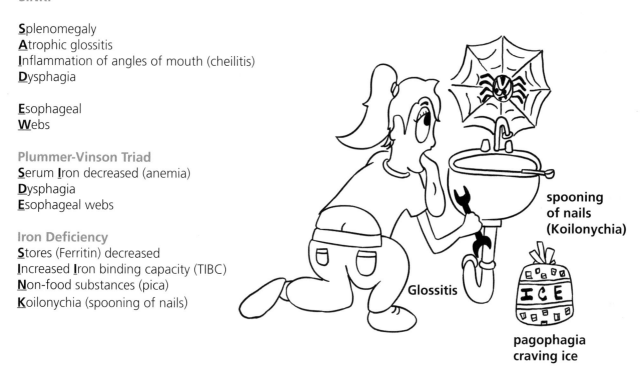

spooning
of nails
(Koilonychia)

Glossitis

pagophagia
craving ice

Figure 3.1 Plummer-Vinson Syndrome

ESOPHAGEAL VARICES
Enlargement of esophageal veins

Etiology/Pathophysiology
- Variceal formation is the main complication of portal vein HTN resulting in dilation of gastroesophageal collaterals

Risk Factors
- Cirrhosis most common cause in adults
- Portal vein thrombosis most common cause in children

Clinical Manifestations/Physical Exam
- Upper GI bleeding: hematemesis, melena, hematochezia

Diagnosis
- EGD: enlarged veins, "red wale" markings, and cherry red spots leads to increased risk of bleeding

Management/Prognosis
- Endoscopic ligation: endoscopic treatment of choice (lower complication rate and fewer re-bleeds) ± sclerotherapy
  - Balloon tamponade: used in fast hemorrhages or second line
  - Surgical decompression: portosystemic shunts (TIPS), devascularization, and embolization
- Prophylaxis:
  - Nonselective BBs (eg, propranolol, nadolol)
  - Long-acting nitrates

EVA continued drinking despite her **HEAVY BLEEDING,** all because she couldn't get her **LOVA** back, even after asking a **PRO** for **TIPS** as a **last resort.**

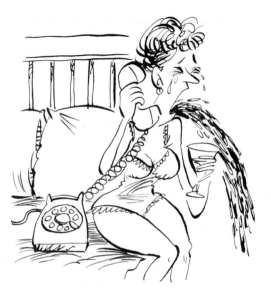

- **E**sophageal **VA**rices usually due to cirrhosis after long history of heavy drinking

Management:
- **L**igation (endoscopic)
- **O**ctreotide
- **Va**sopressin

- **T**ransjugular **I**ntrahepatic **P**ortosystemic **S**hunt (TIPS as last resort)
- **Pro**pranolol as **pro**phylaxis

Figure 3.2 Esophageal Varices

GASTROESOPHAGEAL REFLUX DISEASE

Backflow of stomach acid into esophagus which damages the LES

Etiology/Pathophysiology

- Incompetent LES leads to reflux of gastric acid

Risk Factors

- Pregnancy (progesterone decreases motility), hiatal hernia, obesity, tobacco, and alcohol

Clinical Manifestations/Physical Exam

- Typical symptoms: heartburn (pyrosis) is hallmark; often retrosternal and postprandial; regurgitation (water brash or sour taste in the mouth), dysphagia, nighttime cough
- Atypical symptoms: hoarseness, aspiration, aspiration pneumonia, noncardiac chest pain, "asthma" (bronchospasm and wheezing)
- Alarm symptoms: dysphagia, odynophagia, weight loss, bleeding
- Complications: esophagitis, esophageal stricture, Barrett's esophagus, esophageal adenocarcinoma

Diagnosis

- Clinical/historical diagnosis (especially with classic presentation)
- Endoscopy: often used as first line diagnostic tool if workup needed to rule out complications
- 24-hour ambulatory pH monitoring (gold standard)
- Esophageal manometry: decreased LES pressure

Management/Prognosis

- **Stage 1: lifestyle modification first**
  - Elevate head off the bed by 6 inches
  - Decrease fat intake, lose weight, stop smoking, reduce alcohol consumption, avoid recumbency for 3 hours postprandially
  - Avoid large meals and certain foods (fatty/spicy foods, citrus, chocolate, caffeinated products, peppermint)
- **Stage 2: "as needed" pharmacological therapy**
  - Antacids, histamine (H_2) receptor antagonists
  - If alarm or atypical symptoms, EGD is next appropriate step
- **Stage 3: scheduled pharmacologic therapy**
  - H2 receptor antagonists, PPIs, and prokinetic agents (cisapride)
  - PPIs drug of choice in severe disease
  - Nissen fundoplication in some cases refractory to medicine

PEPTIC ULCER DISEASE (PUD)

Imbalance of decreased mucosal protective factors (mucus, bicarbonate, prostaglandins, blood flow) in gastric ulcers or increased damaging factors (acid, pepsin) in duodenal ulcers

Etiology/Pathophysiology

- *H. pylori* infection most common cause
- NSAIDs inhibit prostaglandin and mucus synthesis
- Others: Zollinger-Ellison syndrome, alcohol, smoking, stress (burns, trauma, surgery, severe illness), male gender, elderly age, corticosteroid use, malignancy

Risk Factors

- 4% of gastric ulcers are caused by gastric cancer or may become malignant

Clinical Manifestations/Physical Exam

- DU usually benign
- Ulcer-like or acid dyspepsia: mid-epigastric pain relieved with food; worse before meals or 2–5 hours after meals, nocturnal symptoms, especially with duodenal ulcers
- Food-provoked dyspepsia/indigestion: worse with meals (especially 1–2 hours after meals), weight loss, associated with gastric ulcer
- GI bleed: peptic ulcer disease most common cause of upper GI bleed

Diagnosis

- Endoscopy ± biopsy (gold standard)
- Upper GI series should be followed by endoscopy (especially with gastric ulcer)
- *Helicobacter pylori* testing:
  - Endoscopy with biopsy (gold standard for diagnosing *H pylori*)
  - Urea breath test: noninvasive testing
  - Stool antigen
  - *H. pylori* is only eradicated when patient's **BREATH** stops smelling like **DUNG**; both urea **BREATH** test and *H. pylori* **STOOL** antigen can confirm diagnosis and eradication of *H. pylori* after treatment

Management/Prognosis

- *H-pylori* positive
  - Bismuth quadruple therapy: bismuth subsalicylate + tetracycline + metronidazole + PPI for14 days
  - Concomitant therapy: clarithromycin + amoxicillin + metronidazole + PPI for 10–14 days
  - Triple therapy: clarithromycin + amoxicillin + PPI for 14 days (if penicillin-allergic, use metronidazole); alternate treatment is bismuth subsalicylate + tetracycline + metronidazole
- *H-pylori* negative
  - Antisecretory therapy (PPIs, H2 receptor antagonists): 4–8 weeks in patients with complicated duodenal ulcers and 8–12 weeks; gastric ulcer may need confirmation of healing via upper endoscopy
  - Misoprostol, antacids, bismuth compounds, sucralfate
- Refractory
  - Parietal cell vagotomy
  - Bilroth II (associated with dumping syndrome)

Table 3.1 Peptic Ulcer Disease

	Duodenal Ulcer (DU)	**Gastric Ulcer (GU)**
Causative Factors	Increased damaging factors	Decreased mucosal protective factors
	• Acid • Pepsin	• Mucus • Bicarbonate • Prostaglandins (eg, NSAID use)
Incidence	• 4 times more common than GU • Almost always benign • Most common in the duodenal bulb	• Less common than DU • 4% due to gastric cancer • Most common in the antrum
Factors	• Better with meals • Worse 2–5 hours after meals	• Worse with meals (esp. 1–2 hours after meals)
Age	• Younger: ages 30–55	• Older: ages 55–70

Gastrointestinal

GASTRIC CARCINOMA

Cancer formed in the mucus-producing cells lining the stomach

Etiology/Pathophysiology

- Adenocarcinoma most common worldwide (90%)
- Lymphomas, leiomyosarcomas

Risk Factors

- Most commonly age >40
- *H. pylori* most important risk factor; salted, cured, smoked food, food containing nitrites (thought to be converted by *H. pylori* into noxious compounds)
- Pernicious anemia, chronic atrophic gastritis
- Smoking, ETOH, blood type A, achlorhydria

Clinical Manifestations/Physical Exam

- Patients usually present in late stage of disease
- Indigestion, weight loss, early satiety, abdominal pain/fullness, nausea, post-prandial vomiting, dysphagia, melena, hematemesis
- METS: **VIRCHOW** and his **SISTER MARY** sold **BLUMER SHELVES** in **KRUKENBERG, IRELAND** until they eventually died of gastric cancer
- Virchow's node: enlarged supraclavicular lymph node
- Sister Mary Joseph's node: enlarged periumbilical lymph node
- Blumer's shelf: mass felt on digital rectal exam
- Krukenberg tumor: ovarian metastases
- Irish node: enlarged left anterior axillary lymph node

Diagnosis

- EGD with biopsy: definitive diagnosis
  - Linitis plastica: thickening of stomach wall due to diffusive cancer infiltration; this is the worst type of gastric cancer
- Iron deficiency anemia is commonly seen

Management/Prognosis

- Gastrectomy, radiation, and chemotherapy (both adenocarcinoma and lymphoma)

DISEASES OF THE GALLBLADDER

Acute Cholecystitis

Cystic duct obstruction (gallstone) causes gallbladder inflammation and infection

- Cystic (gallbladder) duct obstruction leads to inflammation and infection
- 50–80% (*E. coli, Klebsiella, Enterococci, Bacteroides* species: same bacteria in acute cholangitis)
- Risk factors: **5Fs (fat, fair, female, forty, fertile)**, Native Americans, OCP use, bile stasis, chronic hemolysis, cirrhosis, infection, rapid weight loss, IBD, TPN, fibrates, increased triglycerides
- Clinical manifestations: biliary colic (episodic RUQ pain/epigastric pain especially with food); fever/ nausea/vomiting; palpable gallbladder (33%)
- Positive Murphy's sign: acute RUQ pain/inspiratory arrest with gallbladder palpation
- Positive Boas sign: referred pain to right subscapular area
- Diagnosis: U/S initial test of choice: ± thickened gallbladder (>3 mm); distended gallbladder, sludge, gallstones, pericholecystic fluid, positive sonographic Murphy's sign
- Labs: increased WBCs (leukocytosis with left shift); increased bilirubin, increased ALP and LFTs
- HIDA scan (gold standard); positive = nonvisualization of gallbladder
- Management: NPO, IV fluids, antibiotics (eg, ceftriaxone + metronidazole) followed by cholecystectomy, usually within 72 hrs; laparoscopic cholecystectomy preferred when possible
- Cholecystostomy (percutaneous drainage of gallbladder) in nonoperative patients

Acute Acalculous/Chronic Cholecystitis

ACUTE ACALCULOUS CHOLECYSTITIS

- Acute necroinflammatory disease of the gallbladder with a multifactorial pathogenesis; high morbidity/mortality (10%)
- Etiology: gallbladder stasis and ischemia leading to a local inflammatory reaction in gallbladder wall; leads to concentration of bile salts, gallbladder distention, secondary infection, perforation or necrosis of gallbladder tissue
- Risk factors: (current) hospitalization and critically ill status (in critically ill patients, unexplained fever, leukocytosis, jaundice, sepsis or vague abdominal discomfort may be only signs of this condition)
- Because the presentation may be insidious, perforation, gallbladder necrosis, and gangrene may be seen at time of diagnosis
- Diagnosis: based on clinical symptoms in the setting of supportive imaging and the exclusion of alternative diagnoses; ultrasonography
  - If diagnosis remains uncertain, contrast-enhanced abdominal CT
  - If diagnosis remains uncertain after CT, HIDA scan
- Management: supportive care (IV fluids, bowel rest, pain control, correction of electrolytes); broad spectrum antibiotics; definitive management is cholecystectomy or cholecystostomy

CHRONIC CHOLECYSTITIS

- Chronic inflammatory cell infiltration of the gallbladder seen on histopathology
- Etiology: recurrent attacks of acute cholecystitis leading to fibrosis and thickening of gallbladder

HEPATITIS

Inflammatory condition of the liver

Hepatitis A Virus (HAV)

Viral liver disease caused by infected person or contaminated food or water

- Transmission: feco-oral
- Contaminated water/food during international travel (40%), day care workers, shellfish
- Usually asymptomatic in children age <6, mild disease in adults
- Most common source for adults: hepatitis A (only viral hepatitis associated with spiking fevers)
- Acute hepatitis: positive IgM HAV Ab (antibodies)
- Past exposure: positive IgG HAV Ab with negative IgM
- Self-limiting (symptomatic treatment)
- Post exposure prophylaxis for close contacts: immune globulin

Hepatitis C Virus (HCV)

Viral liver disease due to contact with infected blood

- Transmission: parenteral (most common), sexual; increased risk if history of blood transfusion before 1992; no documented cases through breastfeeding
- 85% of patients with HCV develop chronic infection
- Fulminant is rare
- Anti HCV: positive within 6 weeks; does not imply recovery
- HCV-RNA more sensitive than anti HCV
- Screening for HCC via serum alpha-fetoprotein & U/S

	HCV RNA	Anti-HCV
Acute hepatitis	Positive	±
Resolved hepatitis	Negative	±
Chronic hepatitis	Positive	Positive

- Pegylated interferon alfa 2b and ribavirin
- Newer options
  - Genotype 1: ledipasvir-sofosbuvir, elbasvir-grazoprevir, ombitasvir-paritaprevir-ritonavir plus dasabuvir with or without ribavirin, simeprevir plus sofosbuvir, and daclatasvir plus sofosbuvir
  - Genotype 2: sofosbuvir and weight-based ribavirin
  - Genotype 3: daclatasvir plus sofosbuvir (if no cirrhosis), If cirrhosis: daclatasvir plus sofosbuvir plus ribavirin or sofosbuvir plus pegylated interferon or sofosbuvir plus ribavirin
  - Genotype 4: ledipasvir-sofosbuvir, elbasvir-grazoprevir (± ribavirin), ombitasvir-paritaprevir-ritonavir plus weight-based ribavirin

Hepatitis B Virus (HBV)

Viral liver disease due to contact with infected blood or sexual partner

- Transmission: perinatal, percutaneous, sexual, parenteral
- Three possible states
  - Acute (70% subclinical, 30% jaundice, <1% fulminant hepatitis)
  - Chronic (~10% adult acquired; >90% perinatally acquired)
  - Chronic asymptomatic carrier: increased risk for hepatocellular carcinoma; most are asymptomatic
- Serologic Tests
  - HBs**Ag**: first evidence of HBV infection or chronic infection if positive occurs after 6 months, hence **A**ttack is **G**rowing
  - HBs**Ab**: distant resolved infection or vaccination hence **A**ttack **B**locked
  - HBcAb IGM: acute infection; may be the only **M**arker in the window period
  - HBcAB IGG: chronic infection or distant resolved infection; attack is **G**rowing (chronic) or **G**one (resolved)
  - HBe**AG**: increased viral infection and infectivity; **A**ttack is **G**rowing
  - HBe**AB**: indicates waning viral replication, decreased infectivity; **A**ttack getting **B**etter

Diagnosis	HBsAg	anti-HBs	anti-HBc	HbeAg	Anti-Hbe
Window Period	Negative	Negative	IgM	Negative	Negative
Acute hepatitis	Positive	Negative	IgM	±	±
Recovery	Negative	Positive	IgG	Negative	Negative
Immunization	Negative	Positive	Negative	Negative	Negative
Chronic hepatitis replicative	Positive	Negative	IgG	Positive	Negative
Chronic hepatitis nonreplicative	Positive	Negative	IgG	Negative	Positive

- Acute HBV: supportive
- Chronic HBV (positive HBsAg and HBV DNA) if increased ALT or inflammation on biopsy; positive HbeAg leads to interferon α 2b, lamivudine; adefovir, tenofovir, telbivudine, entecavir newer options
- HBV vaccine initiated at 0, 1, and 6 months from initial dose; HBV vaccine contraindicated if allergic to Baker's yeast

Gastrointestinal

ACUTE PANCREATITIS

Sudden inflammatory condition affecting the pancreas

Etiology/Pathophysiology

- Gallstones (most common); ETOH
- Meds: thiazides, protease inhibitors, estrogen, didanosine, etc
- Iatrogenic (ERCP), infections (eg, viral)
- Malignancy, scorpion bites, idiopathic, post traumatic
- Cystic fibrosis; increased triglycerides
- Pathophysiology: acinar cell injury leads to intracellular activation of enzymes, auto-digestion of pancreas, edema, interstitial hemorrhage, coagulation, and cellular fat necrosis

Clinical Manifestations/Physical Exam

- Epigastric abdominal pain: constant, boring (frequently radiating to back or other quadrant)
    - ± exacerbated in supine position and with walking
    - ± relieved with leaning forward, sitting, or fetal position
- Nausea, vomiting, and fever are common symptoms
- Physical exam: ± epigastric tenderness, decreased bowel sounds secondary to adynamic ileus, dehydration, shock, tachycardia, Cullen's sign and Grey Turner's sign are infrequent but if present it suggests necrotizing (hemorrhagic) pancreatitis
- Cullen's sign: periumbilical ecchymosis
- Grey Turner: flank ecchymosis

Diagnosis

- Laboratory values: leukocytosis, increased glucose, hypocalcemia, increased bilirubin, increased triglycerides
    - Lipase: compared to amylase, more specific, rises earlier (4–8 hrs), and stays elevated longer (7–14 days)
    - Amylase: >3x upper limit of normal suggestive of pancreatitis but levels do not equal severity and amylase is not specific for pancreatitis; rises in 6–12 hrs and returns to normal within 3–5 days
    - ALT: increased three-fold highly suggestive of gallstone pancreatitis hypertriglyceridemia
- Abdominal CT: diagnostic test of choice
- Abdominal U/S: used to rule out gallstones, common bile duct dilation, ascites, pseudocysts
- AXR: ± "sentinel loop" (localized ileus—dilated small bowel in LUQ); used to rule out other conditions (perforation); pancreatic calcification suggestive of chronic pancreatitis

Management/Prognosis

- 90% recover without complications within 3–7 days and require supportive measures only ("rest the pancreas")
- Supportive therapy: NPO, IV fluids (up to 10 L/day); analgesia with opioids
- Antibiotics not used prophylactically unless secondary infection occurs; treat with broad spectrum antibiotics: (eg, imipenem/cilastatin)
- Ranson's criteria used to assess severity
- ERCP if biliary sepsis suspected (effective only in obstructive jaundice)

INFLAMMATORY BOWEL DISEASE

- Idiopathic (most likely due to immune reaction to GI tract flora)
- Most common in Caucasians, increased refined sugar intake, decreased fruit/vegetable intake. Smoking increases incidence of CD. Smoking may be associated with reduced incidence of UC.
- Most commonly presents age 15–35
- Manifestations common in both: uveitis, arthritis, erythema nodosum, pyoderma gangrenosum, primary sclerosing cholangitis (more common in UC)

Crohn Disease

Inflammatory condition of the digestive tract

- Any segment of GI tract (from mouth to anus); transmural
- Most commonly involves terminal ileum
- RLQ pain (ileocolitis), diarrhea with no visible blood
- Associated with perianal disease, abscesses, and strictures
- Diagnosis: upper GI series with small bowel follow through: strictures (string sign), abscesses, fistulas; endoscopy (skip lesions, ie, normal areas interspersed with inflamed areas and cobblestone appearance of mucosa); biopsy (transmural inflammation, noncaseating granulomas, microscopic skip lesions); positive ASCA (antibodies vs. saccharomyces cerevisiae)
- Management: corticosteroids with or without aminosalicylates; immunomodulators (eg, 6-mercaptopurine, methotrexate); anti-TNF agents (adalimumab, infliximab, certolizumab); anti-integrins (natalizumab)

Ulcerative Colitis

Digestive tract condition associated with ulcers and inflammation

- Rectum always involved with proximal contiguous spread
- Limited to colon; mucosal and submucosal involvement only
- LLQ pain, diarrhea (may have visible blood), tenesmus, urgency
- Increased incidence of toxic megacolon and colorectal cancer
- Diagnosis: flexible sigmoidoscopy or colonoscopy (uniform inflammation, ulcerations and pseudopolyps); barium enema (loss of haustral markings, ie, stove-pipe sign; biopsy (diffuse nonsegmental inflammation limited to mucosa and submucosa); positive p-ANCA
- Management: topical aminosalicylates (topical corticosteroids may also help); immunomodulators (eg, 6-mercaptopurine, methotrexate, azathioprine); anti-TNF agents (adalimumab, infliximab); anti-integrins (natalizumab); surgery may be curative in some cases

Gastrointestinal

King with **CROWNS** love **BIG MEALS** and **PEACE**.

Crowns = Crohn's

B12 deficiency (due to ileal involvement)
Ileum MC site of involvement
Granuloma formation

Mouth to anus involved
Entire wall (**transmural**)
ASCA positivity
Lesion show **skip pattern**
String sign seen on UGI series

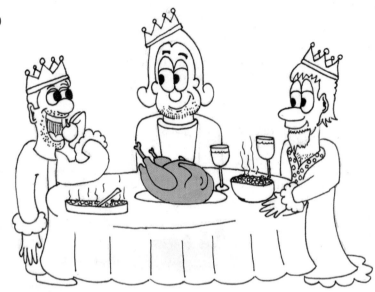

PEACE = No Blood-Non Bloody Diarrhea

Figure 3.3 Crohn's Disease

DISEASES AFFECTING BILIRUBIN

Liver conditions which affect bilirubin, an orange-yellow pigment formed (in the liver) when RBCs undergo the breakdown of hemoglobin

Crigler-Najjar Syndrome

High levels of unconjugated bilirubin in blood

- Increased indirect (unconjugated) hyperbilirubinemia: 0.6–1.0 per million
- UGT
  - Type I: no UGT activity; autosomal recessive
  - Type II: very little UGT activity (≤10% of normal); autosomal dominant
- Type I: jaundice during week 1 of life with severe progression in week 2 leading to kernicterus (increased bilirubin in CNS and basal ganglia lead to hypotonia, deafness, lethargy, oculomotor palsy, and death often by age of 15 months); hyperbilirubinemia usually persists lifelong
- Type II: usually asymptomatic; often an incidental finding on routine lab testing
- Isolated indirect (unconjugated) hyperbilirubinemia with normal LFTs; liver looks normal on biopsy
- CN I: serum indirect bilirubin often 20–50 mg/dL
- CN II: serum indirect bilirubin often 7–10 mg/dL
- Phototherapy, plasmapheresis (in crisis)
- Liver transplant definitive

Budd Chiari Syndrome

Blood flow via hepatic vein is blocked

- Laying in the **SAND** while absorbing **UV radiation** made **BUDD** forget how to play the **HARP**
- **H**epatomegaly, **A**scites, **R**UQ **P**ain
- **U**/S or **V**enography (gold standard)
- **S**hunt, **AN**gioplasty with stent, **D**iuretics

Gilbert's Syndrome

High levels of unconjugated bilirubin in blood

- Common benign hereditary disorder with reduced activity of UGT enzyme (5–10% of U.S. population)
- Reduced UGT activity (10–30% of normal) leads to increased indirect bilirubin; also, due to defective bilirubin uptake mechanism
- Usually asymptomatic but may experience transient episodes of jaundice during periods of stress, fasting, ETOH, or illness
- Usually an incidental finding: slight increased isolated indirect bilirubin level with normal liver function values
- No management needed because it is a mild, benign disease

Dubin Johnson Syndrome

High levels of conjugated bilirubin in blood

- Isolated mild conjugated (direct) hyperbilirubinemia due to inability of hepatocytes to secrete conjugated bilirubin (MRP2 gene mutation)
- Autosomal dominant
- Usually asymptomatic but may present with generalized constitutional symptoms
- Mild conjugated (direct) hyperbilirubinemia (2–5 mg/dL) but can increase with concurrent illness, pregnancy OCPs
- Grossly black liver on biopsy
- No management needed

Dubin Johnson syndrome = **D**irect bilirubin (isolated increased direct bilirubin), autosomal **D**ominant, **D**ark liver on biopsy

Patterns of Liver Disease

> **Alcoholic hepatitis**
> - AST:ALT > 2:1 (**S** for **S**cotch)

> **Viral/toxic/inflammatory processes**
> - ALT > AST (**L** for **L**iver disease)
> - AST and ALT often >1,000 in acute hepatitis (viral, toxic, autoimmune)

> **Biliary obstruction/intrahepatic cholestasis**
> - Increased **GGT** with increased alkaline phosphatase (**GGT** for **G**all **G**ets in **T**rouble)

> **Tests of hepatic synthetic function**
> - During liver damage, **PT**s go before **ALL**. **PT** levels are an earlier indicator of severe liver disease/prognosis than **AL**bumin.

CIRRHOSIS

Liver fibrosis with nodular regeneration that leads to increased portal pressure

Etiology/Pathophysiology

- Alcohol is the most common cause in the United States
- Chronic viral hepatitis (HBV, HCV, HDV), nonalcoholic fatty liver disease, hemochromatosis, autoimmune hepatitis, primary biliary cirrhosis, primary sclerosing cholangitis, and drug toxicity

Risk Factors

- Chronic alcohol use is the most important risk factor

Clinical Manifestations/Physical Exam

- Fatigue, weakness, weight loss, muscle cramps, anorexia
- Ascites, hepatosplenomegaly, gynecomastia, spider angioma/telangiectasias, caput medusa, muscle wasting, bleeding, palmar erythema, jaundice, Dupuytren's contractures
- Hepatic encephalopathy: confusion and lethargy (increased ammonia levels toxic to the brain)
- Asterixis (flapping tremor with wrist extension); fetor hepaticus
- Esophageal varices, spontaneous bacterial peritonitis

Diagnosis

- U/S determines liver size and evaluates for hepatocellular carcinoma
- Liver biopsy definitive
- Child-Pugh classification used for staging

Management/Prognosis

- Encephalopathy: lactulose or rifaximin; neomycin second-line; protein restriction
- Ascites: sodium restriction; diuretics (spironolactone, furosemide); paracentesis
- Pruritus: cholestyramine is a bile acid sequestrant which reduces bile salts in the skin, leading to less irritation from the bile salts
- Screening for hepatocellular carcinoma: U/S and alpha-fetoprotein; the 2017 American Association for the Study of Liver Diseases (AASLD) guideline on the management of hepatocellular carcinoma recommends surveillance using ultrasonography at 6-month intervals

ABCDEs of Cirrhosis

<u>A</u>scites
<u>B</u>12 deficiency
<u>C</u>oagulopathy with advanced disease
<u>D</u>etoxification impaired
<u>E</u>strogen ↑ (gynecomastia)
<u>F</u>lapping tremor (asterixis)
<u>G</u>lucose abnormalities
<u>H</u>emoglobin
<u>I</u>ncreased infections
<u>J</u>aundice
<u>K</u> (vitamin) deficiency
<u>L</u>ethargy (encephalopathy)

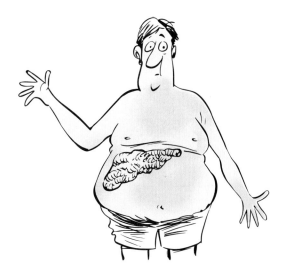

Figure 3.4 Cirrhosis

WILSON'S DISEASE

Free copper accumulation in liver, brain, kidney, cornea

Etiology/Pathophysiology

- Rare autosomal recessive disorder (ATB7B mutation leads to inadequate bile excretion of copper with increased small intestine absorption of copper; copper deposition in tissues causes cellular damage)

Risk Factors

- Most commonly age >40

Clinical Manifestations/Physical Exam

- CNS copper deposits, basal ganglia deposition: Parkinson-like symptoms (bradykinesia, tremor, rigidity), dementia; personality and behavioral changes
- Liver disease: hepatitis, hepatosplenomegaly, cirrhosis, hemolytic anemia
- Corneal copper deposits lead to Kayser-Fleischer rings (brown or green pigment in cornea)

Diagnosis

- Increased urinary copper excretion, decreased ceruloplasmin (the serum carrier molecule for copper)

Management/Prognosis

- Ammonium tetrathiomolybdate: increases urinary copper excretion by binding to copper
- Penicillamine: chelates copper (must give pyridoxine/Vitamin B6 to prevent depletion)
- Zinc: enhances urinary copper excretion and blocks intestinal copper absorption

With **Wilson's disease** treatment, you've got to **ZAP** the copper in order to treat it:

- **Z**inc
- **A**mmonium tetrathiomolybdate
- **P**encillamine

VITAMIN DEFICIENCIES

Diet lacking in specific nutrients lead to insufficient amounts of essential vitamins

Vitamin C (Ascorbic Acid) Deficiency

- **Vitamin C deficiency**: "3 Hs": **h**yperkeratosis, **h**emorrhage, **h**ematologic (anemia)
- Diets lacking raw citrus fruits and green vegetables (excess heat denatures vitamin C), smoking
- Scurvy: malaise, weakness, vascular fragility (due to abnormal collagen production) with recurrent hemorrhage in gums, skin (perifollicular), and joints; impaired wound healing, hyperkeratotic papules

Vitamin D Deficiency

- Rickets (children): softening of the bones leading to bowing deformities (eg, bowed legs), fractures, dental problems, muscle weakness, developmental delays
- Osteomalacia (adults): diffuse body pains, muscle weakness and fractures; looser lines
- Management/Prognosis: ergocalciferol (vitamin D) (treatment of choice)

Vitamin A Deficiency

- Vitamin A function: vision, immune function, embryo development, hematopoiesis, skin and cellular health (epithelial cell differentiation)
- Vitamin A deficiency
  - Visual changes (especially night blindness), impaired immunity (poor wound healing)
  - Squamous metaplasia: conjunctiva, respiratory epithelium, urinary tract
  - Bitot spots (white spots on conjunctiva)
  - Xerophthalmia (dry eye), alopecia, loss of taste

Bitot couldn't see the poorly healing spot on his skin because it was midnight.

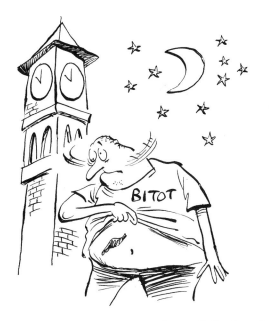

- Visual changes (especially **night blindness**)

- Impaired immunity (poor wound healing)

- **Squamous metaplasia** (conjunctiva, respiratory epithelium, urinary tract)

- **Bitot spots** (white spots on conjunctiva)

Figure 3.5 Vitamin A Deficiency

Vitamin B Deficiency

Thiamine (B1) Deficiency

- ETOH most common cause in United States, decreased thiamine intake (eg, non-enriched cereal)
- Beriberi:
  - "Dry": paresthesias, demyelination leads to peripheral neuropathy, symmetrical peripheral neuropathy characterized by both sensory & motor impairments, mostly of the distal extremities; anorexia, muscle cramps, and wasting
  - "Wet": high output failure, dilated cardiomyopathy, edema
- Wernicke's encephalopathy triad: ophthalmoplegia (paralysis of the ocular muscles), ataxia (difficulty walking and balancing), global confusion
- Korsakoff's dementia: memory loss (especially short-term memory), irreversible confabulation

Korsakoff drank so much he **forgot** that **W**eak-eyed **Wernicke W**addled be**W**ilderly right past him **1** minute **AGO.**

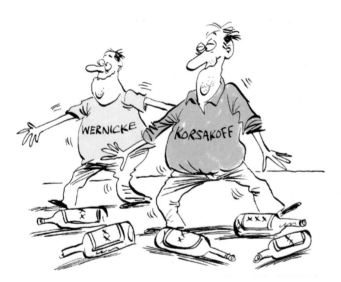

Wernicke's Triad:
- **Ataxia** (waddled)
- **Global confusion** (bewildered)
- **Ophthalmoplegia** (ocular weakness)

Korsakoff's Dementia:
- **Memory loss** (especially short-term memory), confabulation, irreversible

Figure 3.6 Vitamin B1 (Thiamine) Deficiency

Riboflavin (B2) Deficiency

- Oral-ocular-genital syndrome:
  - Oral: lesions of mouth, magenta-colored tongue, angular cheilitis, pharyngitis
  - Ocular: photophobia/corneal lesions
  - Genital: scrotal dermatitis

Niacin/Nicotinic Acid (B3) Deficiency

- Often due to diet high in corn (lacks niacin) or insufficient in tryptophan
- Pellagra "3 Ds": **D**iarrhea, **D**ementia, and **D**ermatitis

Pyridoxine (B6) Deficiency

- Alcoholism, isoniazid, oral contraceptives
- Peripheral neuropathy, flaky skin, headache, anemia, sore tongue, stomatitis, and seizures

B12 (Cobalamine) Deficiency

- Pernicious anemia: autoimmune destruction/loss of gastric parietal cells (parietal cells secrete intrinsic factor needed for B12 absorption from the GI tract)
- Strict vegans with diet lacking alternative B12 sources
- Malabsorption: alcoholism, celiac disease, Crohn's, atrophic gastritis, acid-reducing drugs (PPIs and H2 blockers reduce B12 absorption because intrinsic factor works in an acidic environment), gastric bypass surgery
- Neurologic symptoms: (paresthesias, gait abnormalities, memory loss, dementia) due to degeneration of the posterolateral of spinal cord
- Glossitis
- GI disturbances: anorexia and diarrhea
- Macrocytic anemia with hypersegmented neutrophils
- Schilling test, antibody testing
- Management/Prognosis: IM or oral B12 depending on the cause

INVASIVE DIARRHEA

Shigella Dysenteriae

- Most commonly transmitted feco-orally

Enterohemorrhagic *E. Coli*

- Most commonly transmitted via undercooked ground beef, unpasteurized milk/cider, contaminated water, day care centers

Campylobacter Jejuni

- Associated with contaminated poultry, feco-oral
- Most commonly follows post-infectious Guillain-Barré syndrome

Salmonella

- Nontyphoidal: most common source poultry and reptiles (eg, turtles) associated with "pea soup" colored stools
- Typhi: feco-oral transmission; may be a carrier (eg, Typhoid Mary) or cause typhoid fever:
  - Rose spots most common on abdomen, fever with bradycardia (turtles move slowly)
  - Headache, abdominal pain (mimics appendicitis)

Yersinia Enterocolitica

- Associated with pork, pet feces, day care centers
- Can also mimic appendicitis

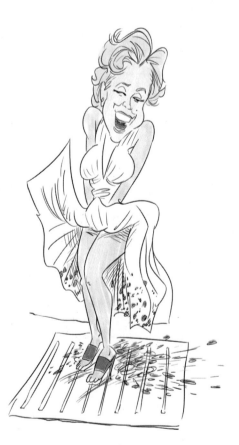

After **entering** the **Barr** in **Camp** and eating fecally contaminated **turtle pea soup, Typhoid Mary** thought she was "**SECSY**" until she had **explosive, watery, bloody diarrhea** that left a **rose-spot** on her **white** dress.

S̲higella dysenteriae: most commonly transmitted feco-orally

E̲nterohemorrhagic *E. Coli*

C̲ampylobacter jejuni associated with contaminated poultry, feco-oral. Most common preceding event in post-infectious Guillain-**Barré**

S̲almonella

Y̲ersinia enterocolitica

White (fecal leukocytes) or blood may be seen in patients with invasive diarrhea

Figure 3.7 Invasive Diarrhea

Chapter 4

Musculoskeletal

SHOULDER DISLOCATION

Anterior Shoulder Dislocations

Usually due to violent external rotation, abduction, and posterior forces; (~95% of all shoulder dislocations)

- Arm abducted, externally rotated; humeral head is located anterior and/or inferior, causing a loss of the deltoid contour
- Emergent reduction required

Posterior Shoulder Dislocations

Forced adduction, internal rotation

- Often associated with seizures, electric shock injuries, direct trauma; 4%
- Arm adducted, internally rotated
- Anterior shoulder appears flat
- Humeral head prominent
- Emergent reduction required

ABE ran to the ER after dislocating his shoulder while shaving his Axillary Hair.

Mechanism:
Forced Abducted and External Rotation

Physical Exam:
- **Shoulder "squared off" loss of deltoid contour**

- **Arm held in Abduction and External Rotation**

- **Rule out Axillary nerve damage pre and post reduction**

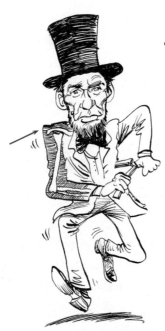

- **Hill-Sachs fracture posterolateral Humerus**

  - **Bankart Lesion: Broken glenoid rim due to injury of anterior (inferior) glenoid labrum**

  - **Shaving axillary hair; patients are instructed not to do overhead movements right after reduction**

Figure 4.1 Anterior Shoulder Dislocation

Posterior shoulder dislocation = when you get an **electric shock** after touching an electrified **post**, you will fly in the **AIR** and have a **seizure**, dislocating your shoulder

Adducted and **I**nternally **R**otated (associated with seizures and shock)

ROTATOR CUFF INJURIES

Inflamed tendons

Etiology/Pathophysiology

- Chronic erosion, ± trauma; affects the supraspinatus, infraspinatus, teres minor, subscapularis
- Tendonitis: inflammation often with subacromial bursitis

Risk Factors

- Rotator cuff tear: most common cause of shoulder pain in patients age >40

Clinical Manifestations/Physical Exam

- Anterior deltoid pain with decreased ROM especially with overhead activities, internal rotation, or abduction (combing hair, reaching for wallet)
- Weakness, atrophy, and continuous pain most commonly seen with tears
- Physical exam:
  - ROM: passive ROM usually greater than active ROM (limited active ROM) of humerus
  - Supraspinatus strength test: "empty can" test
  - Impingement tests of subscapular nerve/supraspinatus:
    - Positive Hawkins-Kennedy test: elbow/shoulder flexed at 90° with sharp anterior shoulder pain with internal rotation
    - Positive drop arm test: pain with inability to lift or hold the arm above shoulder level or severe pain while slowly lowering arm after shoulder abducted to 90°
    - Positive Neer test: arm fully pronated (thumbs down) with pain during forward flexion (while shoulder is held down to prevent shrugging)

Management/Prognosis

- Tendonitis: shoulder pendulum/wall climbing exercises, ice, NSAIDs, physical activity
- Tear: rehabilitation, NSAIDs, intra-articular steroids; surgery for ROM preservation

ABE the MINOR DROPS his EMPTY CAN and quickly SITS down because he almost PASSED out after looking ABOVE and seeing a HAWK leave DROPPINGS NEER him.

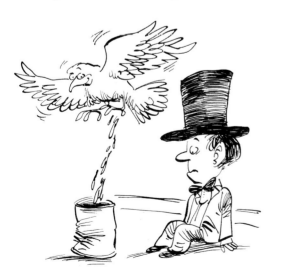

- Pain with **AB**duction and **E**xternal rotation

- Teres **MINOR** is part of the **SITS** muscles

- Above: **SUPRA**spinatus most commonly involved

Physical Examination:
- **Empty Can test**
- **Passive** ROM > active
- **HAWK**INS test
- **DROP** arm test
- **NEER** test

Figure 4.2 Rotator Cuff Injuries

FRACTURES

Proximal Humeral Fracture

Direct blow to arm
- Etiology: FOOSH (fall on outstretched arm)
- Risk factors: metastatic breast cancer (proximal humerus is a common site for pathologic fracture)
- Clinical manifestations: patients usually hold arm in adducted position; check deltoid sensation to rule out brachial plexus injury; ± crepitus/ecchymosis

Proximal Humerus Fracture
- **P**lexus injuries must be ruled out
- **H**eld in adduction (arm position)
- **F**OOSH is most common mechanism

Supracondylar Fracture

FOOSH (fall on outstretched hand) with hyperextended elbow (extra-articular)
- Risk factors: most commonly children age 5–10
- Clinical manifestations: swelling/tenderness at elbow/prominent olecranon with depression proximally
- Complications: median nerve and brachial artery injury leads to Volkmann's ischemic contracture (claw-like deformity from ischemia with flexion/contracture of wrist); radial nerve injury
- Diagnosis: if displaced, abnormal anterior humeral line on lateral view; if non-displaced, leads to positive anterior fat pad sign (supracondylar fracture in children and radial head fracture in adults)
- Management: if displaced, ORIF (all displaced fractures or severe swelling should be admitted for observation with immediate orthopedic consult); if non-displaced, splint

Radial Head Fracture

Fall on outstretched arm resulting in fracture to radial head
- Clinical manifestations: lateral (radial) elbow pain, inability to fully extend elbow
- Diagnosis: notoriously difficult to see; posterior or increased anterior fat pad
- Management: if nondisplaced, sling, long arm splint, 90°; if displaced, ORIF

Monteggia Fracture

Proximal ulnar shaft fracture with anterior radial head dislocation
- Etiology: usually direct blow to forearm
- Clinical manifestations: elbow pain, paresthesias to thumb, radial nerve injury (wrist drop)
- Management: ORIF

Galeazzi Fracture

Mid-distal radial shaft fracture with dislocation of distal radio-ulnar joint
- Etiology: FOOSH or direct blow
- Clinical manifestations: fracture/deformity at radial surface of wrist; additionally, ulnar head will appear prominent at wrist because it is dorsally displaced
- Management: unstable so ORIF required; long arm splint; sugar tong splint for stabilization
- **Type I:** isolated growth plate fracture (may look normal) (best outcome)
- **Type II:** growth plate fracture and fracture of metaphysis (good prognosis) (most common type)
- **Type III:** growth plate fracture and fracture of epiphysis (good prognosis)
- **Type IV:** fracture extending across metaphysis, growth plate, and epiphysis (needs reduction)
- **Type V:** growth plate compression injury (may arrest growth) (worst prognosis)

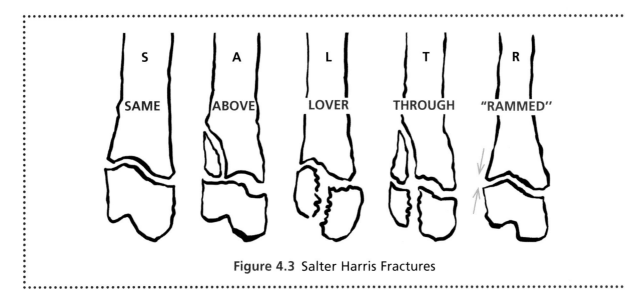

Figure 4.3 Salter Harris Fractures

Monte**GG**ia fracture—**two Gs** represent problem in **two locations**

- Proximal Ulnar shaft fracture
- Anterior radial head dislocation

People usually confuse this with GaleaZZi fracture; **G comes before Z,** so the fracture is **Proximal** with Monte**GG**ia

Galea**ZZ**i fracture—**two Zs** represent a problem in **two locations**

- Distal radial shaft fracture
- Dislocation of distal radio-ulnar joint

Z comes after G, so the fracture is **DISTAL** with Galea**ZZ**i

In an adult, **fat pads** will increase the **RADIUS** of his or her **HEAD**

Anterior fat pad sign: **Radial head** fracture in **adults**

During the history and physical, remember the things you should ask/identify with the mnemonic HAND:

- **H**ow did this injury happen?
- **A**nti-tetanus (Have you received a tetanus shot?)
- **N**ot employed (Are you employed? If yes, what do you do?)
- **D**ominant hand

- **H**urts (Palpate and ask where there is pain)
- **A**ny ROM deficits?
- **N**erves: check radial, ulnar, and median nerve to rule out nerve damage
- **D**iscrimination (2-point discrimination)

EPICONDYLITIS

Inflammation or injury to the epicondyle bone

Lateral Epicondylitis (Tennis Elbow)

Inflammation of tendon insertion of ECRB muscle

- Etiology: repetitive pronation of forearm and excessive wrist extension
- Clinical manifestations: lateral elbow pain especially with gripping, forearm pronation, and wrist extension against resistance; possible radiation down forearm
- Management: RICE (rest, ice, compression, elevation); NSAIDs to reduce inflammation; physiotherapy; bracing; intraarticular corticosteroid injection

Medial Epicondylitis (Golfer's Elbow)

Inflammation of the interface between pronator teres and flexor carpi radialis

- Etiology: repetitive stress at tendon insertion of flexor forearm muscle
- Risk factors: frequent golfing; repetitive household chores
- Clinical manifestations: tenderness over medial epicondyle worse with pulling activities, reproduced by forcefully extending elbow against resistance with forearm supinated and wrist flexion against resistance
- Management: same as lateral epicondylitis (however more difficult to treat)

Lateral Epicondylitis (Tennis Elbow)

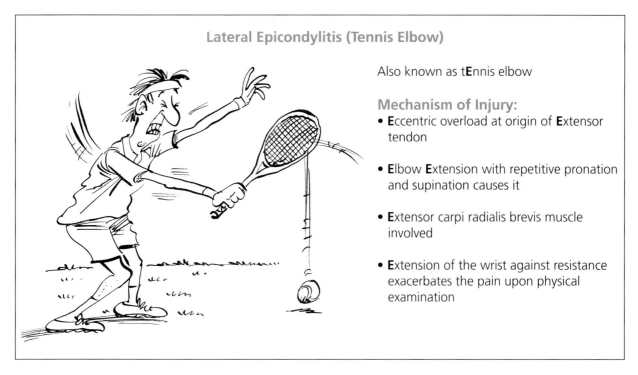

Also known as t**E**nnis elbow

Mechanism of Injury:
- **E**ccentric overload at origin of **E**xtensor tendon

- **E**lbow **E**xtension with repetitive pronation and supination causes it

- **E**xtensor carpi radialis brevis muscle involved

- **E**xtension of the wrist against resistance exacerbates the pain upon physical examination

Figure 4.4 Lateral Epicondylitis (Tennis Elbow)

Medial Epicondylitis (Golfer's Elbow)

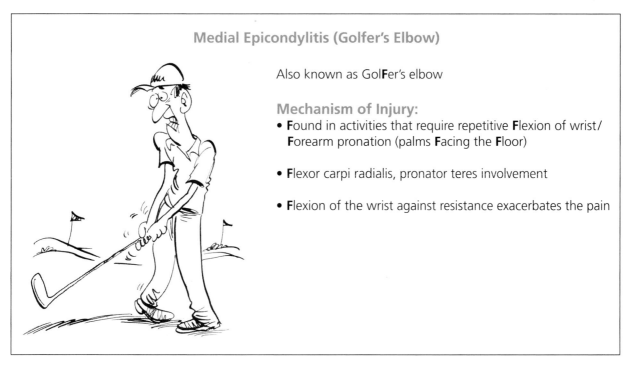

Also known as Gol**F**er's elbow

Mechanism of Injury:
- **F**ound in activities that require repetitive **F**lexion of wrist/**F**orearm pronation (palms **F**acing the **F**loor)

- **F**lexor carpi radialis, pronator teres involvement

- **F**lexion of the wrist against resistance exacerbates the pain

Figure 4.5 Medial Epicondylitis (Golfer's Elbow)

Musculoskeletal

THUMB INJURIES

Skier's/Gamekeeper's Thumb

Ulnar collateral ligamental injury of thumb leading to instability of metacarpophalangeal joint

- Etiology: forced abduction of the thumb
- Clinical manifestations: skier's thumb (acute condition eg, after fall); gamekeeper's thumb (chronic hyperabduction injury); thumb far away from the other digits (especially with valgus stress, pulling thumb away from hand); metacarpophalangeal tenderness; weakness in pinch strength; ± fracture at base of proximal phalanx (if ligamental rupture pulls off piece of bone)
- Management: thumb spica and referral to hand surgeon (because affects pincer function); surgical repair for complete rupture

Bennett Fracture: Dislocation/Rolando Fracture

Fractures at the base of the thumb

- Clinical manifestations: Bennett's fracture: intra-articular fracture through base of first metacarpal bone with the large distal fragment dislocated radially and dorsally by abductor pollicis longus muscle; Rolando's fracture (comminuted Bennett's fracture)
- Management: unstable so ORIF required; thumb spica for stabilization

---

Gamekeeper's thumb:

- Gamers keep their games until they ABuse them
- Chronic hyperABduction injury
- Rolando fracture: Rolls around the base of the thumb (comminuted)

HIP INJURIES

Hip Dislocation

An orthopedic emergency

- Etiology: trauma most common cause (MVA, fall from height); posterior dislocation most common type of hip dislocation (90%); anterior usually secondary to forced hip abduction
- Risk factors: avascular necrosis (reduced with early closed reduction, <6 hrs); sciatic nerve injury, DVT, bleeding
- Clinical manifestations: hip pain with leg shortened; internally rotated and adducted with hip/knee slightly flexed; anterior may be externally rotated

Hip Fracture

Fracture in upper part of the femur

- Etiology: femoral head/neck fracture: high incidence of avascular necrosis with femoral neck fracture (intracapsular and have high association with DVT and PE post-injury); intertrochanteric/subtrochanteric are extracapsular
- Risk factors: elderly age (very common); osteoporosis; decreased bone mass due to minor/indirect trauma; high-impact injury
- Clinical manifestations: hip pain with leg shortened, externally rotated and abducted
- Management: ORIF; observation alone may be indicated for those with minimal pain, high surgical risk, or inability to move independently

If you have a hip dislocation you must POST an AD to help SHORTEN your INTERNAL stay at the hospital.

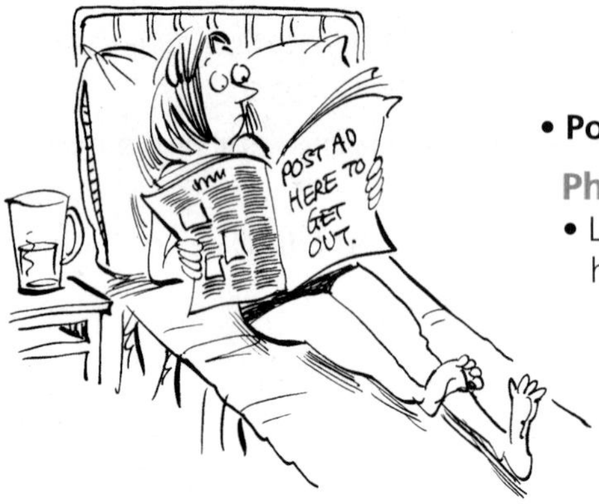

- **Posterior** (most common type)

Physical Exam:
- Leg **Shortened, Internally rotated,** and **Adducted** with hip/knee slightly flexed.

Figure 4.6 Hip Dislocation

Hip fractures SHORTEN your ER visit because you get admitted and abducted to the floor right away.

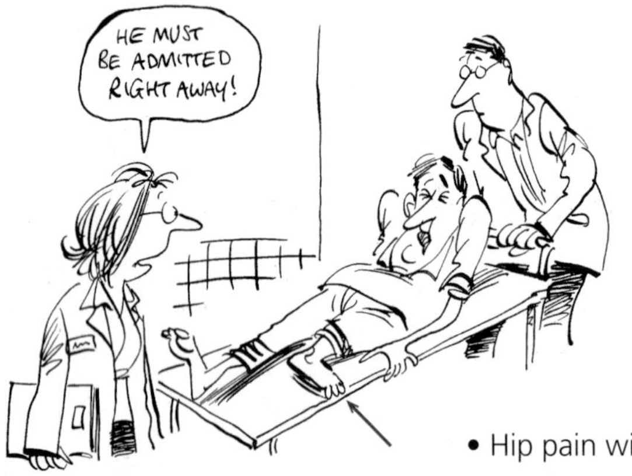

- Hip pain with leg **Shortened** and **E**xternally **R**otated and **abducted**

Figure 4.7 Hip Fracture

LEGG-CALVÉ PERTHES DISEASE

Idiopathic avascular osteonecrosis of the femoral head in children

Etiology/Pathophysiology

- Ischemia of capital femoral epiphysis

Risk Factors

- Most commonly affects children age 4–10; boy > girls (4:1)
- Low incidence in African Americans

Clinical Manifestations/Physical Exam

- Painless limping (worsened with continued activity especially at the end of the day), hip pain may radiate to thigh, knee, or groin; restricted ROM (loss of abduction and internal rotation)

Diagnosis

- Early: Increased density of femoral head, widening of cartilage space
- Advanced: deformity, crescent sign (subchondral fracture)

Management/Prognosis

- Observation: children age <5 or patients with <50% femoral involvement, NSAIDs; bedrest; self-limiting with revascularization within 2 years usually (depends on age)
- Abduction bracing: children age >5 or patients with significant loss of abduction
- Pelvic osteotomy

ABE had to stop for AIR because his painless LIMPING got worse as the CRESCENT moon lit up the sky.

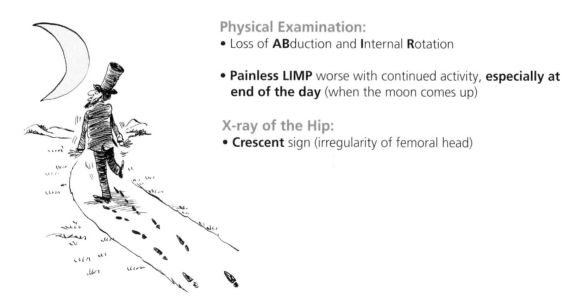

Physical Examination:
- Loss of **AB**duction and **I**nternal **R**otation

- **Painless LIMP** worse with continued activity, **especially at end of the day** (when the moon comes up)

X-ray of the Hip:
- **Crescent** sign (irregularity of femoral head)

Figure 4.8 Legg-Calvé Perthes Disease

Musculoskeletal

SLIPPED CAPITAL FEMORAL EPIPHYSIS

Femoral head (epiphysis) slips posterior and inferior at growth plate

Risk Factors

- Most commonly affects age 7–16, obese boys during growth spurt due to weakness of growth plate (due to hormonal changes at puberty)
- Hypothyroidism or hypopituitarism in childhood if it develops before puberty

Clinical Manifestations/Physical Exam

Hip, thigh, or knee pain, painful limping, external rotation of affected leg

Management/Prognosis

- ORIF because of increased risk of avascular necrosis
- Non-weight-bearing (crutches)

After the OBESE boy slipped on a cap, HE PAINFULLY LIMPED to the ER.

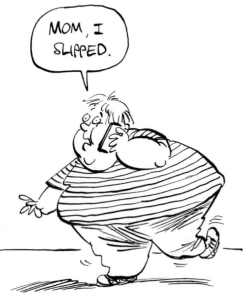

- MC in **obese male children.**

- Hip, thigh, or knee **pain with Limping**

- **E**xternal **R**otation of affected leg

- May be seen with **H**ypothyroidism (**E**levated TSH)

Figure 4.9 Slipped Capital Femoral Epiphysis

COLLATERAL LIGAMENT INJURY

Overstretched or torn ligaments in the knee

Medial (MCL) and Lateral (LCL)

- Valgus stress with rotation (most common)
- LCL: varus stress without rotation
- Localized pain, swelling, ecchymosis, and stiffness
- Most common VaLGus stress (ideally with knee at 30°); the lower part of the L in VaLgus points outward so valgus stress is where the Lower part of the Leg is pushed Laterally (outward) while a medial force is applied at the knee; the feet Go away from the body
- LCL: VaRus stress; the lower part of the leg is pushed inward (the feet Return to the body) while an outward (lateral) pressure is applied to the knee (to mimic a bow-leg seen in Rickets)
- Management for grades I (sprains) & II (incomplete tears): conservative (pain control, physical therapy to restore ROM and muscle strength, RICE, NSAIDs)
- Management for grade III (complete tears): surgical repair

Ottawa Knee Rules: **O** zero ability to flex knee to 90°, **T**enderness to patella, **T**enderness to fibular head, **A**ge >55, **W**alking not possible in ER (4 steps), or **A**fter injury occurred, unable to walk (4 steps)

Anterior Cruciate Ligament (ACL)

- Noncontact pivoting injury (deceleration, hyperextension, internal rotation)
- Most common injured knee ligament (± be associated with meniscal tears)
- 70% associated with sports
- ACL laxity: Lachman's test (most sensitive); pivot shift test; anterior drawer test (least reliable because spasm may stabilize knee)
- ± Segond fracture: avulsion of lateral tibial condyle with varus stress to knee; if present, ligamental injuries are most likely present; Segond fracture is pathognomonic for ACL tear
- Associated with "pop" and swelling leads to hemarthrosis
- ± knee buckling, inability to bear weight
- Patient usually does not actively extend knee
- Management is controversial; depends on activity level of patient (therapy vs. surgical)

ACL Injuries: **A**nterior drawer test, **C**ommon (most common injured knee ligament), **L**achman's test (most sensitive)

Posterior Cruciate Ligament (PCL)

- Dashboard injury (most common): anterior force to proximal tibia with knees flexed or direct blow injury; fall on flexed knee
- Usually associated with other ligamentous injuries
- Physical exam: pivot shift test, posterior drawer test
- Anterior bruising especially anteromedial aspect of proximal tibia; large effusion
- Almost always treated operatively (± lead to degenerative changes)

PCL Injuries: **P**ivot shift test (posterior drawer test), **Ca**r related injury (commonly a dashboard injury), **L**ots of **L**igamental injuries (if PCL is present, look for other ligamental injuries)

MENISCAL TEARS

Tears in knee cartilage

Etiology/Pathophysiology

- Degenerative (squatting, twisting, compression, or trauma with rotation)

Clinical Manifestations/Physical Exam

- Usually complaining of locking, popping, giving way, effusion after activities
- Medial tears are 3x more common than lateral (because of more bony attachments)
- Positive McMurray's sign (pop or click while tibia is externally and internally rotated)
- Apley test
- Joint line tenderness
- Effusion

Management/Prognosis

- NSAIDs; partial weight-bearing until orthopedic follow-up

Meniscal Tears

- **M** comes before **L** in the word **MeniscaL**
- Therefore, **M**edial tears are 3x more common than **L**ateral tears

---

OSGOOD-SCHLATTER DISEASE

Osteochondrosis of patellar tendon at tibial tuberosity from overuse

Etiology/Pathophysiology

- Repetitive stress or small avulsions due to quadriceps contraction on patellar tendon insertion into tibia

Risk Factors

- Most common cause of chronic knee pain in young active adolescents
- Most commonly affects boys ages 10–15, athletes with "growth spurts" (bone growth faster than soft tissue growth so quadriceps contraction transmitted through patellar tendon to the tuberosity; usually resolves with time)

Clinical Manifestations/Physical Exam

- Activity-related knee pain/swelling (running, jumping, kneeling); painful lump below knee, tenderness to the anterior tibial tubercle

Diagnosis

- X-ray: prominence or heterotopic ossification at tibial tuberosity

Management/Prognosis

- RICE, NSAIDs, quadriceps stretching
- Surgery in some cases only after growth plate has closed

If you are in high school and you want to GO PRO, you must play AS GOOD as you always do even when your knee is in pain and swells during activities.

AS GOOD = OSGOOD
- **G**rowth spurt related
- **O**steochondrosis

- **P**atellar tendon traction on tibial tubercle ossification center
- **R**unning and activity-**R**elated pain
- **O**ssification at tibial tuberosity seen on radiographs

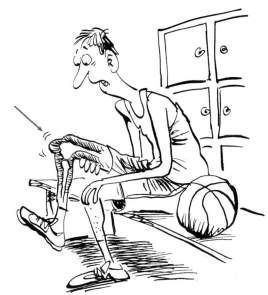

Figure 4.10 Osgood-Schlatter Disease

ANKLE SPRAINS

Ankle ligaments that are overstretched or torn

After tripping over an **ANT'S TALE** you will need to **CALL** for a **CANE** in order to avoid an ANKLE SPRAIN.

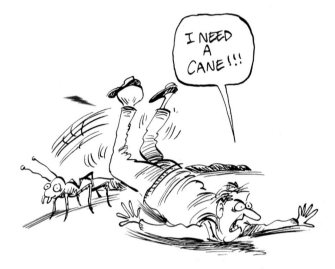

Most common sprained ligaments:
- **Ant**erior **Tal**ofibular (most common)

- **CALCANE**ofibular (second most common)

Figure 4.11 Ankle Sprain

> **OTTAWANs Must Obey the Ottawa Ankle Rules for Ordering X-rays**
>
> **O**uch: pain in malleolar zone
>
> **T**enderness along posterior edge or tip of lateral malleolus
>
> **T**enderness along posterior edge or tip of medial malleolus
>
> **A**fter the injury occurred, the patient is unable to walk or
>
> **W**alking is not possible for >4 steps in the ER
>
> Foot x-rays are required if:
>
> **A**long the fifth metatarsal area there is tenderness or
>
> **N**avicular tenderness (midfoot)

ACHILLES TENDON RUPTURE

Lower leg tendon at back of leg that is torn

Etiology/Pathophysiology

- Mechanical overload from eccentric contraction of gastrocsoleus complex

Risk Factors

- 75% occur as a sports-related injury
- Most commonly ages 30–50

Clinical Manifestations/Physical Exam

- Sudden heel pain after push-off movement, "pop," sudden, sharp calf pain
- Positive Thompson test: weak, absent plantar flexion (when the gastrocnemius muscle is squeezed) (perform Thompson test in prone position)

Management/Prognosis

- Surgical repair allows for early ROM
- Splint initially with some plantar flexion with subsequent changes in angle; gradual dorsiflexion toward neutral position

---

ATR

- **A**cute sharp calf pain
- **T**hompson test positive
- **R**epair surgically

JONES FRACTURE AND PSEUDOJONES FRACTURE

Fracture of the fifth metatarsal bone

Etiology/Pathophysiology

- Jones fracture: transverse fracture through diaphysis of fifth metatarsal
- PseudoJones fracture: transverse avulsion fracture at base (tuberosity) of fifth metatarsal due to plantar flexion with inversion; much more common and less serious than a true Jones fracture

Management/Prognosis

- Jones fracture
  - Non-weight bearing for 6–8 weeks, followed by repeat x-rays because it is often complicated by nonunion/malunion
  - Frequently requires ORIF/pinning
- PseudoJones fracture
  - Walking cast over a period of 2–3 weeks
  - ORIF if displaced

As per their **bad union,** lifeguards **cannot walk,** swim, or **dive for** 6 minutes at **JONES** beach after **5** P.M. or they don't get paid for **6–8 weeks.**

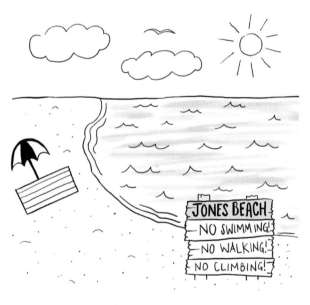

- **Transverse fracture through diaphysis of 5th metatarsal**

Treatment:
- **Non-weight bearing (cannot walk) for 6–8 weeks, followed by repeat x-rays, as often complicated by malunion.**

Figure 4.12 Jones Fracture

BACK PAIN

Evaluation

- Standing:
  - Observation: gait, ambulation assessed as patient walks on toes and heels; ROM, posture, and abnormal curvature is observed
  - Palpation: palpate spine, assess for infection or fracture (use gentle impact with closed fist to evaluate for tenderness)
- Sitting:
  - Sitting SLR
  - L4: diminished knee jerk reflex, ankle dorsiflexion, anterior thigh pain and/or sensory loss (as well as medial ankle)
  - L5: weakness with big toe extension, walking on heels more difficult than walking on toes. Pain and/or sensory loss on lateral thigh/leg, hip, groin, dorsum of the foot (especially between 1st and 2nd toes)
  - S1: diminished ankle jerk reflex, weakness with plantar flexion, pain and/or sensory loss posterior leg, calf, gluteus, foot plantar surface; walking on toes more difficult than walking on heels
- Supine:
  - Straight leg raise (SLR): ipsilateral pain down back of leg, below knee, when leg is raised 30–70°; 80% sensitivity
  - Crossover SLR: pain in affected leg when unaffected leg is raised; increased specificity for sciatic nerve lesions
  - Abdominal exam: inguinal area (for masses, femoral pulses, bruits); distal vascular status

---

You can assess reflexes by starting from the ankles and going up to the triceps while saying **12345678!**
- **S1-S2** loss of ankle jerk
- **L3-L4** loss of knee jerk
- **C5-C6** loss of biceps jerk
- **C7-C8** loss of triceps jerk

Herniated Disk (Nucleus Pulposus)

- Clinical Manifestations
  - Pain in a dermatomal pattern; increased pain with coughing, straining, bending, sitting
  - Most commonly at L5-S1 (it is the junction between mobile and non-mobile spine); also L4-L5
  - Sciatica: back pain radiating through thigh/buttock to lower leg (below knee) down L5-S1 dermatome (increased with Valsalva)
  - Positive SLR, positive crossover test; strength, reflex, and sensibility deficits

Cauda Equina Syndrome

- Clinical Manifestations
  - Central disc herniation compressing nerve roots of cauda equina
  - New onset of urinary or bowel retention/incontinence with saddle anesthesia, uni/bilateral leg radiation, decreased anal sphincter tone on rectal exam
- Management: a neurosurgical emergency

Lumbosacral Sprain/Strain

- Clinical Manifestations
  - Acute strain/tear of paraspinal muscles especially after twisting or lifting injuries
  - Back muscle spasms, loss of lordotic curve, decreased ROM, no neurologic changes (no sensory loss, paresthesias etc.), no pain below knee
- Management: NSAIDs/analgesics, ± muscle relaxers (metaxalone, cyclobenzaprine, methocarbamol); prompt return to activity recommended; ± need brief bed rest if severe

Spinal Stenosis (Pseudoclaudication) (Neurogenic)

- Clinical Manifestations/Physical Exam
  - Narrowing of spinal canal with impingement of the nerve roots and cauda equina; seen especially age >60
  - Back pain with paresthesias in one or both extremities
  - Worsened with extension: prolonged standing/walking
  - Relieved with flexion: sitting/walking uphill (unlike claudication); lumbar flexion leads to increased canal volume
- Management: Lumbar epidural injection of corticosteroids, decompression laminectomy

Spinal Compression Fracture

- Clinical Manifestations/Physical Exam
  - Lumbar compression fracture (osteoporosis), chronic corticosteroid use, systemic illness
  - Pathologic fractures in patients with malignancy or trauma
  - Back pain and point tenderness at level of compression
- Management: orthopedic and neurosurgery consult; analgesics; observation, kyphoplasty/vertebroplasty

After **Saddling** her horse to go **STAR**gazing, **Caud**et had **incontinence** to the point where she felt a **shock go down her legs** and was **rushed to the OR.**

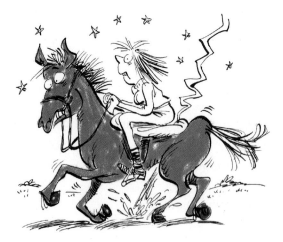

Clinical Manifestations:
- New onset of bowel retention/ urinary **Incontinence**

- **Saddle anesthesia**

- **Pain radiating to unilateral or bilateral leg(s)**

- **Sphincter Tone of Anus Reduced (STAR)**

- **Neurosurgical emergency!**

Figure 4.13 Cauda Equina Syndrome

Spondylolysis

- Clinical Manifestations
  - Defect (either failure of fusion or stress fracture) in pars interarticularis usually from repetitive microtrauma (especially hyperextension injuries)
  - Usually asymptomatic
  - Can occur in children who play football because it is an inherent weakness of bone

Spondylolisthesis

- Clinical Manifestations
  - Slippage of anterior portion of one vertebral body on another; 50% symptomatic
  - Best seen on lumbosacral film; 25–50% of affected patients will develop back/leg pain (± associated with sciatica)

Ankylosing Spondylitis

- Clinical Manifestations
  - Progressive stiffening of spine especially in men age >40
  - Insidious onset of morning stiffness decreased with exercise (decreased ROM)
  - HLA B27 inflammatory arthropathy
  - "Bamboo spine" seen on x-ray; sacroiliitis
- Diagnosis:
  - Lumbosacral x-ray: extremes of age, trauma, unresolved pain, pain for >4–6 weeks, suspected complication or history of malignancy
  - CT scan: bony disease (superior to MRI), better detail of disk and soft tissue surrounding the spine
  - MRI: vertebral neoplasm, disk herniation, and disc infection
  - ESR: patients at risk for malignancy, infection, ankylosing spondylitis

Musculoskeletal

Emergency Back Pain

Must-know medical diagnoses that are emergencies and commonly associated with back pain

- **AAA (abdominal aortic aneurysm):** age >50, abdominal/flank pain, hematuria, palpable abdominal mass, diminished lower extremity pulses, history of HTN, syncope
- **Vertebral osteomyelitis:** h/o TB, ETOH, elderly, IVDU, malaise, fever, weight loss, corticosteroid use; *S. aureus* most common pathogen
- **Epidural abscess:** history of epidural anesthesia, back surgery, trauma, DM, IV drug use, ETOH. Similar presentation to epidural hematoma but occurs more slowly
- **Spinal malignancy:** metastatic lesions most common (eg, prostate, lung, breast, kidney, thyroid); multiple myeloma most common primary malignancy
  - Risk factors: prior malignancy, age >50, intractable pain, increased ESR
- **Cauda equina:** condition causing back pain

"When a patient has severe back pain, he will FAINT on a MAT!"

<u>F</u>ever
<u>A</u>ge (>60y)
<u>I</u>V drug user
<u>N</u>euro deficits
<u>T</u>uberculosis (Pott's disease)

<u>M</u>idline vertebral tenderness or <u>M</u>alignancy history
<u>A</u>lcohol (intoxicated, alcoholic)
<u>T</u>rauma

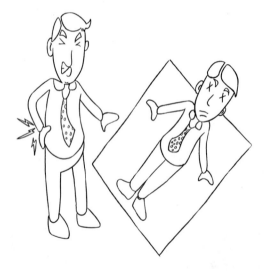

Diagnoses Not To Be Missed!
AAA my BACK!

<u>AAA</u> Abdominal Aortic Aneurysm
<u>B</u>one (bony metastases, vertebral osteomyelitis)
<u>A</u>bscess (epidural)
<u>C</u>auda equina
<u>K</u>idney (pyelonephritis)

Figure 4.14 Criteria for Imaging Patient With Back Pain

SARCOMA

Osteosarcoma

Cancer affecting large bones of the extremities

- Risk factors: bone malignancy (most common); most commonly adolescents (80% age <20), with second peak age 50–60, especially if there is a history of Paget's or radiation
- Clinical manifestations: 90% in metaphysis of long bones (most common in femur, then tibia, humerus); commonly metastasizes to lungs (usually the cause of death); bone pain/joint swelling, palpable soft tissue mass
- Diagnosis: x-ray "hair on end" or "sun ray/burst" appearance of soft tissue mass; mixed sclerotic/lytic lesions; periosteal bone reactions; Codman triangle: ossification of raised periosteum
- Management: limb-sparing resection (if not neovascular); radical amputation (if neovascular); chemotherapy as adjuvant treatment

> Osteo**SARCOMA**
>
> - **S**unray/burst on x-ray
> - **A**djuvant chemotherapy
> - **R**adiation history increases risk
> - **C**odman triangle seen on x-ray
> - **O**steoid production (immature bone)
> - **M**etastasis to the lungs/**M**alignant
> - **A**dolescents most commonly affected

Ewing's Sarcoma

Cancer of the bones or soft tissue

- Risk factors: giant cell tumor (most common in children); most commonly males age 5–25
- Clinical manifestations: femur and pelvis (most common locations); bone pain, ± palpable mass, possible joint swelling; ± fever
- Diagnosis: x-ray: lytic lesion with layered periosteal reaction "onion peel" appearance
- Management: chemotherapy; surgery, radiation

> **Onion peels** helped **Ewing** protect his **children** from **Femur and Pelvic** injuries.

Musculoskeletal

OSTEOCHONDROMA

Overgrowth at the growth plates

Risk Factors

- Most common benign bone tumor
- Most common in males age 10–20
- Begins in childhood and grows until skeletal maturity
- May precede chondrosarcomas

Diagnosis

- Often pedunculated, grows away from growth plate and involves medullary tissue

Management/Prognosis

- Observation; resection if becomes painful, located in the pelvis (most common site of malignant transformation)

OsteoCHONdroma: this tumor "CHONS" you into thinking it is malignant when it is not!

- It starts off with the word -osteo, as in "osteosarcoma"
- Then it "cons" you because osteochondroma is benign while osteosarcoma is not.

SCLERODERMA (SYSTEMIC SCLEROSIS)

Systemic connective tissue disorder

Etiology/Pathophysiology

- Thickened skin (sclerodactyly) with multisystemic involvement (eg, lung, heart, kidney, GI tract)

Clinical Manifestations/Physical Exam

- Tight, shiny, thickened skin (localized or generalized)
- Limited cutaneous systemic sclerosis "**CREST** syndrome"
    - **C**alcinosis cutis
    - **R**aynaud's phenomenon
    - **E**sophageal motility disorder
    - **S**clerodactyly (claw hand)
    - **T**elangiectasias
- Diffuse cutaneous systemic sclerosis: skin thickening: trunk and proximal extremities, trunk involvement

Diagnosis

- Antinuclear antibodies (ANA)
- Anti-Scl-70 (topoisomerase I) antibodies: diffuse disease
- Anticentromere antibodies—associated with limited disease (CREST syndrome); associated with a better prognosis

Management/Prognosis

- Disease-modifying antirheumatic drugs
- Corticosteroids
- Raynaud's: vasodilators (CCBs, prostacyclin)

AntiCentromere AB—associated with limited disease C for CREST syndrome and it is NOT CENTral (no proximal involvement).

Musculoskeletal

SYSTEMIC LUPUS ERYTHEMATOSUS

Chronic systemic, multi-organ autoimmune disorder of connective tissues

Etiology/Pathophysiology

- Type III hypersensitivity reaction

Risk Factors

- Young women age 20–40 (9:1), African American, Hispanic, Native American
- Genetic, environmental sun exposure, infections, hormonal (estrogen)
- Drug-induced lupus: procainamide, hydralazine, INH, quinidine

Clinical Manifestations/Physical Exam

- Joint pain (90%), fever, and malar "butterfly" rash
- Discoid lupus: annular, erythematous patches on face and scalp heals with scarring
- May be ANA negative in some cases
- Systemic: CNS, cardiovascular, glomerulonephritis, retinitis, oral ulcers, alopecia

Diagnosis

- Positive antinuclear antibodies (Ab): initial test (nonspecific)
- Positive rheumatoid factor
- Positive anti-double-stranded DNA and anti-Smith Ab are 100% specific for SLE (not sensitive)
- Antiphospholipid Ab syndrome (APLS): increased risk of arterial and venous thrombosis
  - Anticardiolipin Ab, anti-beta 2 glycoprotein antibodies, and lupus anticoagulant are paradoxically associated with increased PTT
  - $\pm$ false positive syphilis test (VDRL, RPR) in antiphospholipid syndrome
- Positive anti-histone bodies with drug-induced lupus (not associated with kidney/CNS damage)

Management/Prognosis

- Sun protection
- Hydroxychloroquine for skin involvement
- NSAIDs or acetaminophen for arthritis
- May use pulse dose steroids; cytotoxic drugs (methotrexate, cyclophosphamide)

ANA SMITH woke up with JOINT PAIN, a FEVER, and a RASH on a STRANDED sunny island.

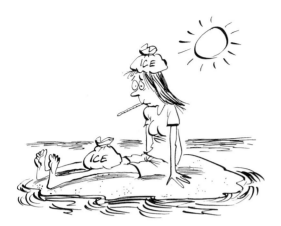

Triad:

- **JOINT PAIN**, **FEVER**, and **RASH** (includes butterfly/malar rash)

- **ANA** initial screening test (non-specific).

- ⊕ anti-double **STRANDED DNA** and/or **anti-SMITH antibodies; 100% specific for SLE**

Figure 4.15 Systemic Lupus Erythematosus

QUIN hurt his HIP when he lifted up HIS STONED wife.

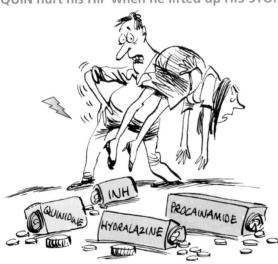

- **QUINidine**

- **Hydralazine**
- **INH**
- **Procainamide**

- Patient will have ⊕ **anti-HISTONE** bodies

- Usually doesn't present with neurological or renal complications as seen with SLE

Figure 4.16 Drug-Induced Lupus

Musculoskeletal

SJÖGREN'S SYNDROME

Autoimmune disorder attacking the exocrine glands

Etiology/Pathophysiology

- Primary: occurs alone
- Secondary: associated with other autoimmune disorders

Clinical Manifestations/Physical Exam

- Salivary glands: xerostomia (dry mouth)
- Lacrimal glands: dry eyes (keratoconjunctivitis sicca)
- Parotid enlargement
- Dyspareunia due to decreased vaginal secretions

Diagnosis

- ANA (especially anti-Ro and anti-La antibodies)
- Schirmer test (decreased tear production)

Management/Prognosis

- Artificial tears
- Pilocarpine (cholinergic) for xerostomia

Because you are so **dry**, you must **RO**w to **L.A** while eating **CARP** on a **large Parrot.**

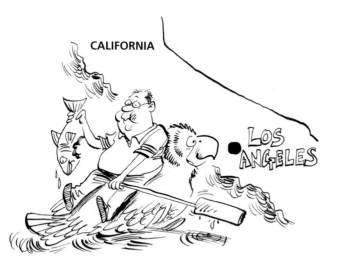

CALIFORNIA

LOS ANGELES

Clinical Manifestations:
Dry mouth, dry eyes
Parotid En**large**ment

Diagnosis:
ANA:⊕ **antiSS-A (RO)** and/or
⊕ **antiSS-B (LA)**
⊕ **Schirmer test**

Management: Pilo**carp**ine

Figure 4.17 Sjogren Syndrome

POLYMYALGIA RHEUMATICA

Idiopathic inflammatory condition causing synovitis, bursitis, and tenosynovitis

Etiology/Pathophysiology

- Aching/stiffness of proximal joints (shoulder, hip, neck)
- Closely related to giant cell arteritis

Risk Factors

- Age >50

Clinical Manifestations/Physical Exam

- Bilateral proximal joint aching/stiffness usually lasting longer than 30 minutes (in morning)
- Difficulty with combing hair, putting on a coat, getting out of chair
- No muscle weakness

Diagnosis

- Clinical diagnosis
- Increased ESR
- Normochromic normocytic anemia
- ± increased platelets (acute phase reactant)

Management/Prognosis

- Corticosteroids (low dose)
- Methotrexate

Giant cells in the **proximal** joints start **aching** due to the **stiff ROOMS** in the **ATTIC**.

- Closely related to **giant cell** ARTERITIS
- Bilateral **proximal joint aching/morning stiffness** of the pelvic and shoulder girdle >30 min

ROOM ATTIC = rheumatica

GOUT

Uric acid deposition in the soft tissue, joints, and bone

Etiology/Pathophysiology

- Secondary to longstanding hyperuricemia many people are hyperuricemic
- Etiologies of exacerbation:
  - Purine-rich food (alcohol, liver, oily fish, yeasts) causing rapid change in uric acid concentration
  - Acute episodes can occur with acute increase or decrease in uric acid level
  - Medications: diuretics (thiazides, loop), ACE inhibitors, pyrazinamide, ethambutol, aspirin

Risk Factors

- Most commonly men (especially age >30)
- Postmenopausal women

Clinical Manifestations/Physical Exam

- Acute gouty arthritis: (80% monoarthropathy) with severe joint erythema, swelling, and stiffness (often extends past affected joint); podagra (often first metatarsophalangeal joint but also knees/ankles/feet)
- Tophi deposition: solid uric acid in soft tissues (eg, helix of ear)
- Uric acid nephrolithiasis and nephropathy; uric acid stones associated with low urine volume and acidic pH; may cause glomerulonephritis

Diagnosis

- Arthrocentesis: negatively birefringent needle-shaped urate crystals
- X-ray: "mouse/rat bite," "punched-out" erosions if severe; ± tophi

Management/Prognosis

- Acute: NSAIDs drug of choice; colchicine second line; corticosteroids; avoid aspirin as it is associated with increased serum uric acid
- Chronic: allopurinol first line in long-term management; febuxostat/probenecid; colchicine

People with **GOUT** want to **THRO**W out the painful **NEEDLES** in their **TOES**.

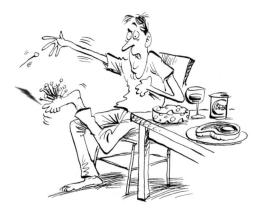

- **Podagra:** first MTP joint (**big TOE**) most common

  Diagnosis: Ar**thro**centesis- **negatively** birefringent **NEEDLE**-shaped **urate crystals** (knee joint)

Figure 4.18 Gouty Arthritis

Gouty arthritis

Oxidase inhibitors (allopurinol)

Uric acid

Tophi deposition

RHEUMATOID ARTHRITIS

Chronic inflammatory disease with persistent symmetric polyarthritis plus bone erosion, cartilage destruction, and joint structure loss

Etiology/Pathophysiology

- Destruction by pannus

Risk Factors

- Women, smoking

Clinical Manifestations/Physical Exam

- Prodrome: constitutional systemic symptoms: fevers, fatigue, weight loss, anorexia; decreased ROM
- Small joint stiffness: (wrist, PIP, knee, MTP, shoulder, ankle) worse with rest; morning joint stiffness >30 min; after initiating movement, improves later in day
- Arthritis: swollen, tender, erythematous, "boggy" joint; boutonniere deformity (flexion at PIP, hyperextension of DIP); swan neck deformity (flexion at DIP, hyperextension of PIP; ulnar deviation at most common joint; rheumatoid nodules
- Felty's syndrome (rare): RA and splenomegaly with decreased WBC and repeated infections
- Caplan syndrome: pneumoconiosis and RA

Diagnosis

- Positive rheumatoid factor (best initial test); sensitive, not specific
- Anti-citrullinated peptide antibody (most specific for RA)
- Increased C-reactive protein and ESR
- Arthritis in ≥3 joints, morning stiffness, disease duration >6 weeks
- X-rays: symmetric, narrowed joint space (osteopenia/erosions), subluxation, deformities, ulnar deviation of hand

Management/Prognosis

- NSAIDs; low-dose corticosteroids
- Prompt initiation of DMARDs: (eg, methotrexate, hydroxychloroquine, leflunomide, azathioprine)

Morning **Wood (STIFFNESS)** is usually **SYMMETRICAL** until it gets **BOGGY** after you urinate.

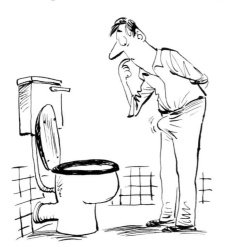

- Soft, warm **BOGGY** joints on physical examination
- **MORNING STIFFNESS** of joints > 60 min
- **SYMMETRICAL** joint narrowing on x-ray

Figure 4.19 Rheumatoid Arthritis

OSTEOARTHRITIS

Chronic disease due to articular cartilage damage and degeneration

Risk Factors

- Obesity is a big risk factor
- Most common in weight-bearing joints (knees, hips, spine, hip)
- Narrowed joint space (loss of articular cartilage), sclerosis, and osteophyte formation

Clinical Manifestations/Physical Exam

- Evening joint stiffness decreases with rest, worsens throughout the day and changes in weather, decreases ROM, crepitus; no inflammatory signs "hard bony joint"
- Heberden's node (palpable osteophytes at DIP joints); Bouchard's node: PIP osteophytes

Diagnosis

- Asymmetric joint space loss, osteophytes, subchondral bone cysts/sclerosis

Management/Prognosis

- Acetaminophen preferred initial treatment
- NSAIDs (more effective), corticosteroid injections, sodium hyaluronate, glucosamine and chondroitin, knee replacement

GRANULOMATOSIS WITH POLYANGIITIS

Formerly called Wegener's, a small vessel vasculitis with granulomatous inflammation and necrosis of nose, lungs, and kidney

Clinical Manifestations/Physical Exam

- TRIAD:
  - Upper respiratory tract/nose (ENT): nasal congestion, saddle nose deformity (cartilage involvement), epistaxis, otitis media, mastoiditis, stridor, sinusitis often refractory to treatment; constitutional: fevers, migratory arthralgias, malaise, weight loss; episcleritis, conjunctivitis
  - Lower respiratory tract (lung): parenchymal involvement results in cough, dyspnea, hemoptysis (pulmonary hemorrhage), wheezing, pulmonary infiltrates, cavitation
  - Renal: rapidly progressing/crescentic glomerulonephritis: hematuria, proteinuria

Diagnosis

- Positive increased C-ANCA
- Chest x-ray: infiltrates, nodules, masses, or cavities (nonspecific)

Management/Prognosis

- Corticosteroids and cyclophosphamide
- Methotrexate alternative to cyclophosphamide

Due to constant **SINUSITIS, COUGH,** and **GLOMERULONEPHRITIS, WEGENER** couldn't maintain a **C** and **rapidly progress** to a low **GPA.**

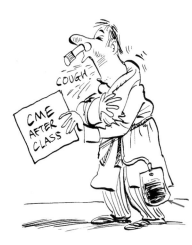

- **Triad:** upper respiratory tract, lower respiratory tract, and kidney involvement

- **Biopsy:** granulomatous vasculitis

- ⊕ **C-ANCA**

- Kidney involvement often leads to **rapidly-progressing glomerulonephritis**

Figure 4.20 Granulomatosis with Polyangiitis

Musculoskeletal

Chapter 5

EENT

EYE DISORDERS

Blepharitis

Inflammation of both eyelids

- Anterior: *Staph. aureus*, viral or seborrheic infection
- Posterior: dysfunction of meibomian gland, rosacea, and allergic dermatitis
- Eye irritation/itching, burning to eyelid, erythema, crusting, scaling, red rimming of eyelid, and eyelash flaking
- Anterior: eyelid hygiene
- Posterior: eyelid massage/expression of meibomian gland regularly

> **BLE**pharitis: inflammation of **B**oth **L**ids of the **E**yes

Hordeolum (Stye)

Local infection of the eyelid margin (external sebaceous gland)

- *Staph. aureus* (90–95%)
- Focal abscess: painful, warm, swollen red lump on eyelid
- Warm compresses are a mainstay of treatment (most eventually point and drain without treatment)
- Topical antibiotic ointment (erythromycin, bacitracin) if actively draining
- Incision and drainage if no drainage occurs within 48 hours

> Hordeo**LUM**: painful, warm, swollen red **LUMP** on eyelid

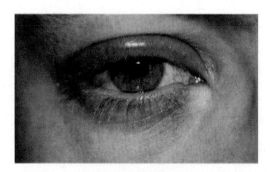

Figure 5.1 Blepharitis

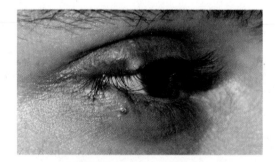

Figure 5.2 Hordeolum

EENT

Chalazion

Painless granuloma of the internal meibomian sebaceous gland results in focal eyelid swelling

- Hard, nontender eyelid swelling on conjunctival surface of eyelid
- Granuloma tends to be larger, firmer, slower growing, and less painful than hordeolum
- Eyelid hygiene, warm compresses; antibiotics usually not necessary
- Injection of corticosteroid or incision and drainage may be necessary if distorting vision

> **Chalazion**: **C** for Chronic, and **LAZI** (it is too **lazy** to cause pain).

Pterygium and Pinguecula

Growths of the conjunctiva

- Associated with increased UV exposure in sunny climates as well as sand, wind, dust
- Pterygium: elevated, superficial, fleshy, triangular-shaped "growing" fibrovascular mass
- Most commonly found in the inner corner/nasal side of eye and extends laterally
- Management: observation in most cases (artificial tears); removal if growth affects vision

> **Pterygium** grows like the triangular wing of a pterodactyl: **F**leshy, **T**riangular-shaped **G**rowing fibro-vascular mass

> **Pinguecula**: yellow elevated nodule on nasal side of eye does not grow (**PINS** are pinned down to one place and don't move!)

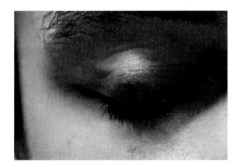

Figure 5.3 Chalazion

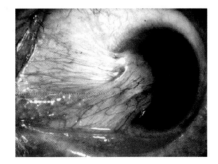

Figure 5.4 Pterygium

OPHTHALMIA NEONATORUM

Eye infection that infants contract during delivery; requires specific treatment approach

Management

- Day 1: chemical conjunctivitis due to silver nitrate; artificial tears may be helpful
- Days 2–5: gonococcal infection most likely cause; presents with purulent conjunctivitis with exudate and swelling of the eyelids; IM or IV ceftriaxone needed once infection has occurred; use topical erythromycin prophylactically to prevent infection
- Days 5–7: *Chlamydia trachomatis* most likely cause; may occur up to 23 days after birth; use oral erythromycin
- Days 7–11: HSV conjunctivitis

Prophylaxis

- Standard neonatal prophylaxis against gonococcal conjunctivitis given immediately after birth is erythromycin ointment 0.5%; other options include topical tetracycline 1.0%, silver nitrate, and povidone-iodine 2.5%
- Neonatal ocular prophylaxis is not effective in preventing neonatal chlamydial conjunctivitis

> **SILVER GOO CLINGS to HER** eyes: day 1 use **Silver** nitrate (prophylaxis) or erythromycin; days 2–5 treat for **Go**nococcal; days 5–7 treat for **Ch**lamydia; days 7–11 treat for **Her**pes

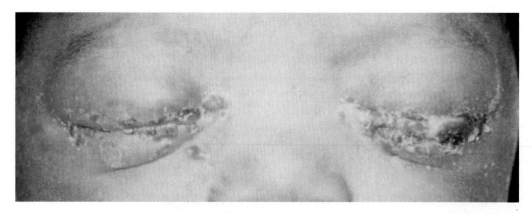

Figure 5.5 Conjunctivitis Neonatorum

ORBITAL FLOOR "BLOWOUT" FRACTURE

Blunt trauma to the orbital bone

Clinical Manifestations/Physical Exam

- Decreased visual acuity (trapped orbital tissue); enophthalmos
- Diplopia especially with upward gaze (due to inferior rectus muscle entrapment)
- Orbital emphysema (eyelid swelling with blowing of the nose)
- Epistaxis, dysesthesias, hyperalgesia, anesthesia to anteromedial cheek (due to stretch of infraorbital nerve)

Diagnosis

- CT scan

Management/Prognosis

- Nasal decongestants to reduce pain (avoid blowing nose)
- Prednisone to reduce edema
- Antibiotics: ampicillin, sulbactam and/or clindamycin
- Surgical repair

Blowout fractures won't allow you to see the vowels A, E, I, O, and U.

- **<u>A</u>cuity of vision may be decreased**

- **<u>E</u>nophthalmos**

- **<u>I</u>nferior rectus muscle entrapment, Infraorbital nerve injury (cheek numbness)**

- **<u>O</u>rbital emphysema**

- **<u>U</u>pward gaze causes diplopia**

- **And sometimes Y antibiotics: clindam<u>Y</u>cin and/or Unas<u>Y</u>n**

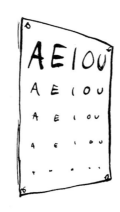
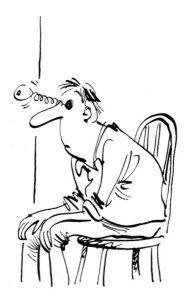

Figure 5.6 Orbital Blowout Fractures

GLOBE RUPTURE

Outer membranes of eye that are disrupted by blunt or penetrating trauma; an ophthalmologic emergency

Clinical Manifestations/Physical Exam

- Ocular pain (but may be absent), diplopia
- Misshapen pupil with prolapse of ocular tissue from sclera
- Visual acuity markedly reduced (may be light perception only)
- Orbits: enophthalmos (recession of the globe within the orbit), foreign body may be present, may have exophthalmos; severe conjunctival hemorrhage (360° bulbar)
- Corneal/sclera: prolapse of the iris through the cornea; positive Seidel's test (parting of the fluorescein dye by a clear stream of aqueous humor from anterior chamber); obscured red-reflex; irregular pupil (may be teardrop-shaped); hyphema

Management/Prognosis

- Rigid eye shield (protect eye from applied pressure, impaled object should be left undisturbed)
- Immediate ophthalmology consult
- IV antibiotics
- Avoid topical eye solutions
- Hyphema: blood in anterior chamber; place at 45 degrees to keep RBCs from staining cornea

When the **GLOBE RUPTURES,** you need a **RIGID SHIELD** to prevent **TEAR DROPS** in the **SIDE** of your eyes.

- **RIGID SHIELD to protect eye and ophthalmology consult**

- **Irregular pupil-teardrop** shaped

- **Positive SeIDEL test** (side)

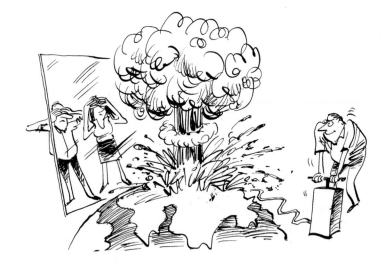

Figure 5.7 Globe Rupture

MACULAR DEGENERATION

Deterioration of the macula (retina) which controls central vision and leads to eventual vision loss; most common cause of legal blindness in those age ≥ 75

Etiology/Pathophysiology

- DRY (atrophic): gradual breakdown of macula cells leads to gradual blurring of central vision; presence of drusen bodies
- WET (exudative or neovascular): new, abnormal vessels grow underneath the central retina leading to vision loss

Risk Factors

- Age ≥ 50, Caucasian, women
- Smoking

Clinical Manifestations/Physical Exam

- Bilateral blurred or loss of central vision (including detailed and colored vision), scotomas, metamorphopsia, micropsia

Management/Prognosis

- Dry: Amsler grid at home to monitor stability, vitamin A, C, and E may slow progression
- Wet: anti-angiogenics in wet (eg, bevacizumab)

Macular Degeneration

- **DRY**: Drusen bodies
- **WET**: neovascular (new abnormal blood vessels grow underneath central retina; lots of new blood vessels so it gets WET)

RETINAL DETACHMENT

Retinal tear detaches the retina from the choroid plexus (rhegmatogenous most common type); an ophthalmologic emergency

Etiology/Pathophysiology

- Exudative (serous): subretinal fluid accumulates, detaching retina (HTN, central retinal vein occlusion, papilledema)
- Traction: adhesions separate retina (eg, proliferative diabetic retinopathy, sickle cell disease, trauma)

Clinical Manifestations/Physical Exam

- Progressive unilateral vision loss: shadow "curtain" in peripheral visual field
- Photopsia (flashing lights), floaters, no pain/redness

Diagnosis

- Fundoscopy: retina hanging in the vitreous
- Positive Shafer's sign (clumping of pigment cells in the anterior vitreous [sometimes called the tobacco dust sign])

Management/Prognosis

- Laser, cryotherapy ocular surgery; keep the patient supine
- Miotics are contraindicated

When police pull you over, you must ask your **Shafer (chauffeur)** to pull the **CURTAIN** on the **SIDE** window in order to see the **flashing lights and floaters.**

Clinical Manifestations:

- **Photopsia (Flashing lights)** and **Floaters**

- **Unilateral** vision loss **"curtain"** down on the eye that blocks peripheral vision then progresses to central vision loss

- **Shafer's sign:** clumping of pigment cells in the anterior vitreous

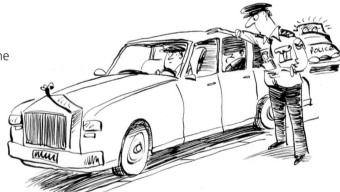

Figure 5.8 Retinal Detachment

FOREIGN BODY (OCULAR) AND CORNEAL ABRASION

Material trapped under the upper eyelid resulting in corneal injury

Clinical Manifestations/Physical Exam

- Foreign body sensation, tearing, red, painful eye

Diagnosis

- Corneal abrasions are "ice-rink"/linear abrasions seen especially with foreign body under eyelid (so evert the eyelid to look for it)

Management/Prognosis

- Check visual acuity first
- Foreign body removal; avoid sending patients home with topical ophthalmic anesthetics
- Antibiotics ophthalmic drops with 24-hour ophthalmology follow up (antipseudomonal fluoroquinolones preferred if contact lens wearer)
- Rust ring: remove rust ring at 24 hours by ophthalmologist

If you don't get your **eyes checked first**, you will definitely **cut the cornea** when you get on the **ICE RINK.**

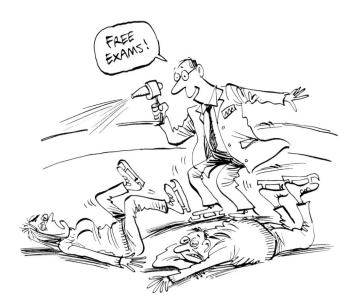

Figure 5.9 Foreign Body/Corneal Abrasion

CHEMICAL BURN
Ophthalmologic emergency

Etiology/Pathophysiology

- **Alkali burns:** worse than acids (liquefactive necrosis), denatures proteins and collagen, causes thrombosis of vessels (eg, fertilizers, household cleaners, drain cleaners)
- **Acid burns:** coagulative necrosis (H^+ precipitates protein barrier); eg, industrial cleaners

Management/Prognosis

- **Immediate irrigation** (greatest impact on prognosis)
  - LRS or normal saline (with pH 6–7.5, LRS is closer to normal saline pH 7.1 than is normal saline, which has pH 4.5–7.0)
  - LRS is less irritating than normal saline
  - Irrigate for minimum 30 min or at least 2 liters of fluid
- Check pH after irrigation: continue irrigation for 30 min until eye pH 7.0–7.3; check visual acuity once pH is normal
- Broad spectrum antibiotics (eg, moxifloxacin) and cycloplegic agents (eg, 0.25% atropine drops) with ophthalmology referral

---

CHEMICALS BURN the eyes:

- **CH**ECK **PH** (after irrigation)
- **E**mergency
- **M**oxifloxacin (broad spectrum antibiotics)
- **I**mmediate **I**rrigation
- **C**all ophthalmology
- **A**cuity checked **A**fter irrigation
- **L**actated ringers first line for irrigation
- **S**aline second line for irrigation

ACUTE NARROW ANGLE CLOSURE GLAUCOMA

Increased intraocular pressure leading to optic nerve damage; an ophthalmologic emergency

Etiology/Pathophysiology

- Leading cause of preventable blindness in the United States
- Decreased drainage of aqueous humor via trabecular meshwork and canal of Schlemm Mydriasis (pupillary dilation further closes the angle); eg, dim lights, sympathomimetics, and anticholinergics

Risk Factors

- Patients with preexisting narrow angle or large lens—elderly, hyperopes (far-sighted), and Asians

Clinical Manifestations/Physical Exam

- Severe, sudden onset of unilateral ocular pain; nausea, vomiting, headache; vision changes: halos around lights, loss of peripheral vision (tunnel vision)
- Conjunctival erythema, cloudy "steamy" cornea, mid-dilated fixed, nonreactive pupil, eye hard on palpation

Diagnosis

- Increased intraocular pressure by tonometry (>21 mm Hg)
- Funduscopy: optic disc blurring or "cupping" of optic nerve (thinning of the outer rim of the optic nerve head)

Management/Prognosis

- Combination of topical agents (eg, BB [timolol], alpha-2 agonist [apraclonidine, brimonidine], prostaglandin [latanoprost], miotic/cholinergic [pilocarpine or carbachol]) often with a systemic agent to lower intraocular pressure (eg, PO/IV acetazolamide or IV mannitol)
- Laser iridotomy is definitive management

Treat Glaucoma with ABCs!

- **A**cetazolamide first-line agent: **decreased A**queous humor production results in decreased IOP
- **B**eta-**B**lockers (eg, timolol): **B**rings down the IOP without affecting visual acuity
- **C**holinergics (**C**arbachol/pilocarpine): **C**onstricts pupil and reduces intraocular pressure by increasing aqueous humor drainage

Chronic Open Angle Glaucoma:

In order to see, you must keep **both** entrances of the **tunnel** open at all times!

Progressive **bilateral** peripheral vision loss: **tunnel vision**

CONJUNCTIVITIS (RED EYES)

Inflammation of the outermost layer of the sclera and inner surface of the eyelid

Etiology/Pathophysiology

- Three types: viral, allergic, bacterial
- Bacterial causes include *Staphylococcus aureus*, *Streptococcus pneumoniae*, *H. influenzae*, *M. catarrhalis*, *N. gonorrhoeae*, and *Chlamydia trachomatis*

Risk Factors

- Viral (most common in children): highly contagious from direct contact; often starts unilaterally and progresses to bilateral involvement in 1–2 days; swimming pools are most common source of outbreaks
- Allergic: response to an allergen
- Bacterial: transmitted by direct contact and autoinoculation

Clinical Manifestations/Physical Exam

- Viral: foreign body sensation, conjunctival erythema, and itching; normal vision; possible viral symptoms; ipsilateral preauricular lymphadenopathy, copious watery discharge (may be mucoid), punctate staining on slit lamp examination
- Allergic: conjunctival erythema; normal vision; other allergic symptoms (eg, nasal congestion, marked itching); often bilateral; cobblestone mucosa appearance to inner upper eyelid, erythema, stringy or watery discharge, chemosis (conjunctival swelling)
- Bacterial: purulent discharge, lid crusting (eye "stuck shut" in the morning), conjunctival erythema, usually no significant visual changes

Diagnosis

- Direct visualization and slit lamp examination

Management/Prognosis

- Viral: supportive; warm to cool compresses; artificial tears; antihistamines for itching and redness (eg, olopatadine); antihistamines with decongestants (eg, pheniramine-naphazoline)
- Allergic: symptomatic: topical antihistamines (H1 blockers): olopatadine (antihistamine/mast cell stabilizer), pheniramine-naphazoline (antihistamine and decongestant), emedastine; topical NSAID: ketorolac
- Bacterial: topical antibiotics: erythromycin, fluoroquinolones (eg, moxifloxacin) and sulfonamides; if contact lens wearer, cover *Pseudomonas* (eg, topical ciprofloxacin or aminoglycoside)

Having **RED EYES** can make you **"C" FUNKE.**

Etiologies:

- **C**onjunctivitis
- **F**oreign body (ocular)
- **U**veitis (Iritis)
- **N**arrow angle closure glaucoma
- **K**eratitis (corneal ulceration)
- **E**piscleritis

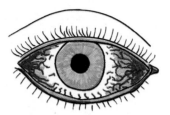

Figure 5.10 Red Eyes

OPTIC NEURITIS

Acute inflammatory demyelination of CN II (optic nerve)

Etiology/Pathophysiology

- Multiple sclerosis
- Medications: ethambutol, chloramphenicol
- Autoimmune

Risk Factors

- Mostly commonly age 20–40

Clinical Manifestations/Physical Exam

- Painful loss of vision; decrease in color vision desaturation; visual field defects: central scotoma (blind spot) over hours to a few days; usually unilateral
- Ocular pain worse with eye movement, Marcus-Gunn pupil (relative afferent pupillary defect); during swinging-flashlight test from unaffected eye into the affected eye, pupils appear to dilate

Diagnosis

- Funduscopy: 2/3 normal disc/cup (retrobulbar neuritis) or 1/3 optic disc swelling/blurring (papillitis)

Management/Prognosis

- IV glucocorticoids followed by oral corticosteroids
- Vision usually returns with treatment

Marcus shot himself with the **Gun multiple** times until he finally **Died** from **pain**.

- Can be a presentation of **Multiple sclerosis**

Physical Exam:
- **Marcus Gunn pupil**—when bright light is shone from unaffected eye to affected eye, the pupils **di**late rather than constrict.

- **Pain with ocular movement**

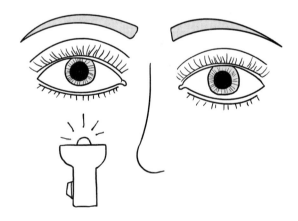

Figure 5.11 Optic Neuritis

CENTRAL RETINAL ARTERY OCCLUSION

Retinal artery embolus

Etiology/Pathophysiology

- Most commonly due to atherosclerotic disease

Clinical Manifestations/Physical Exam

- Acute, sudden monocular vision loss, usually preceded by amaurosis fugax

Diagnosis

- Fundoscopy:
  - Pale retina with cherry-red macula (red spot) due to obstruction of retinal blood flow
  - Vessels may show "box car appearance"
- Emboli (20% of patients); usually no hemorrhage

Management/Prognosis

- Decrease intraocular pressure to prevent anterior chamber involvement (acetazolamide)
- No treatment has been shown effective
- Lay patient flat on back, massage orbit to dislodge clot

After eating a fatty steak she crashed her cherry red car into a pale pole because she suddenly lost vision in one eye.

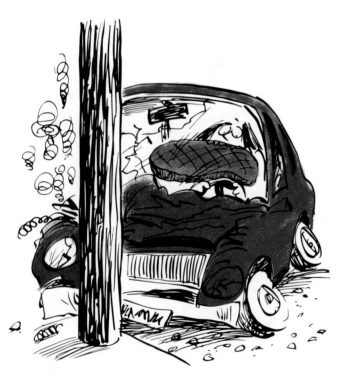

Associated with **Atherosclerotic disease (fatty steak)**

Manifestations: acute **sudden monocular vision loss**

Fundoscopy: **pale retina** with **cherry red macula** (red spot) due to obstruction of retinal blood flow

Vessels may show segmentation **boxcar** appearance

Figure 5.12 Central Retinal Artery Occlusion

CATARACTS

Lens opacification (thickening)

Risk Factors

- Aging (most commonly age ≥60)
- Cigarette smoking
- Congenital: ToRCH syndrome (toxoplasmosis, rubella, CMV HSV)
- Corticosteroids
- Diabetes mellitus
- Malnutrition
- UV light

Clinical Manifestations/Physical Exam

- Usually bilateral
- Blurred vision over months to years, halos around lights
- Physical exam: absent red reflex, opaque lens

Management/Prognosis

- Cataract removal

Diabetes, steroids, aging, and TORCHing cigarettes will eventually lead to **bilateral** cataracts.

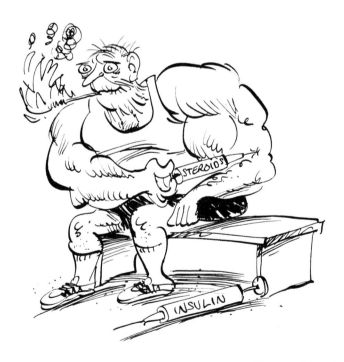

- Lens opacification usually **bilateral**

Risk Factors:
- **Smoking cigarettes, corticosteroids, diabetes, aging,** UV light, and malnutrition

- Congenital: **TORCH syndrome: T**oxoplasmosis, **O**ther (syphilis), **R**ubella, **C**MV, and **H**SV

Figure 5.13 Cataracts

OTITIS EXTERNA
Swimmer's ear

Etiology/Pathophysiology
- *Pseudomonas* (most common type)
- *Staph* and *Strep*
- *Aspergillus* (fungal)

Clinical Manifestations/Physical Exam
- Ear pain (otalgia), pruritus in ear canal, auricular discharge, ear
- Physical exam: pain on traction of the ear canal/tragus, external auditory canal erythema/edema/debris

Management/Prognosis
- Protect ear against moisture
- Ciprofloxacin/dexamethasone otic
- Aminoglycoside otic suspension: neomycin/polymixin-B/hydrocortisone otic (except if tympanic membrane perforation is suspected because aminoglycosides are ototoxic)

While **swimming**, microbes **PASS** through the **outer ear**.

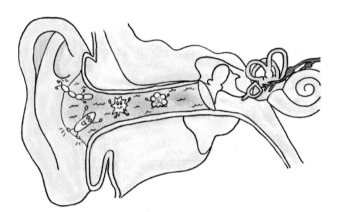

Swimming is the most common cause of outer ear infection.

Common Organisms
_P__seudomonas_ most common
_A__spergillus_ (if fungal)
_S__taphylococcal aureus_
_S__treptococcal spp._

Figure 5.14 Otitis Externa

ACUTE OTITIS MEDIA

Inflammation of middle ear

Etiology/Pathophysiology

- *Strep. pneumo (most common), H. influenza, Moraxella catarrhalis, Strep. pyogenes*
- Often preceded by URI

Risk Factors

- Young children, eustachian tube dysfunction, day care, pacifier/bottle use, parental smoking, not being breastfed

Clinical Manifestations/Physical Exam

- Fevers, otalgia, ear tugging in infants, conductive hearing loss, stuffiness
- If TM perforation, rapid relief of pain (usually heals in 1–2 days)
- Physical exam:
  - Bulging, erythematous TM with effusion and decreased TM mobility on pneumatic otoscopy
  - Loss of landmarks on TM

Management/Prognosis

- Amoxicillin over 10–14 days is treatment of choice; cefixime in children; amoxicillin/clavulanic acid second line
- If penicillin-allergic, use erythromycin-sulfisoxazole, azithromycin, or TMP/SMX
- Myringotomy (surgical drainage) if severe otalgia or if severe mastoiditis
- Tympanostomy if recurrent

Acute Otitis Media (**AOM**)

- **A**moxicillin treatment of choice
- **O**talgia
- **M**obility of TM decreased (gold standard for diagnosis)

EENT

ACOUSTIC (VESTIBULAR) NEUROMA

Benign tumor of Schwann cells

Etiology/Pathophysiology

- CN VIII schwannoma (Schwann cells produce myelin sheath)

Clinical Manifestations/Physical Exam

- Unilateral sensorineural hearing loss
- Tinnitus, headache
- Facial numbness
- Continuous disequilibrium

Diagnosis

- MRI or CT scan

Causes of Sensorineural Hearing Loss Auditory Physical Exam Findings

SensoriNeural has lateralization to Normal ear and Normal AC > BC

When **Men** wearing construction **Vests Drill (loud noise exposure)** outside of **Presby**terian Church, the people **Inside** will eventually stop hearing the **Acoustic** guitar.

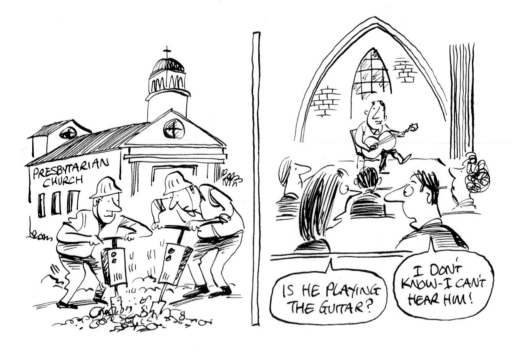

Figure 5.15 Auditory Physical Exam Findings

VERTIGO

Loss of balance or dizziness

Clinical Manifestations/Physical Exam

- **Ben**ign positional vertigo: episodic vertigo no hearing loss
- **Men**iere's: episodic vertigo with hearing loss
  - People with **Meniere's** won't be able to **fully hear** the **TV**
  - Hearing and balance disorder characterized by: episodic ear **Fullness, Hear**ing loss, **T**innitus, and **V**ertigo
- **Vest**ibular neuritis: Continuous vertigo, no hearing loss
  - **V**estibular **N**euritis: vertigo only, no hearing loss; due to inflammation of vestibular portion of CN8 in the inner ear; most common after viral infection
- **Labyrinth**itis: continuous vertigo with hearing loss
  - Labyrinthitis: **L**oss of hearing with vertigo/tinnitus due to cochlear involvement

Management/Prognosis

- **Block histamine** and **acetylcholine** before "**doping** up" on **benzos**.
  - Antihistamines: first-line, block histamine (and acetylcholine)
  - Anticholinergics: block acetylcholine
  - Dopamine blockers
  - Benzodiazepines: used in refractory patients

Ben and his **Men** wore **Vests** before they went into the **peripheral labyrinth.**

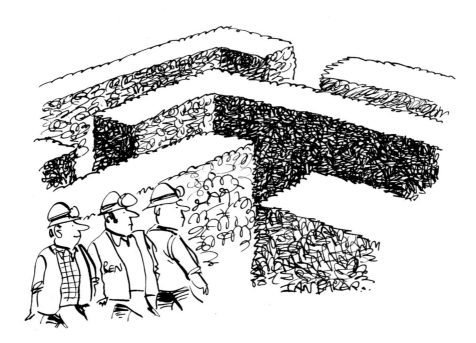

Figure 5.16 Vertigo

CHOLESTEATOMA
Abnormal growth of squamous epithelium causing mastoid bony erosion

Etiology/Pathophysiology
- Chronic eustachian tube dysfunction (chronic negative pressure pulls part of the tympanic membrane causing granulation tissue that over time, erodes ossicles leading to conductive hearing loss)

Clinical Manifestations/Physical Exam
- Painless otorrhea (brown/yellow auricular discharge with strong odor)
- Peripheral vertigo
- Conductive hearing loss

Diagnosis
- Granulation tissue seen with otoscope

Management/Prognosis
- Surgical excision and reconstruction of the ossicles

Cholest**EATO**ma

- **C** for **C**onductive hearing loss
- Granulation tissue that, over time, **EATs** away the ossicles

---

Mucormycosis will leave a **Black MARC** on your **face!**

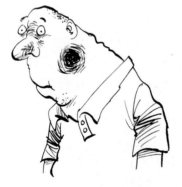

Mucor
Absidia
Rhizopus
Cunninghamella

May cause **Black eschar** on face.

Figure 5.17 Mucormycosis

Chapter 6

Reproductive

AMENORRHEA

Absence of menses

Etiology/Pathophysiology

- Etiologies of secondary amenorrhea: workup includes pregnancy test, serum prolactin, FSH, LH, TSH
  - Unexpected pregnancy most common cause of secondary amenorrhea; first step in amenorrhea workup is to rule out pregnancy
  - Hypothalamic dysfunction: 35%
    - Etiologies: hypothalamic disorders, anorexia (or weight loss 10% below IBW), exercise, stress, nutritional deficiencies, systemic disease (eg, celiac disease)
    - Diagnosis: normal/low FSH and/or LH; low estradiol, normal prolactin levels
    - Management: stimulate gonadotropin secretion: clomiphene, menotropin
  - Pituitary dysfunction: 19% (eg, prolactinoma, pituitary infarction [Sheehan's syndrome])
    - Diagnosis: decreased FSH, decreased LH, increased prolactin (galactorrhea) if prolactinoma; MRI of pituitary sella
    - Management: transsphenoidal surgery (tumor removal)
  - Ovarian disorders: 40%; PCOS; premature ovarian failure: follicular failure or follicular resistance to LH and/or FSH; Turner's syndrome
    - Clinical manifestations: symptoms of estrogen deficiency (similar to menopause)
    - Diagnosis: increased FSH and LH, decreased estradiol: ovarian abnormalities; normal or decreased FSH, LH (pituitary or hypothalamus)
    - Progesterone challenge test: positive withdrawal bleeding (ovarian); no withdrawal bleeding: other causes
  - Uterine disorder: scarring of the uterine cavity (Asherman's syndrome)
    - Diagnosis: pelvic U/S: absence of normal uterine stripe; hysteroscopy may be used to diagnose and treat
    - Management: estrogen

Clinical Manifestations/Physical Exam

- Primary amenorrhea is failure of onset of menarche (menstruation) by:
  - Ages 15–16 in the presence of normal growth and secondary sex characteristics
  - Age 13 in the absence of secondary sex characteristics or if height is less than the third percentile
  - Ages 12–13 in the presence of breast development and cyclic pelvic pain
- Secondary amenorrhea is absence of menses for:
  - Greater than 3 cycle intervals or 6 months in a woman with previously normal menstruation; the absence of menstruation for ≥ 3 in this population should prompt an evaluation as to the etiology
  - 9 months in a woman who was previously oligomenorrheic

Primary Amenorrhea

	Uterus Present	Uterus Absent
Breast Present	Outflow obstruction • Transverse vaginal septum • Imperforate hymen	• Mullerian agenesis • Androgen insensitivity
Breast Absent	Elevated FSH, LH • Turner's syndrome • Premature ovarian failure Normal/low FSH, LH • Hypothalamus or pituitary failure • Puberty delay (athletes, illness, anorexia)	Rare

The Second Pregnancy will bring out the HIPO in U.

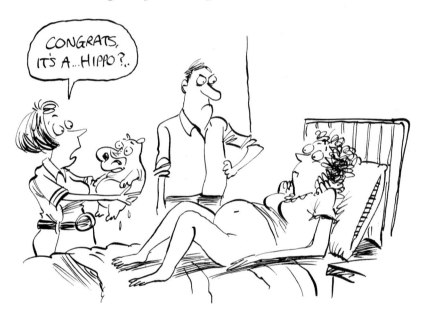

Rule out **pregnancy.** If negative, then look for potential issues in:

• **Hi**pothalamus
• **Pi**tuitary
• **O**varies
• **U**terus

Figure 6.1 Secondary Amenorrhea

Secondary amenorrhea will cause a **STOPP** in **MENSES**:

• **S**econdary
• **T**hyroid
• **O**varian failure
• **P**COS
• **P**rolactinoma

• **M**enopause
• **E**ffects of medication
• **N**ervosa (anorexia)
• **S**carring of **E**ndometrium;
• **S**topping medications (OCPs)

Reproductive

DYSMENORRHEA

Painful menstruation that affects normal activities

Etiology/Pathophysiology

- Primary dysmenorrhea: due to increased prostaglandins
- Secondary dysmenorrhea: due to pelvic pathology (endometriosis, adenomyosis, leiomyomas, adhesions, PID, etc.)

Risk Factors

- Primary dysmenorrhea: pain usually 1–2 years after onset of menarche in teenagers
- Secondary dysmenorrhea: most commonly women age ≥25

Clinical Manifestations/Physical Exam

- Diffuse pelvic pain with onset of menses (± lower abdomen, suprapubic or pelvic with onset of menses or may radiate to lower back and legs)
- Pain may be intermittent and associated with headache, nausea, vomiting; often lasts 1–3 days
- Physical exam: normal (may have uterine tenderness); associated findings depend on cause

Management/Prognosis

- NSAIDs: inhibits prostaglandin-mediated uterine activity; supportive: application of heat, rest, vitamin E
- Hormonal contraception: estrogen-progestin, progestin
- Laparoscopy: if treatment for primary fails (done to rule out secondary causes)

Dysmenorrhea: **P**rimary dysmenorrhea **due to Prostaglandins**

The **Pain** of secondary dysmenorrhea will leave a girl **PALE.**

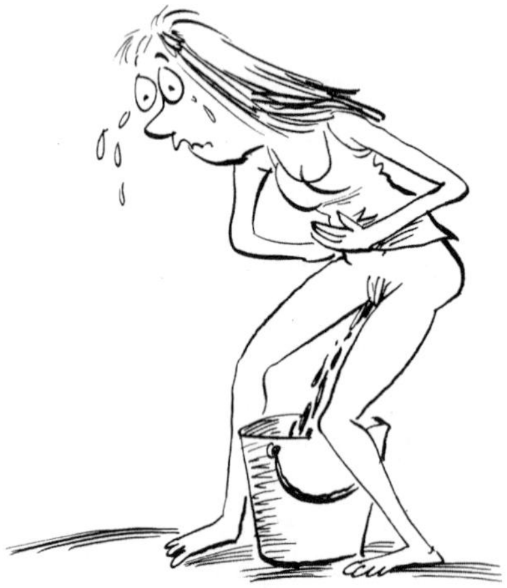

Must r/o PALE:

Pelvic Inflammatory Disease
Adenomyosis
Leiomyoma
Endometriosis

Management: The **PALE** girl was crying **N-Said** that her menses is causing her extreme **pain.**

NSAIDS to suppress prostaglandin mediated uterine activity

Figure 6.2 Secondary Dysmenorrhea

Reproductive

ADENOMYOSIS

Islands of endometrial tissue which make up the uterine lining within the myometrium (muscle layer) of the uterus

Risk Factors

- Most commonly women in the later reproductive years

Clinical Manifestations/Physical Exam

- Dysmenorrhea (worsens with menses), progressive heavier menstrual blood loss, ± infertility
- Physical exam: tender, symmetrically enlarged, "boggy" uterus

Diagnosis

- Diagnosis of exclusion of secondary amenorrhea
- Post-TAH examination of uterus: definitive diagnosis

Management/Prognosis

- Total abdominal hysterectomy (TAH): only effective therapy
- Conservative treatment to preserve fertility: analgesics, low dose OCPs

After bleeding profusely and having intense pain, Adena got into the TUB and said AH with relief from the hysteria.

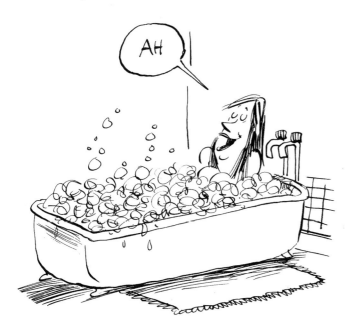

Clinical Manifestations:

- **Menorrhagia**
  bleeding

- **Dysmenorrhea**
  painful bleeding

- **T**ender **U**terus with **B**ogginess

Abdominal **H**ysterectomy-Definitive Management

Figure 6.3 Adenomyosis

ENDOMETRIOSIS

Presence of endometrial tissue outside of the uterus

Risk Factors

- Most commonly in ovaries, posterior cul de sac, broad and uterosacral ligaments, rectosigmoid colon, bladder, and distal ureter
- 10% incidence in women; 15% of U.S. population
- Onset usually age $\geq$35
- Nulliparity, family history, early menarche

Clinical Manifestations/Physical Exam

- Classic triad:
  - Cyclic premenstrual pelvic pain $\pm$ low back pain
  - Dysmenorrhea
  - Dyspareunia (painful intercourse)
- Dyschezia (painful defecation); pre-post menstrual spotting
- Infertility (most common cause of infertility, 25%), asymptomatic in one-third of patients
- Physical exam: usually normal; $\pm$ fixed tender adnexal masses, nodular thickening of the uterosacral ligament, fixed retroverted uterus

Diagnosis

- Transvaginal U/S: homogeneous echo-pattern ("ground-glass" appearance) of the endometrioma cyst
- Laparoscopy with biopsy: definitive diagnosis
  - Can appear dark blue, powder-burn black, red, white, yellow, brown, or non-pigmented lesions on visual inspection
  - Endometrioma: large endometriosis involving the ovaries classified as a benign tumor: usually filled with old blood appearing chocolate-colored (chocolate cyst)

Management/Prognosis

- Medical (conservative) ovulation suppression
  - Combined OCPs and NSAIDs; progesterone: suppresses GnRH
  - Leuprolide, danazol
- Surgical
  - Conservative laparoscopy with ablation: used if fertility desired
  - Total abdominal hysterectomy with salpingoophorectomy: if no desire to conceive (TAH-BSO)

After eating <u>chocolate prunes,</u> <u>Avery</u> developed <u>pelvic pain</u> with <u>painful spotting</u> <u>N SAID,</u> "I need to start taking my <u>OCPs."</u>

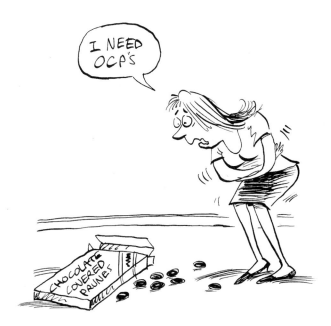

Classic Triad:
- **Pelvic pain**

- **Dysmenorrhea** Painful spotting

- Dys**pareun**ia

Most common site of ectopic endometrial tissue: **Ovaries** (Avery)

Chocolate cysts

Management: **NSAIDs +**
Oral contraceptives
Conservative laparoscopy c ablation
Progesterone
Surgery definitive management

Figure 6.4 Endometriosis

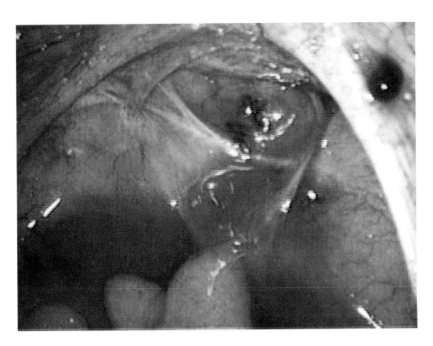

Figure 6.5 Endometriosis

LEIOMYOMATA (UTERINE FIBROIDS)

Benign uterus smooth muscle tumor (leiomyoma: fibromyoma)

Risk Factors

- 30% of U.S. population; most commonly women in their 30s (especially age >35)
- 5× more common in African Americans
- Hormonal: growth related to estrogen production; may increase with pregnancy or may change in size with menstrual cycles; often regresses after menopause

Clinical Manifestations/Physical Exam

- Most common benign gynecologic lesion
- Often asymptomatic but bleeding most common presenting symptom: menorrhagia, dysmenorrhea
- Abdominal pressure/pain related to size of tumor and location; bladder frequency/urgency
- Large, irregular hard palpable mass in abdomen, pelvis, or mobile uterus with irregular contour on bimanual exam

Diagnosis

- Pelvic U/S: hypoechoic, well-circumscribed round masses, frequently with shadowing

Management/Prognosis

- Treatment rarely needed; determined by size, symptoms, rate of growth, and desire for fertility
- Medical: inhibition of estrogen (decreases endometrial growth)
  - Leuprolide: GnRH agonist that causes inhibition when given continuously; used if near menopause or preoperatively for hysterectomy (makes the uterus smaller)
  - Progestins (eg, medroxyprogesterone)
- Surgical
  - Myomectomy: used especially to preserve fertility
  - Artery embolization
  - Hysterectomy: definitive treatment in women who completed childbearing; fibroids most common cause for hysterectomy

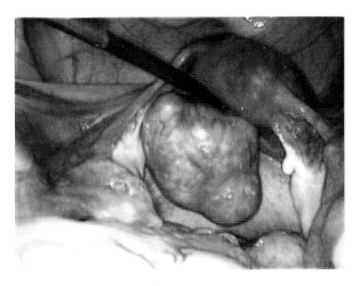

Figure 6.6 Leiomyoma

LEIOMYOMA:

- **L**arge palpable mass
- **E**strogens increase growth
- **I**rregular mass
- **O**besity
- **M**enorrhagia
- **Y**ears (age ≥35)
- **O**bservation done in many cases
- **M**yomectomy done to preserve fertility
- **A**frican Americans (5x more common)

PREMENSTRUAL SYNDROME

Physical, behavioral, and mood changes seen with cyclical occurrence during the luteal phase of the menstrual cycle

Etiology/Pathophysiology

- Unknown; possible correlation with hormones and neurotransmitters

Clinical Manifestations/Physical Exam

- Somatic: bloating, breast swelling/pain, headache, changes in bowel, fatigue, muscle/joint pain
- Emotional: depression, hostility, irritability, libido changes
- Behavioral: food cravings, poor concentration, noise sensitivity, loss of motor senses
- Premenstrual dysphoric disorder: severe PMS with functional impairment

Diagnosis

Clinical manifestations, plus:

- Pain for 7–14 days before onset of menses
- Pain relieved within 2–3 days of onset of menses
- At least 7 days symptoms-free during follicular phase

Management/Prognosis

- Mood symptoms: SSRIs (often first line) given daily or in luteal phase (starting on day 14 of cycle) depending on severity; oral contraception therapy (eg, monophasic)
- Breast pain: ± danazol, bromocriptine
- Bloating: ± spironolactone, calcium carbonate, low-salt diet

Girls become Lunatics in the Luteal phase due to PMS.

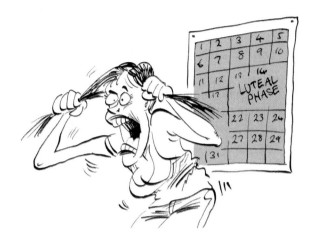

Cluster of physical, behavioral mood changes with cyclic occurrence during **luteal phase** of menstrual cycle

Figure 6.7 Premenstrual Syndrome

Premenstrual dysphoric disorder (severe PMS with functional impairment) = **DISPHORIC**

- **D**epressed
- **I**nterest decreases
- **S**ad
- **P**ain
- **H**ypersomnia
- **O**verwhelmed
- **R**age
- **I**ncreased appetite
- **C**oncentration decreases

ENDOMETRITIS

Pregnancy-related infection of the uterus postpartum or post abortion

Etiology/Pathophysiology

- Etiology: postpartum uterine infection, eg post C-section (often due to retained products of conception)
- Pathophysiology: (acute) often an ascending infection from normal vaginal flora; often polymicrobial including group A beta (*hemolytic Streptococcus*), group B (*Streptococcus, S. aureus, Ureaplasma urealyticum, Peptostreptococcus, Gardnerella vaginalis, B. fragilis, C. trachomatis*)

Clinical Manifestations/Physical Exam

- Postpartum fever (>38°C (>100.4°F), chills
- Abdominal pain
- Vaginal bleeding/discharge; foul smelling lochia
- Endometritis may be associated with salpingitis and oophoritis

Diagnosis

- Clinical: patients with fever and abdominal pain especially after a C-section or post abortion

Management/Prognosis

- Prevention prior to C-section: first generation cephalosporin (eg, cefazolin); 1 dose within 60 min of C-section; if beta-lactam allergy, clindamycin and gentamicin can be used
- Infection post C-section: clindamycin and gentamicin; ampicillin-sulbactam
- Infection post vaginal delivery: ampicillin and gentamicin

When you have <u>fever, abdominal pain, and tenderness,</u> you will be classified in <u>group A</u> and you will <u>C</u> the <u>staff</u> in the ER before being treated by the <u>Gentlemen</u> in the <u>Clinic</u>.

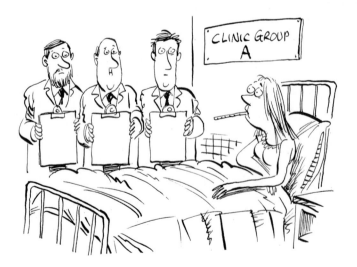

- **Fever, abdominal pain, and uterine tenderness** especially after **C-section**

- **Group:** MC polymicrobial including group A strep, group B strep, *S. Aureus*

- **Treatment** (infection after C-section): clindamycin + gentamycin

Figure 6.8 Endometritis

MENOPAUSE

Cessation of menses for >1 year due to loss of ovarian function

Risk Factors

- In the United States, typically ages 50–52; may occur earlier in those with DM, smokers, vegetarians, and malnourished patients
- Premature menopause occurs age <40
- Without the protective benefits of estrogen, these patients are at increased risk for heart disease and osteoporosis

Clinical Manifestations/Physical Exam

- Estrogen deficiency changes: menstrual cycle alterations, vasomotor instability (including hot flashes), mood changes, skin/nail/hair changes, dyspareunia (painful intercourse), osteoporosis, urinary incontinence hyperlipidemia, increased cardiovascular events
- Irregular menstrual cycles
- Physical exam:
  ◦ Decreased bone density; skin: thin/dry decreased elasticity
  ◦ Vaginal: atrophy thin mucosa; pH >7.0

Diagnosis

- Increased serum FSH, increased LH
- Decreased estrogen: predominant estrogen at menopause
- Androstenedione levels are unchanged

Management/Prognosis

- Vasomotor insufficiency/hot flashes: estrogen, progesterone, clonidine, SSRIs gabapentin
- HRT: estrogen and progesterone or estrogen only; must consider risks versus benefits

Women with menopause have <u>heat flashes, mood changes, and skin dryness</u> but once they take <u>estrogen</u> they will be blissful at <u>HeaRT!</u>

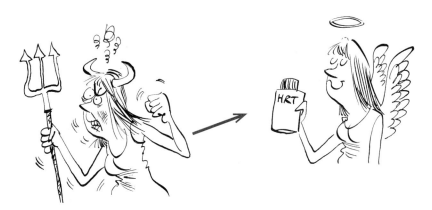

Estrogen deficiency changes: **heat flashes, mood changes, skin/vaginal dryness**
Treatment: **estrogen/ progesterone; HRT** (**H**ormone **R**eplacement **T**herapy)

Figure 6.9 Menopause

POLYCYSTIC OVARIAN SYNDROME (PCOS)

Endocrine syndrome characterized by triad of amenorrhea (chronic anovulation), obesity, and hirsutism (increased androgen)

Etiology/Pathophysiology

- Insulin resistance which results in an insulin-facilitated and luteinizing hormone-driven increase in ovarian androgen production

Clinical Manifestations/Physical Exam

- Menstrual irregularities: oligomenorrhea (70%), secondary amenorrhea (50%), dysfunctional uterine bleeding
- Increased androgens: hirsutism (50%—coarse hair growth along midline structures (face, neck, abdomen), acne, ± male pattern baldness
- Insulin resistance: type II DM, obesity (80%), acanthosis nigricans, HTN
- Physical exam:
  - Bilateral enlarged smooth mobile ovaries on bimanual examination
  - Signs of hirsutism, acanthosis nigricans

Diagnosis

- Exclude other disorders: thyroid (TSH), pituitary adenoma (prolactin levels), ovarian tumors, Cushing's syndrome (dexamethasone suppression test)
- Labs: increased testosterone, increased DHEA-S (intermediate of testosterone); LH:FSH ratio $\geq$3:1 (normal 1.5:1)
- Pelvic U/S: bilateral enlarged ovaries with peripheral cysts (not necessary for diagnosis)
- GnRH agonist stimulation test: rise in serum hydroxyprogesterone
- Lipid panel, glucose tolerance test (for DM)

Management/Prognosis

- Lifestyle changes: diet, exercise, weight loss
- OCPs suppress androgen, decreases LH production
- Metformin: in patients with insulin resistance, may also help to induce ovulation in anovulatory patients
- Clomiphene induces ovulation for desired fertility
- Spironolactone blocks testosterone but is also teratogenic

Hairy women with PCOS must avoid endometrial CA by combining their SCILS to get highLy increased test scores.

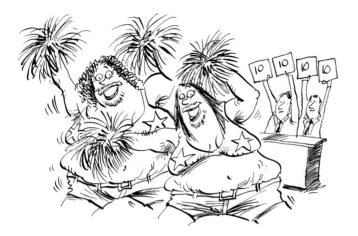

Hallmarks:
Hirsutism (hairy)
Amenorrhea (anovulation)
Insulin Resistance

Figure 6.10 Polycystic Ovarian Syndrome (PCOS)

Clinical manifestations due to **PCOS**:

- **P**roduction of androgens
- **C**hronic anovulation
- **O**besity
- **S**ugar (DM)

Diagnosis: high **LH**:FSH ratios, increased **Test**osterone

Management: Combination OCPs

- **S**pironolactone
- **C**lomiphene for **I**nfertility
- **L**ifestyle modifications
- **S**urgery (wedge resection)

SPONTANEOUS ABORTION

Non-elective termination of a pregnancy before 20 weeks' gestation

Etiology/Pathophysiology

- Chromosomal abnormalities most common reason 50%
- Others: maternal infection, physical trauma, uterine defects, endocrine abnormalities, malnutrition, maternal drug use, immunologic (antiphospholipid syndrome), infections (toxoplasmosis, rubella, CMV, HSV— ToRCH)

Risk Factors

- Risk factors include: increased maternal (or paternal) age, increased parity

Clinical Manifestations/Physical Exam

- Most common during the first 7 weeks of gestation
- Classifications:
  - Threatened: may be viable or abortion may follow; no products of conception expelled from the uterus with cervical os closed; threatened is the only type associated with possible fetal viability
    - Bloody vaginal discharge, uterus size compatible with dates; may have uterine contractions
  - Inevitable: no products of conception (POC) expelled, progressive cervical dilation, $\pm$ rupture of membranes
    - Moderate bleeding, moderate to severe uterine cramping; uterus size compatible with dates
  - Incomplete: some POC expelled, some POC still retained; cervical os is dilated
    - Heavy bleeding, moderate to severe cramping, retained tissue, boggy uterus
  - Complete: all products of conception expelled from the uterus; cervical os usually closed
    - Pain, cramps, and bleeding usually subside; pre-pregnancy size of uterus
  - Missed: embryo not viable but retained in the uterus; no POC expelled, cervical os closed
    - Loss of pregnancy symptoms; may have brown discharge
  - Septic: retained POC becomes infected leading to maternal infection; cervical os closed (usually with cervical motion tenderness)
    - Vaginal bleeding, fevers, chills, brownish discharge, uterine tenderness

Diagnosis

- Pelvic U/S (most useful test)
  - Negative factors include: $\geq$25 mm gestational sac in the absence of a yolk sac or embryo, absence of fetal cardiac activity in an embryo with any crown rump length, fetal heart rate (<100 bpm), abnormal gestational sac, yolk sac
- Human chorionic gonadotropin/hCG
  - At a baseline, serum hCG level of 500 IU/L; a drop in hCG of >21% is strongly suggestive of miscarriage
  - At a baseline, serum hCG of 5000 IU/L; a drop in hCG of >35% is strongly suggestive of miscarriage
- Blood type Rh(D) and antibody screening
- Serum progesterone <5 ng/mL is associated with a nonviable pregnancy

Reproductive

Management/Prognosis

- Observation: threatened, completed
- Scheduled surgical evacuation: missed
- Emergent surgical evacuation: inevitable, incomplete, septic:
  - Suction curettage in first semester
  - Dilation and evacuation in second trimester
- RhoGAM if mother is Rh− (and father is Rh+ or unknown); must be given to prevent isoimmunization from maternal-fetal blood contact to prevent complications during subsequent pregnancies if subsequent pregnancies include a fetus that is Rh positive
- Elective Abortion:
  - Medical: Mifepri**stone** and **Miso**prostol
    - Mifepri**stone** will turn the fetus into "**stone**" by inhibiting progesterone receptors thus stopping growth of fetus
    - **Mis**oprostol will make you **miss** the baby after it contracts out of the uterus—causes uterine contractions

---

Spontaneous Abortion

- The abortions that start with *I* have a **DILATED OS** (inevitable and incomplete abortions)
- The rest usually have a closed **OS**
- Once they are **DILATED**, the treatment is **Dilation** and evacuation (or **D**ilation & **C**urettage)

ECTOPIC PREGNANCY

Pregnancy outside the uterine cavity, most commonly in the fallopian tube (ampulla 75%), isthmus (14%), fimbria (14%), and then abdomen, ovarian, cervix

Risk Factors

- High risk: previous ectopic (biggest factor), PID (second biggest factor), history of tubal ligation, endometriosis, IUD use, assisted reproduction, advanced maternal age
- Middle risk: infertility, history of genital infections, multiple partners; African Americans, Hispanics

Clinical Manifestations/Physical Exam

- **Classic triad:** unilateral pelvic/abdominal pain, vaginal bleeding, amenorrhea (pregnancy); these symptoms can also be seen with threatened abortion (more common than ectopic)
- Ruptured/rupturing ectopic
  - Severe abdominal pain
  - Dizziness
  - Nausea, vomiting
  - Syncope, hypotension, signs of shock (from hemorrhage)
  - Atypical: vague symptoms, menstrual irregularities
- Cervical motion tenderness, adnexal mass
- $\pm$ mild uterine enlargement

Diagnosis

- Serial quantitative β-hCG:
  - Should double every 24–48 hrs; in ectopic, serial β-hCG rises <66% expected, decreases, or plateaus
  - If initial value <1500 mIU/mL, repeat q 2–3 days
- Transvaginal U/S:
  - Presence (or absence) of pregnancy within or outside uterus
  - Absence of gestational sac with levels β-hCG >2,000 strongly suggests ectopic or nonviable IUP
- Culdocentesis: $\pm$ nonclotted blood present
- Laparoscopy: to diagnose and treat (rarely used)

Management/Prognosis

- Stable ectopic pregnancies: methotrexate
  - Indications: gestation <3–4 cm, β-hCG <5,000
  - Contraindications: ruptured ectopic, β-hCG >5,000, + fetal heart activity, history of TB
- All other ectopics: surgical (eg, laparoscopic)
- RhoGAM: given to all Rh-negative mothers
- Follow up: serial β-hCG levels to confirm complete removal of all trophoblastic tissue
- Contraception for a limited time afterward may be suggested

Reproductive

Ectopic Pregnancy

If HCG is positive, you **must rule out** an ectopic with an U/S or that baby will never sing the ABCs:

- **A**menorrhea
- **B**leeding
- **C**onstant unilateral pain

When a stable, <4 cm ectopic is found without activity in either PAIR of your TUBALS, you can pay less than $5,000 Bucks for Magic PILLS or else you have to pay more than $5,000 bucks for surgery.

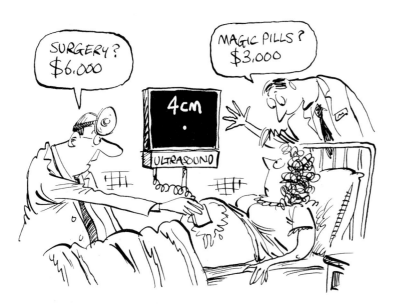

Classic Triad:
- **P**ain
- **A**menorrhea
- **I**rregular bleeding
  in women of
- **R**eproductive age

Magic PILLS (Methotrexate)

Indications:
- Pregnancy outside the uterus seen on U/S
- Inactivity of fetal heart
- <4 cm size of ectopic in tube
- <5,000 beta HCG
- Stable patient

Figure 6.11 Ectopic Pregnancy: Medical vs Surgical

For all other patients, surgery is usually indicated (eg, hCG >5,000).

Ectopic Pregnancy

- **T**enderness (cervical motion) on examination
- **U**/S shows absence of uterine gestation
- **B**eta hCG used in both diagnosis and monitoring post-treatment
- **A**dnexal mass on examination
- **L**aparoscopic
- **S**yncope, shock, severe abdominal pain, swooning (dizziness), sinking BP (hypotension), sick (nausea and vomiting) are **Signs of InStability**

OVARIAN CANCER

Tumor which forms in the ovaries (second most common gynecologic cancer after endometrial but ovarian has highest mortality of all gynecological cancers)

Risk Factors

- Positive family history, increased number of ovulatory cycles (infertility, nulliparity, age ≥50)
- BRCA1 and BRCA-2
- Peutz Jeghers, Turner syndrome
- Fifth most common cancer of all in women; most commonly age 40–60

Clinical Manifestations/Physical Exam

- Rarely symptomatic until late in disease (extensive metastasis)
- Abdominal fullness/distention, back or abdominal pain; urinary frequency
- Irregular menses, menorrhagia, postmenopausal bleeding
- Physical exam:
    - Abdominal or ovarian mass (solid, fixed, irregular), ascites
    - Sister Mary Joseph's node: METS to umbilical lymph nodes
    - Constipation (secondary to intestine compression)

Diagnosis

- Pelvic U/S; CT abdomen/pelvis, CT chest (staging)
- Histology: 90% epithelial (especially if postmenopausal); germ cell increased incidence in patients age ≥30
- Mammography to assess for metastasis or primary tumor in breast

Management/Prognosis

- Protective factors: OCPs (decrease number of ovulatory cycles), high parity, total abdominal hysterectomy
- Poor prognosis
- Surgery: tumor debulking
- Chemotherapy: paclitaxel and cisplatin or carboplatin
- Serum CA-125 levels used to monitor treatment progress

People with ovarian <u>CA</u> have <u>less time</u> or seconds to pay <u>taxes</u> to buy <u>platinum</u> or sing the <u>ABCDEs.</u>

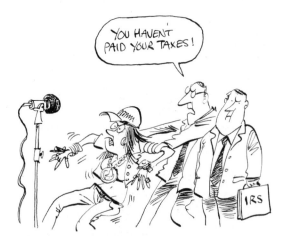

CA = CA-125 tumor marker

Management: Pacli**Tax**el, **Platin drugs**
Ascites, **B**RCA-1/2, **C**onstipation, **D**oppler, **E**pithelial (most common type)

Figure 6.12 Ovarian Cancer

ENDOMETRIAL CANCER

Endometrial hyperplasia from unopposed estrogen usually precedes endometrial cancer

Etiology/Pathophysiology

- Estrogen-dependent cancer

Risk Factors

- Mostly postmenopausal (75%), peaking at ages 50–60, perimenopausal (25%), premenstrual (5–10%)
- **ENDOMETRIUM**:
  - **E**strogen (endometrial cancer is estrogen-dependent); associated with antecedent endometrial hyperplasia
  - **N**o kids (nulliparity) or no ovulation (anovulation)
  - **D**M (diabetes mellitus)
  - **O**besity
  - **M**enopause (late age, ≥ 52)
  - **E**lderly (mostly commonly postmenopausal)
  - **T**amoxifen
  - **R**ising BP (HTN)
  - **I**n the myometrium (adenomyosis)
  - **U**nmanaged PCOS
  - **M**enarche (early)

Clinical Manifestations/Physical Exam

- Most common gynecologic malignancy in United States; fourth most common malignancy incidence in women overall (first: breast, second: lung, third: colorectal)
- Abnormal vaginal bleeding: postmenopausal bleeding, pre- or perimenopausal leads to menorrhagia or metrorrhagia

Diagnosis

- Endometrial biopsy: adenocarcinoma (>80%), sarcoma (5%)
- Pelvic U/S: if endometrial stripe is >4 mm, significant for hyperplasia and possibly malignancy

Management/Prognosis

- Stage I: hysterectomy (TAH-BSO) $\pm$ post-op radiation treatment; most are well-differentiated (one of the most curable gynecologic cancers)
- Stage II: TAH-BSO and lymph node excision (pelvic and para aortic) $\pm$ post-op radiation treatment

PELVIC ORGAN PROLAPSE (POP)

Coughing or laughing more than <u>2/3</u> of the time increases <u>I</u>ntraabdominal pressure causing a P<u>OP</u>, sending your uterus into the vagina.

Grade 1: descent into upper **2/3** of vagina

Grade 2: cervix approaches **I**ntroitus

Grade 3: **O**utside introitus

Grade 4: complete **P**rolapse

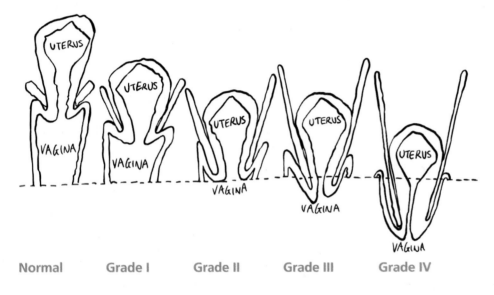

Normal   Grade I   Grade II   Grade III   Grade IV

Figure 6.13 Pelvic Organ Prolapse

GESTATIONAL TROPHOBLASTIC DISEASE

Hydatidiform mole (molar pregnancy); neoplasm due to abnormal placental development with trophoblastic tissue proliferation

Etiology/Pathophysiology

- Complete molar pregnancy: an egg with no DNA is fertilized by 1 or 2 sperm (46 chromosomes); higher risk of malignant potential
- Partial molar pregnancy: an egg is fertilized by two sperm (or one sperm that duplicates its chromosomes); there may be fetal development but is always malformed and nonviable

Clinical Manifestations/Physical Exam

- 80% benign; choriocarcinoma is malignant
- Painless vaginal bleeding in month 4 or 5 of pregnancy ($\pm$ brownish discharge)
- Uterine size/date discrepancies (usually larger than expected)
- Hyperemesis gravidarum
- Preeclampsia (<20 weeks)

Diagnosis

- U/S: "snowstorm" or "cluster of grapes" appearance and absence of fetal parts/heart sounds; cluster of grapes indicates enlarged cystic chorionic villi
- β-HCG: very high >100,000 (especially with complete molar pregnancy)
- Maternal serum α-fetoprotein: very low

Management/Prognosis

- Uterine suction or surgical curettage; patients are followed until β-hCG falls to undetectable level
- METS: chemotherapy (eg, methotrexate) destroys trophoblastic tissue

Date = DilATE and suction or curettage

Give **MET**hotrexate for **METS**

Even in the <u>snowstorm</u>, the groom fed the bride a <u>cluster of grapes</u> under the <u>CHUPA</u> and remembered the date when they first **MET**.

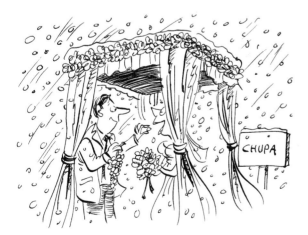

Clinical Manifestations:
CHUPA (Hebrew word for canopy):
Choriocarcinoma (malignant form)
Hyperemesis gravidarum
Uterine size/date discrepancies
Painless vaginal bleeding/
   Preeclampsia before 20 weeks' gestation

Snowstorm/cluster of grapes appearance on U/S

Figure 6.14 Gestational Trophoblastic Disease (Molar Pregnancy)

GESTATIONAL DIABETES MELLITUS

Glucose intolerance or DM during pregnancy leading to hyperglycemia

Etiology/Pathophysiology

- Placenta release of human placental lactogen (HPL) leads to maternal insulin resistance

Risk Factors

- Family or prior history of gestational DM, spontaneous abortion, history of infant with macrosomia, multiple gestations, obesity, maternal age $\geq$30

Clinical Manifestations/Physical Exam

- Usually asymptomatic and found on routine screening; usually subsides postpartum
- $\pm$ hyperglycemia, hypoglycemia, recurrent infections
- Fetal complications: fetal demise, congenital malformation, abruption placentae, premature labor, neonate hypoglycemia (from abrupt removal of maternal glucose)

Diagnosis

- Prenatal screening usually done at 24–28 wks' gestation: 50 g oral glucose challenge test; if $\geq$140 mg/dL after 1 hr, perform 3-hour oral GTT
- 3-hour oral GTT (gold standard); positive if >180 mg/dL at 1 hr, >155 mg/dL at 2 hrs, >140 mg/dL at 3 hrs

Management/Prognosis

- Strict adherence to ADA diet
- Insulin (most oral anti-hyperglycemics are contraindicated)
- Early delivery at 38 weeks; consider C-section if child is macrosomic (4,000–5,000 g)

Gestational Diabetes Mellitus

- Fetal complications (**NIBS**): **N**eonatal hypoglycemia; **I**njury to brachial plexus; **B**loody (placentae abruptio); **S**houlder dystocia and macrosomia
- If the mother takes **in** too much **NIBS** after 3 hours, it will lead to **macrosomia**.
- Insulin treatment of choice (does not cross placenta); glybu**ride** does not **ride** on the placenta: oral hypoglycemic that does not cross the placenta

---

Cardinal Movements of Labor

In order to get **Engaged**, you **Flex** on one leg to present the ring, then you **Descend** down the aisle. During your first dance, you **internally rotate, extend** your hand then **externally rotate** her onto the dance floor.

- Engagement
- Flexion
- Descent
- Internal rotation
- Extension
- External rotation

ABRUPTIO PLACENTAE
Premature separation of the placenta from the uterine wall

Risk Factors
- Maternal HTN (most common cause), smoking, cocaine use, folate deficiency, abdominal trauma, high parity, increased age, hypercoagulable states, premature rupture of membranes

Clinical Manifestations/Physical Exam
- Third trimester bleeding
- Severe abdominal pain (painful uterine contractions), rigid uterus
- Complications: DIC (10%); hemorrhagic shock

Diagnosis
- Transabdominal/transvaginal U/S:
  - Fetal distress often presents (fetal bradycardia)
  - May show retroplacental clot
- Differential diagnosis placenta previa:
  - Abnormal placenta implantation on or close to the cervical os; may also present with painless third trimester bleeding

Management/Prognosis
- Immediate delivery if fetal distress, severe abruption

Abruptio Placentae = Abdominal Pain

Placenta Previa = Painless vaginal bleeding

Chapter 7

Endocrine

HYPOTHYROIDISM

Decreased levels of the thyroid hormones levothyroxine (free T4) and/or triiodothyronine (free T3)

Etiology/Pathophysiology

- Hashimoto's thyroiditis, diet deficient in iodine, medication-induced (eg, amiodarone, lithium, and alpha-interferon), and Riedel's thyroiditis
- Later stages of inflammatory thyroiditis: silent lymphocytic thyroiditis, postpartum thyroiditis, and subacute (de Quervain) thyroiditis

Risk Factors

- History of other autoimmune disorders and medications

Clinical Manifestations/Physical Exam

- Decreased metabolic rate leads to cold intolerance, weight gain despite decreased appetite, fatigue, depression, decreased DTR, constipation, anorexia, bradycardia, decreased cardiac output, dry, thickened rough skin, hypoglycemia, and menorrhagia

Diagnosis

- Primary hypothyroidism: decreased free T4 and increased TSH
- Secondary or tertiary hypothyroidism: decreased free T4 and decreased TSH

Management/Prognosis

- Hashimoto's thyroiditis: thyroid hormone replacement
- Iodine deficiency: iodide replacement
- Inflammatory thyroiditis: symptomatic treatment
- Medication induced: patients often become euthyroid once the medication is discontinued
- Riedel's thyroiditis: surgery may be needed in some cases

With hypothyroidism, you become as **cold as a hippo with thick skin in the winter** that is always **bleeding.**

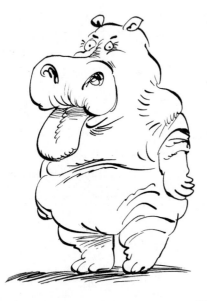

- **Cold intolerance**

- **Weight gain**

- **Dry, thickened skin** (hippo)

- **± goiter, hoarseness of voice, puffy face, periorbital edema, myxedema, enlargement of tongue, loss of outer-third of eyebrows**

- **Menorrhagia and menstrual irregularities**

- **Bradycardia**

Figure 7.1 Hypothyroidism

Hashimoto's Thyroiditis

Most common cause of hypothyroidism in the United States

- Autoimmune thyroid cell destruction by circulating auto-antibodies and lymphocytic infiltration leads to hypothyroidism
- Most commonly age 30–50, far more common in women than in men (10x)
- Clinical manifestations: signs of hypothyroidism
- Diagnosis: positive antithyroid peroxidase and antithyroglobulin antibodies
- Biopsy usually not needed but if done: lymphocytes, germinal follicles, and Hürthle cells
- Thyroid hormone replacement: levothyroxine
- Indications: first-line management of Hashimoto thyroiditis and subclinical hypothyroidism with TSH $\geq$10 mIU/L
- Mechanism: synthetic thyroxine (T4); half-life 7 days
- Monitoring: monitor TSH level at 6-wk intervals when initiating or changing dose
  - Increase dose if TSH is high and decrease dose if TSH is low
  - With the elderly and those with cardiovascular disease, initiate therapy with small, incremental increases
  - During pregnancy, increase dose
- Interactions: best taken AM on empty stomach for optimal absorption; take multivitamins, aluminum, iron/calcium, and PPIs 4 hours apart from levothyroxine (can reduce effectiveness); may need to reduce dose with anticoagulants, insulin, and oral hypoglycemic; cholestyramine may increase T4 requirements
- Side effects: overshoot can have adverse cardiovascular effects and cause osteoporosis

Iodine Deficiency/Nontoxic Goiter

Most common cause of hypothyroidism (worldwide)

- Clinical manifestations: signs of hypothyroidism, goiter, dyspnea (tracheal compression), hoarseness (laryngeal nerve compression)
- Management: iodine replacement; levothyroxine; iodine therapy for compressive goiter

Cretinism (Congenital Hypothyroidism)

Severe mental retardation, increased weight gain, short stature

- Lack of maternal iodine intake during pregnancy or acquired (eg, if mother had TSH-receptor blocking antibodies passed into fetal circulation via the placenta)
- Agenesis of the thyroid gland
- Physical exam: coarse facial features, macroglossia, umbilical hernia, hypotonia, prolonged jaundice, feeding problems, congenital malformations
- Hypothyroid profile: increased TSH and decreased free T4/T3
- Management: levothyroxine (synthetic T4)

Iatrogenic Hypothyroidism

Inadequate secretion of thyroid hormone; often due to treatment for hyperthyroidism with radioactive iodine or surgery (total or subtotal thyroidectomy) without subsequent thyroid hormone replacement

- Amiodarone: contains iodine and may induce hypothyroidism (by the Wolff-Chaikoff effect) or hyperthyroidism (by the Jod-Basedow phenomenon) depending on the underlying state of the patient
- Alpha-interferon: by stimulating the immune system in patients with baseline thyroid autoimmune predisposition (eg, patients with anti-TPO or anti-TG antibodies)
- Lithium: mechanism that causes hypothyroidism in patients taking lithium is poorly understood (may affect the colloid)

HYPERTHYROIDISM

Increased levels of the thyroid hormones levothyroxine (free T4) and/or triiodothyronine (free T3)

Etiology/Pathophysiology

- Graves' disease, toxic adenoma, toxic multinodular goiter, TSH-secreting pituitary adenoma
- Early stages of inflammatory thyroiditis: silent lymphocytic thyroiditis, postpartum thyroiditis, and subacute (de Quervain) thyroiditis

Risk Factors

- History of other autoimmune disorders and medications such as amiodarone

Clinical Manifestations/Physical Exam

- Increased metabolic rate leads to heat intolerance, weight loss despite increased appetite, warm, moist skin, tremors, nervousness, fatigue, weakness, increased sympathetic output, diarrhea, tachycardia, palpitations, high-output heart failure, scanty periods, and hyperglycemia

Diagnosis

- Primary hyperthyroidism: increased free T4 and decreased TSH
- Secondary or tertiary hypothyroidism: increased free T4 and increased TSH

Management/Prognosis

- Graves' disease: radioactive iodine therapy (most common), antithyroid medications (methimazole or propylthiouracil) or thyroidectomy if compressive symptoms or no response to medications; BBs can be used for the symptoms of thyrotoxicosis
- Toxic multinodular goiter and toxic adenoma: radioactive iodine therapy (most common), antithyroid medications (methimazole or propylthiouracil) or thyroidectomy if compressive symptoms or no response to medications; BBs can be used for the symptoms of thyrotoxicosis
- TSH-secreting adenoma: transsphenoidal surgery to remove the pituitary adenoma

With hyperthyroidism you are so hyper you have no time to bleed.

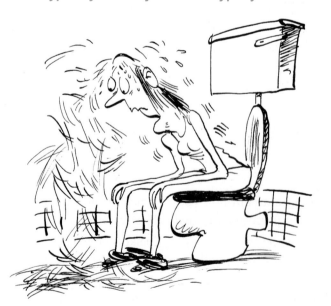

- **Weight loss, diarrhea, heat intolerance**

- **Warm and moist skin, fine hair, alopecia, easy bruising, tachycardia, ± goiter**

- **Mental psychosis, scanty periods**

- **Hyperactivity: tremors, fatigue, nervousness, increased sympathetic output**

Figure 7.2 Hyperthyroidism

Graves' Disease

Most common cause of hyperthyroidism

- Circulating auto-antibodies (TSH receptor antibodies) that actually stimulate the thyroid hormone production leads to hyperthyroidism
- Most commonly women, age 20–40
- Increased association with HLA-DRB1*08 and DRB3*0202
- Thyrotoxicosis: signs of thyroid hormone excess
- Diffusely enlarged goiter (± thyroid bruits due to increased blood flow to thyroid)
- Ophthalmopathy: photophobia, visual loss, diplopia, proptosis/exophthalmos, lid lag
- Pretibial myxedema: swollen red/brown patches on legs with non-pitting edema
- Serum studies show decreased TSH and increased free T4/T3; positive thyroid-stimulating immunoglobulins specific for Graves'; ± other markers of autoimmunity (positive anti-thyroglobulin and/or positive anti-thyroid peroxidase may be seen)
- Radioactive iodine uptake scan shows increased diffuse iodine uptake
- Management: radioactive iodine ablation (most common therapy) (induces hypothyroidism and may transiently worsen ophthalmopathy); thioamides (prevent thyroid hormone synthesis, eg, methimazole and propylthiouracil; will often achieve a euthyroid state within 3-8 wks; side effects include agranulocytosis, aplastic anemia, fulminant hepatitis; methimazole generally preferred (fewer side effects but teratogenic in first trimester of pregnancy; propylthiouracil preferred for first trimester and thyroid storm); beta-blockers (rapid relief of hyperadrenergic symptoms eg, tremor, hypertension, aFib, and tachycardia (propranolol); glucocorticoids for ophthalmopathy (best initial therapy); decompressive therapy; thyroidectomy

In order to avoid the **grave,** you must keep your **eyes wide open, stimulate** yourself by staying **hyper,** and **take up as much iodine** as possible.

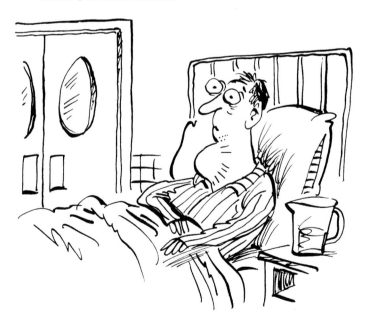

- Graves' disease is caused by **thyroid stimulating antibodies** that increase thyroid hormone synthesis

Clinical Manifestations:
- **Exophthalmos, proptosis** (eyes wide open)

- **Hyper:** tachycardia, anxiety, tremors, nervousness, etc.

Diagnosis:
- + Thyroid-**stimulating** immunoglobulins

- RAI scan: **diffuse increased uptake**

Figure 7.3 Graves' Disease

SUBACUTE GRANULOMATOUS THYROIDITIS

Type of thyroiditis characterized by granulomatous inflammation of the thyroid gland due to viral infection or postviral inflammatory process; also known as de Quervain, nonsuppurative, or giant cell thyroiditis

Etiology/Pathophysiology

- Classic progression is hyperthyroidism (usually when they present); leads to hypothyroidism resulting in resolution with subsequent normal thyroid function (euthyroidism)

Risk Factors

- Most common following a flu-like illness

Clinical Manifestations/Physical Exam

- Signs of hyperthyroidism initially (if presents later in the disease process may have signs and symptoms of hypothyroidism)
- Painful thyroid gland (neck pain) with tenderness on palpation, sore throat; may complain of jaw pain

Diagnosis

- Clinical diagnosis
- Labs: hyperthyroid profile classic: increased free thyroxine (T4) and triiodothyronine (T3), decreased TSH
- Increased ESR
- Biopsy: granulomatous inflammation (biopsy usually not needed)
- Radioactive uptake scan: diffuse decreased iodine uptake

Management/Prognosis

- Usually self-limiting (resolves within weeks to months of presentation)
- Acetylsalicylic acid (eg, aspirin) or NSAIDs; prednisone can be an alternative to NSAIDs
- Corticosteroids for severe cases

She has Dquer**PAINS**

She (most common in women)

Decreased uptake of iodine on radioactive uptake scan

Painful thyroid gland (may present as sore throat)

After viral illness

Increased ESR

Negative thyroid antibodies

Self-limiting (**s**alicylates or other NSAIDs for pain)

PAPILLARY THYROID CANCER

Well-differentiated epithelial-derived thyroid cancer characterized by the presence of papillae

Etiology/Pathophysiology

- Mutations or rearrangements in genes encoding for the proteins in the mitogen-activated protein kinase pathway are critical to the development and progression of differentiated thyroid cancer
- Localized (cervical metastasis) most common; distant METS uncommon

Risk Factors

- Most common after radiation exposure and with family history
- Least aggressive; most common in young females

Clinical Manifestations/Physical Exam

- Usually presents as a painless thyroid nodule without symptoms

Diagnosis

- Biopsy: classically unencapsulated and may be partially cystic; presence of papillae consisting of 1–2 layers of tumor cells surrounding a well-defined fibrovascular core
- Follicles and colloid are usually absent

Management/Prognosis

- Two surgical options: total or subtotal thyroidectomy
- May monitor thyroglobulin levels 6 months after thyroidectomy to look for residual cells

- **P**apillary is most **Popular** (most common thyroid carcinoma)

- **F**ollicular: **Far** in other areas (distant metastasis is common)

- **M**edullary: you will **"C" M**edullary with **M**en-2 (arises from **C** cells and secretes **C**alcitonin)

- Ana**plastic** will turn your **rocks into plastic** (rapid growth and most aggressive); **rock hard nodule** on exam

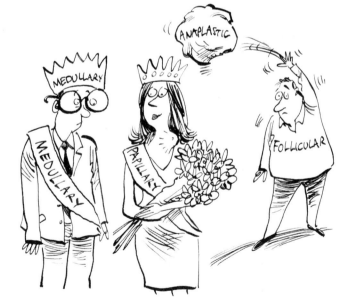

Figure 7.4 Thyroid Cancer

PRIMARY HYPERPARATHYROIDISM

Excess parathyroid production

Etiology/Pathophysiology

- Parathyroid adenoma most common cause overall (85%)
- Parathyroid gland hyperplasia (enlargement) (10%)
- Occurs in 20% of patients taking lithium (lithium increases PTH production)
- Malignant tumor (rare causes; eg, parathyroid carcinoma), multiple endocrine neoplasia (MEN) syndrome

Clinical Manifestations/Physical Exam

- Asymptomatic in many cases
- Signs of hypercalcemia:
  - Stones: kidney stones, nephrogenic diabetes insipidus
  - Bones: painful bones, fractures
  - Abdominal groans: ileus, constipation, nausea, vomiting
  - Moans: weakness, fatigue, altered mental status, depression, psychosis

Diagnosis

- **Triad**: increased serum calcium; increased intact serum PTH; decreased (or normal) serum phosphate
- Increased 24-hour urine calcium
- Osteitis fibrosis cystica: on x-ray (including "salt-and-pepper" appearance of skull) PTH stimulates osteoclast activity and leads to loss of bone mass, cystic bone spaces "brown tumors" (not actual tumors)

Management/Prognosis

- Parathyroidectomy; subsequent hypocalcemia may occur as a result of parathyroidectomy
- Acute hypercalcemia: IV fluids and loop diuretics (to promote renal calcium excretion)

Deno the 1st lost faith in his chef and broke his bones with stones after he became PALE and got abdominal groans while eating rotten raMEN noodles.

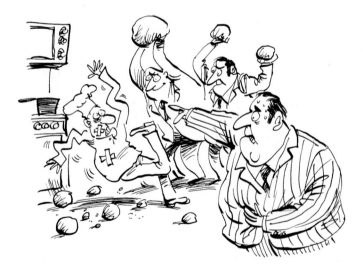

- Adenoma **MC cause of primary (1st) hyper PTH**

Etiologies:
- Parathyroid Adenoma, Lithium Enlargement (hyperplasia)
- May be associated with **MEN** syndrome (I, IIa)

Clinical Manifestations:
- Signs of **Hypercalcemia: stones, bones, abdominal groans, psychic moans**

Diagnosis:
- Hypercalcemia, increased PTH, **decreased phosphate (lost his faith)**

Figure 7.5 Primary Hyperparathyroidism

HYPOPARATHYROIDISM

Injury to parathyroid gland leads to decreased release of PTH

Etiology/Pathophysiology

- Rarely occurs; if present, usually due to low PTH secretion or insensitivity to PTH
- Accidental: damage/removal of parathyroid most common (during thyroidectomy or treatment for cancer in the neck)
- Others:
  - Autoimmune destruction of parathyroid gland
  - Hereditary
  - Radiation treatment
  - Hypomagnesemia (magnesium required for PTH production)

Clinical Manifestations/Physical Exam

- Signs of hypocalcemia: increased muscle contraction (hypocalcemia decreases excitation threshold)
  - Paresthesias in fingers, toes, and lips, muscle cramps, spasm, tetany, carpopedal spasm, increased deep tendon reflexes
  - Positive Trousseau sign (carpopedal spasm), positive Chvostek sign (facial spasm with tapping of cheek)
- Seizures, arrhythmias, hypotension
- Psychiatric symptoms due to hypocalcemia: depression, anxiety, instability
- Cataracts

Diagnosis

- **Triad**: decreased serum calcium; increased serum phosphate; decreased intact serum PTH

Management/Prognosis

- Calcium and vitamin D supplementation (ergocalciferol)
- IV calcium gluconate (acute symptomatic hypocalcemia)

HYPERCALCEMIA

Elevated levels of calcium in the blood

Etiology/Pathophysiology

- Primary hyperparathyroidism (most common cause, 90%) or malignancy
- Parathyroid hormone related:
  - Primary hyperparathyroidism: most common cause overall
  - Familial hypocalciuric hypercalcemia:
  - Lithium therapy
- Malignancy related: due to parathyroid-hormone-related protein (eg, lung, kidney), hematologic malignancies that cause bone damage (eg, multiple myeloma, leukemia)
- High bone turnover: thiazide diuretics, hyperthyroidism, vitamin A intoxication, fat necrosis
- Vitamin D related: intoxication, granulomatous diseases

Clinical Manifestations/Physical Exam

- Most patients are asymptomatic
- Stones: kidney stones, nephrogenic diabetes insipidus; bones: painful bones, fractures; abdominal groans: ileus, constipation, nausea, vomiting; moans: weakness, fatigue AMS, depression, or psychosis

Diagnosis

- Increased ionized calcium >5.6 mg/dL (>1.31 mmol/L) more accurate or serum total calcium >10.5 mg/dL (2.62 mmol/L)
- ECG: may show shortened QT interval, prolonged PR interval, QRS widening

Management/Prognosis

- Mild: observation, seek underlying cause
- Moderate: IV saline, furosemide (promote Ca^{+2} excretion)
- Severe: bisphosphonates, calcitonin; dialysis
- Glucocorticoids may be helpful in granulomatous diseases

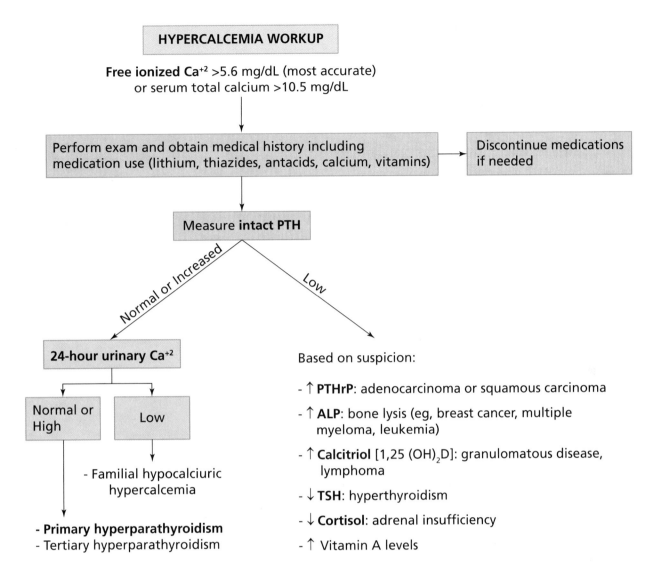

Figure 7.6 Hypercalcemia Workup

Physiology of Calcium

- Hormones that **increase serum calcium concentration**:
  - Parathyroid hormone: para**thy makes it high!**
  - Vitamin D (calci**triol**): **tri**es its **all** to increase calcium
- Hormones that **decrease serum calcium concentration**:
  - Cal**ci**tonin takes **calc**ium from the serum and puts **it o**ut via the **nephrons** and **in** the bones (increases urinary calcium excretion and osteoblastic activity)

HYPOCALCEMIA

Decreased levels of calcium in the blood

Etiology/Pathophysiology

- Hypoparathyroidism: most common cause overall
- Chronic renal disease most common cause if serum PTH is increased
- Vitamin D deficiency: osteomalacia and rickets
- Increased PTH in response to hypocalcemia
- Hypomagnesemia, hyperphosphatemia; hypoalbuminemia
- Others: high citrate states (eg, blood transfusion), severe burns, acute pancreatitis, liver disease

Clinical Manifestations/Physical Exam

- Most patients are asymptomatic
- **So She's Got No Calcium:**
    - **S**keletal: abnormal dentition, osteomalacia, osteodystrophy
    - **S**kin: dry skin, psoriasis
    - **G**I: diarrhea, abdominal pain/cramps
    - **N**euromuscular: muscle cramping, bronchospasm, syncope, seizures, finger/circumoral paresthesias; tetany: Chvostek sign: facial spasm with tapping facial nerve; increased DTR; Trousseau's sign: inflate BP cuff above systolic causes carpal spasm
    - **C**ardiovascular: CHF, arrhythmias

Diagnosis

- Decreased free ionized calcium <4.65 mg/dL (1.16 mmol/L) more accurate or serum total calcium <8.5 mg/dL
- Albumin levels may be needed to correct calcium for hypoalbuminemia
- ECG: ± prolonged QT interval

Management/Prognosis

- Mild: PO calcium and vitamin D (ergocalciferol)
- Potassium and magnesium repletion may be needed in some cases
- Severe/symptomatic: IV calcium gluconate or carbonate

OSTEOMALACIA AND RICKETS

Defect in bone mineralization

Etiology/Pathophysiology

- Vitamin D deficiency leading to decreased calcium and phosphate, thus resulting in demineralization and "soft bones"
- Before epiphyseal closure, rickets; after epiphyseal closure, osteomalacia

Clinical Manifestations/Physical Exam

- Rickets (children): delayed fontanelle closure, growth retardation, delayed dentition costal cartilage enlargement (rachitic rosary), bowing of long bones, spinal kyphosis; epiphyseal plates appear "fuzzy"
- Osteomalacia (adults): asymptomatic initially; diffuse bone pain, muscular weakness (proximal); hypocalcemia; hip pain may cause antalgic gait; bowing of long bones

Diagnosis

- Decreased vitamin D; decreased calcium; decreased phosphate; increased alkaline phosphatase
- Looser lines (zones): transverse "pseudo fracture" lines (visible demineralized osteoids)

Management/Prognosis

- Vitamin D supplementation (ergocalciferol) and calcium supplementation

---

Osteomalacia and Rickets

You are a **looser** if you **bow** out the fight and allow **calcium**, phosphate, and vitamin D to deplete in your body.

- Physical exam: **bow**ing of long bones
- Diagnosis: **decreased calcium, phosphate**, and **vitamin D**
- X-ray: **looser lines** (pseudo-fracture lines)

RENAL OSTEODYSTROPHY

Osteitis fibrosis cystica and osteomalacia present in patients with chronic kidney disease

Etiology/Pathophysiology

- Poor elimination of phosphate and synthesis of vitamin D by failing kidneys, leading to hypocalcemia; results in compensatory increased PTH and eventual osteoid formation (decreased mineralization)

Clinical Manifestations/Physical Exam

- Bone and proximal muscle pain, ± pathologic fractures

Diagnosis

- Secondary hyperparathyroidism: decreased calcium, increased phosphate, increased PTH
- Osteitis fibrosis cystica: subperiosteal erosions, cystic (brown tumor), osteopenia, skull: "salt-and-pepper" appearance

Management/Prognosis

- Phosphate binders: calcium carbonate, calcium acetate; sevelamer used if high calcium
- Vitamin D (ergocalciferol) and calcium

Adding <u>salt and pepper</u> to the food will win you a <u>local TROPHY</u>.

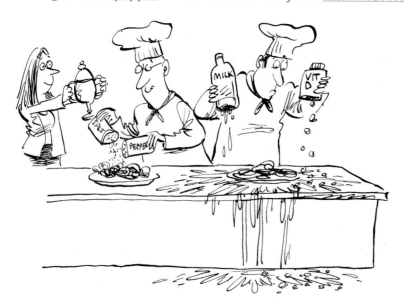

- **Salt-and-Pepper** appearance of skull on x-ray

- **Lo-cal**cium (hypocalcemia)

TROPHY:
  Tumors (**cystic brown** on biopsy)
  Renal failure is the cause
  Osteitis fibrosis cystica on x-ray
  Phosphate is **Hy** (**elevated**)

Figure 7.7 Renal Osteodystrophy

CHRONIC ADRENOCORTICAL INSUFFICIENCY

Inadequate production of cortisol and aldosterone (primary form) and cortisol (secondary form)

Etiology/Pathophysiology

- Primary (Addison's disease): adrenal cortex destruction leads to lack of cortisol, aldosterone (and sex hormones in women)
  - Autoimmune: most common in industrialized countries (70–90%)
  - Infection (most common worldwide): tuberculosis, HIV, etc.
  - Vascular: hemorrhage, thrombosis, trauma
  - Drugs: ketoconazole, rifampin, phenytoin, barbiturates
- Secondary: exogenous steroid use (most common cause); hypopituitarism (rare)

Clinical Manifestations/Physical Exam

- Weakness, muscle aches, fatigue, weight/appetite loss, anorexia, nausea and vomiting, abdominal pain, loss of libido in women
- Hypotension; hyperpigmentation in primary adrenal insufficiency (due to increased ACTH)

Diagnosis

- Labs: hyperkalemia, hyponatremia, low BUN, hypoglycemia, non-anion gap metabolic acidosis
- High dose ACTH (cosyntropin) stimulation test: screening test (little or no increase in cortisol)
- CRH stimulation test: differentiates the causes of adrenal insufficiency
  - Primary (adrenal) leads to high ACTH but low cortisol
  - Secondary (pituitary) leads to low ACTH and low cortisol
  - Tertiary (hypothalamus): delayed, prolonged, or exaggerated ACTH response
- CT of adrenal glands: atrophy of adrenal glands (autoimmune); calcification of adrenal glands (infection); bleeding within adrenal glands (vascular)

Management/Prognosis

- Synthetic glucocorticoids: hydrocortisone, prednisone, dexamethasone
- Synthetic mineralocorticoids: fludrocortisone for primary (Addison's disease only)
- Androgen (DHEA) replacement may improve quality of life and improve bone density

Addison lost her AVID sex drive and became static due to the hyperpigmentation of her skin and lack of sugar and salt in her diet.

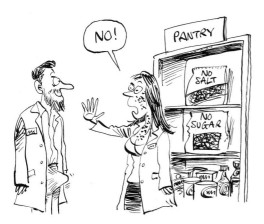

Etiologies:
- **Autoimmune** (most common cause in industrialized countries)
- **Vascular**, eg, hemorrhage
- **Infection**: TB, HIV, etc. (most common cause worldwide)
- **Drugs**: ketoconazole, rifampin, phenytoin, barbiturates

- **Hyperpigmentation of skin**
- **Hypoglycemia**
- **Hypotension** (± orthostatic)
- **Decreased total body sodium (hypovolemia)**

Figure 7.8 Primary Adrenal Insufficiency (Addison's Disease)

Endocrine

CUSHING'S SYNDROME

Disorder caused by exposure to excess cortisol

Etiology/Pathophysiology

- Iatrogenic: long-term high dose corticosteroid therapy (most common cause overall)
- Cushing's disease: pituitary adenoma or hyperplasia
- Ectopic ACTH: ACTH-secreting small-cell lung cancer, medullary thyroid cancer
- Adrenal tumor: cortisol secreting adrenal adenoma

Clinical Manifestations/Physical Exam

- Weakness, depression, psychosis, osteoporosis, weight gain oligo/amenorrhea, DM (polyuria, polydipsia)
- Physical exam: HTN, central obesity with thin extremities, moon facies, buffalo hump, supraclavicular fat pads, skin atrophy, easy bruising, striae, hyperpigmentation, acanthosis nigricans, oily face/acne, hirsutism, virilization

Diagnosis

- Labs: hypokalemia and hyperglycemia; metabolic alkalosis hypernatremia (less common)
- Screening: low dose dexamethasone suppression test (no suppression), elevated salivary cortisol, 24-hour urinary free cortisol leads to increased cortisol
- High dose dexamethasone suppression: positive suppression in Cushing's disease only
- CT or MRI to localize the lesions

> **Cushing's disease** is the only cause of Cushing's syndrome that **suppresses during high-dose dexamethasone suppression testing.**

Management/Prognosis

- Cushing's disease (pituitary): transsphenoidal surgery, radiation therapy
- Ectopic or adrenal tumors: tumor removal; ketoconazole or metyrapone if inoperable (decreases cortisol production)
- Iatrogenic steroid therapy: gradual steroid withdrawal with tapering (to prevent Addisonian crisis)

When smoking **CUSH** that is **LACE**D, you start with **low-doses** and then you get **high.**

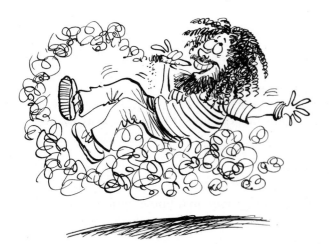

Screening:
- **Low-dose** dexamethasone suppression test
- Salivary or urine cortisol levels
- **High-dose** dexamethasone suppression test **to differentiate**

Etiologies:
- **L**ong-term corticosteroid use (most common)
- **A**drenal tumors
- **C**ushing's disease: pituitary adenoma (ACTH)
- **E**ctopic ACTH-producing tumors

Figure 7.9 Cushing Syndrome

HYPERALDOSTERONISM

Excess aldosterone produced by the adrenal glands

Etiology/Pathophysiology

- Primary hyperaldosteronism: renin independent
  - Idiopathic or bilateral adrenal hyperplasia (60%); most common in women
  - Conn syndrome: adrenal aldosteronoma (40%)
  - Unilateral adrenal hyperplasia (rare)
- Secondary hyperaldosteronism: due to increased renin (via RAAS)
  - Renal artery stenosis (most common), CHF, hypovolemia, nephrotic syndrome

Clinical Manifestations/Physical Exam

- Usually asymptomatic
  - Hypokalemia: proximal muscle weakness, decreased DTR, polyuria
  - HTN (especially in primary hyperaldosteronism): may manifest as headaches, flushing of face
  - Metabolic alkalosis may present with muscle cramps

Diagnosis

- Labs: hypokalemia with metabolic alkalosis (due to aldosterone mediated dumping of K^+ and H^+ in exchange for Na^+ retention)
- Aldosterone-to-renin ratio (ARR) screening:
  - Increased ARR (>20), increased plasma aldosterone (>20), and decreased plasma renin (negative feedback) indicate primary hyperaldosteronism
  - Increased renin indicates secondary hyperaldosteronism
- CT/MRI to look for adrenal or extra-adrenal mass; ECG may show signs of hypokalemia

Management/Prognosis

- Surgical intervention: excision of adrenal aldosteronomas; angioplasty if renovascular HTN
- HTN: spironolactone (blocks aldosterone), ACE inhibitors, CCBs
- Correct electrolytes

> Hyperaldosteronism is a cause of **secondary hypertension**.

Idiots like hyper AL allow themselves to be conned and lose their potassium for alkahol under high pressure.

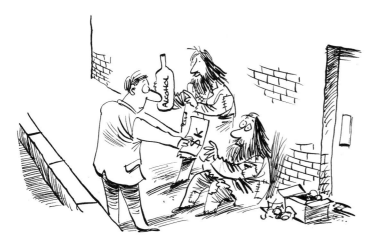

Etiologies:
Idiopathic

Conn syndrome (adrenal adenoma)

Labs show **hypokalemia** and metabolic **alkalosis**

Figure 7.10 Primary Hyperaldosteronism

PHEOCHROMOCYTOMA

Catecholamine-secreting adrenal tumor (enterochromaffin cells)

Etiology/Pathophysiology

- Paraganglioma refers to similar tumors in other sites of the body (extra-adrenal)
- Rule of 10s leads to 10% malignant, 10% bilateral, 10% extra-adrenal (eg, aorta), 10% seen in children
- May be associated with MEN syndrome IIA & IIB, neurofibromatosis (von Hippel Lindau syndrome)

Clinical Manifestations/Physical Exam

- HTN (most consistent finding): may be temporary, sustained, or cause HTN crisis
- Diastolic HTN
- Palpitations, headaches (paroxysmal), excessive sweating; chest or abdominal pain, weakness, fatigue, weight loss (despite increased appetite), anxiety

Diagnosis

- Increase 24-hour urinary catecholamines and their metabolites (metanephrine and vanillylmandelic acid)
- Increased plasma free metanephrines (best test)
- MRI or CT to visualize tumor

Management/Prognosis

- Complete adrenalectomy: definitive management
- Preoperative α-blockade: phenoxybenzamine or phentolamine, followed by BB or CCB (do not start with BB [to prevent unopposed alpha constriction/excess HTN from catecholamine release])

PHEochromocytoma

Palpitations

Headaches

Excessive sweating

You must medicate **PHEO** with **PHEOS**:
(nonselective alpha blockade)

- **Phe**noxybenzamine or **phe**ntolamine
- Followed by BB

DIABETIC KETOACIDOSIS

Serious life-threatening complication of diabetes

Etiology/Pathophysiology

- Part of a spectrum representing the metabolic consequences of insulin deficiency and excess of counterregulatory hormone in response to stressful triggers
- Common in patients with type I DM

Risk Factors

- Stressful triggers (eg, infections) (most common cause)
- Noncompliance with insulin
- Myocardial infarction

Clinical Manifestations/Physical Exam

- Hyperglycemia: thirst, polyuria, polydipsia, nocturia
- Generalized weakness, confusion, weight loss, nausea/vomiting, chest pain, abdominal pain
- Tachycardia, tachypneic hypotension, fever if infection, decreased skin turgor; Kussmaul respirations (deep, rapid breaths), ketotic breath (fruity, acetone odor); acetone is the chemically neutral byproduct of fatty acid metabolism; acids produced are acetoacetate and β-hydroxybutyrate

Diagnosis

- Serum glucose >250 mg/dL; increased serum osmolarity; serum bicarbonate <15 mEq/L
- Arterial pH: <7.3 (high anion gap metabolic acidosis)
- Ketonuria and ketonemia

Management/Prognosis

- IV fluids; treat underlying cause
- Regular insulin until anion gap closes; add glucose when serum glucose <250 to prevent hypoglycemia
- Potassium replacement to prevent hypokalemia

DKA (characterized by **D**ehydration **4K**s and **A**cidosis)

- 4Ks of DKA: **K**etonemia, decrease in total body **K**+, **K**etotic breath, **K**ussmaul respirations
- Management: must **SIP** to survive the dehydration of DKA
  - **S**aline first step
  - **I**nsulin
  - **P**otassium

Anatomy of Adrenals = ACE

- Zona glomerulos**a**: **A**ldosterone
- Zona fasciculata: **C**ortisol
- Zona reticularis: **E**strogen/androgens
- The **pituitary gland** secretes hormones from 2 locations: the anterior and posterior pituitary gland. Most hormones are secreted from the anterior portion, but 2 hormones are secreted from the posterior pituitary.
  - Oxytocin and anti-diuretic hormone (ADH)
  - High school students must **post** an **AD** to go to **Ox**ford!
  - **Post**erior secretes **AD**H and **Ox**ytocin (ADH is made in the hypothalamus but is stored and secreted from the posterior pituitary)

Complications of insulin therapy for diabetes include the **dawn** phenomenon (as the sun comes up at dawn, glucose increases) and the s**O**mogyl effect (hyp**O**glycemia followed by **i**ncrease in glucose (hyperglycemia).

DIABETES INSIPIDUS

Condition whereby impairment of antidiuretic hormone leads to an inability to concentrate urine

Etiology/Pathophysiology

- Central DI: decreased ADH production, idiopathic (most common); autoimmune destruction of posterior pituitary, head trauma, tumor (brain or pituitary), infection, sarcoid granuloma
- Nephrogenic DI: partial or complete insensitivity to ADH
  - Medications: lithium, amphotericin B, demeclocycline
  - Electrolytes: hypercalcemia ($>$11 mg/dL), hypokalemia
  - Intrinsic renal disease (ATN), hyperparathyroidism

Clinical Manifestations/Physical Exam

- Polyuria, polydipsia, nocturia (enuresis in children)
- Hypernatremia if severe or decreased oral water intake

Diagnosis

- Fluid deprivation test establishes a diagnosis of DI: continued production of dilute urine; decreased Uosm ($<$200); and low specific gravity ($<$1.005)
- Desmopressin (ADH) stimulation test differentiates nephrogenic from central DI
  - Nephrogenic DI: continued production of dilute urine (indicates no response to ADH)
  - Central DI: reduced production of urine output (increased Uosm) (indicates a response to ADH)

Management/Prognosis

- Central DI: desmopressin/DDAVP (synthetic ADH); carbamazepine, chlorpropamide (increases ADH)
- Nephrogenic DI: sodium/protein restriction, increased water intake leads to hydrochlorothiazide, indomethacin; difficult to treat

Presence of ADH
due to hyperosmolarity or hypovolemia

- **Thirst stimulated**
- **Decreased urine volume**

Absence of ADH
due to hypoosmolarity

- **Thirst inhibited**
- **Increased urine volume**

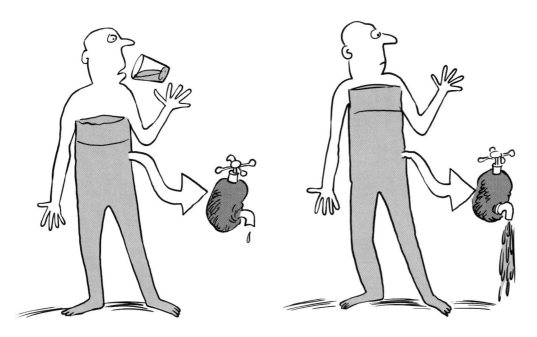

Figure 7.11 Normal Physiology of ADH

DIABETES INSIPIDUS

If you keep saying **NA** to **ADH,** you will **pee and drink** so much that you will **DI**.

The body keeps saying **NA** to **ADH,** due either to deficiency of **ADH** (central) or insensitivity to **ADH** (nephrogenic).

HyperNAtremia **polyuria and polydipsia**

Chapter 8

Genitourinary

NEPHROTIC SYNDROME

Kidney disease characterized by proteinuria, hypoalbuminemia, hyperlipidemia, and edema due to glomerular damage

Etiology/Pathophysiology

- Primary (idiopathic) causes:
  - Minimal change disease (Nil disease): 80% of nephrotic syndrome occurring in children, 20% in adults; no significant visible cellular changes seen on simple light microscopy (minimal change); podocyte damage seen on electron microscope
  - Focal segmental glomerulosclerosis (FSGS): seen in patients with reflux nephropathy, heroin abuse, and HIV
  - Membranous nephropathy: thickened glomerular basement membrane; seen in systemic lupus erythematosus, viral hepatitis, malaria, drugs, hypocomplementemia
- Secondary causes: systemic disorders extrinsic to kidney that affect other organs in addition to kidney (eg, DM)

Clinical Manifestations/Physical Exam

- Edema: peripheral and periorbital edema (especially in pediatric patients); characteristically worse in the morning
- Anemia, DVT, frothy urine, pleural effusions

Diagnosis

- 24-hour urine protein collection: >3.5 g/24 hours in adults; children: total protein/creatinine ratio on spot urine >3 mg protein/mg creatinine (300 mg protein/mmol creatinine)
- Urinalysis: proteinuria (3+ or 4+ on dipstick); oval fat bodies "maltese cross" appearance seen with polarized light
- Hypoalbuminemia, hyperlipidemia; increased BUN and creatinine
- Renal biopsy may differentiate the types in some patients

Management/Prognosis

- Corticosteroids: minimal change disease and FSGS
- Edema reduction: diuretics (thiazides if mild, loop diuretics if severe); fluid restriction, decreased sodium/increased protein diet
- Proteinuria: ACE inhibitors or angiotensin II receptor antagonists
- Hyperlipidemia reduction: diet and medications

If a **child's** **weight** increases by only **3,** this **minimal change** can be due to the loss of **proteins**.

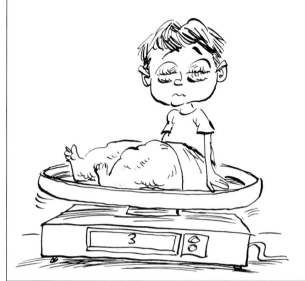

• **Minimal change** (most common cause in **children**)

• **Periorbital edema**

Diagnosis:
• **Urinalysis:** oval **fat bodies** (shaped like Maltese cross seen with polarized microscopy)

• 24-hour urine **protein** collection **>3.5 grams;** >3 mg protein/mg creatinine spot urine in children

Figure 8.1 Nephrotic Syndrome

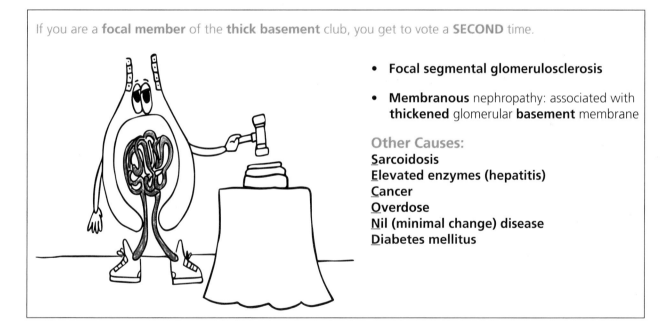

If you are a **focal member** of the **thick basement** club, you get to vote a **SECOND** time.

• **Focal segmental glomerulosclerosis**

• **Membranous** nephropathy: associated with **thickened** glomerular **basement** membrane

Other Causes:
Sarcoidosis
Elevated enzymes (hepatitis)
Cancer
Overdose
Nil (minimal change) disease
Diabetes mellitus

Figure 8.2 Other Causes of Nephrotic Syndrome

GLOMERULONEPHRITIS

Immunologic inflammation of the glomeruli (causes protein and blood leakage into urine) causing HTN, hematuria (proteinuria), and azotemia

Etiology/Pathophysiology

- IgA nephropathy (Berger's disease): most common cause in adults (worldwide); often affects young males within days (24–48 hours) after upper respiratory or GI infection
  - Diagnosis: IgA deposits in mesangium
  - Management: ACE inhibitors and corticosteroids
- Post-infectious: most common after Group A streptococcal infection; commonly age 2–14 with puffy eyelids, facial edema up to 3 weeks after strep infection with scanty, dark (cola-colored) urine
  - Diagnosis: antistreptolysin titers; low complement, biopsy: hypercellularity, increased mono-/lymphocytes
  - Management: supportive, antibiotics
- Membranoproliferative/mesangiocapillary: due to SLE, viral hepatitis, hypocomplementemia; usually present with a mixed nephritic-nephrotic picture
- RPGN is associated with rapid progression to end-stage renal disease. Any can present in RPGN but the following conditions only present with RPGN:
  - Goodpasture's syndrome: anti-glomerular basement membrane antibodies lead to kidney failure and hemoptysis
    - Diagnosis: linear IgG deposits; often occurs after URI
    - Management: high-dose steroid immunosuppression and cyclophosphamide and plasmapheresis (removes antibodies)
  - Vasculitis:
    - Microscopic polyangiitis
    - Granulomatosis with polyangiitis

Clinical Manifestations/Physical Exam

- Hematuria: microscopic or macroscopic
- HTN (80%): secondary to fluid overload
- Edema (85%): peripheral, periorbital
- Fevers, abdominal pain, flank pain, malaise; oliguria

Diagnosis

- Urinalysis: hematuria including RBC casts; proteinuria (usually <3 g/day but may be in nephrotic range); high specific gravity >1.020; possible WBCs
- Increased BUN/creatinine: varying degrees
- Renal biopsy (gold standard) (not needed if post-strep suspected)

Management/Prognosis

- Berger's disease or proteinuria: ACE Inhibitors
- Edematous, hypervolemia or hypertensive: diuretics (eg, loop)
- HTN: BBs, CCBs
- Poststreptococcal glomerulonephritis: supportive and antibiotics
- RPGN or severe disease: corticosteroids and cyclophosphamide
- Lupus nephritis: corticosteroids or cyclophosphamide

Adults that go out to BERGER King rapidly progress and become PIMPS.

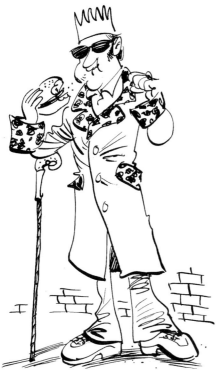

- **Berger disease,** also known as **IgA nephropathy,** most common cause of acute glomerulonephritis in **Adults**

- **P**ost **I**nfectious: MC after GABHS infection

- **M**embrano **P**roliferative

Rapidly progressive glomerulonephritis: associated with poor prognosis; crescents seen on renal biopsy

Figure 8.3 Etiologies of Glomerulonephritis

Clinical Manifestations of Glomerulo**nephr**itis

Nephron damage (oliguria)

Edema

Proteinuria

Hypertension

RBC casts in urine (hematuria)

ACUTE KIDNEY INJURY

Rise in serum creatinine (>50%) or azotemia (rise in blood urea nitrogen concentration)

Intrinsic Injury

- ATN
  - Ischemic: prolonged prerenal, hypotension or post-op
  - Nephrotoxic: aminoglycosides, contrast dye, cyclosporine, medications, rhabdomyolysis, multiple myeloma, etc.
  - Urinalysis: epithelial cell casts and muddy brown casts, low specific gravity
  - Management: remove offending agent(s), supportive treatment
- AIN
  - Inflammatory or allergic response in interstitium
  - Drug hypersensitivity (70%): penicillins, NSAIDs, sulfa drugs, cephalosporins, ciprofloxacin, allopurinol, rifampin; infections: streptococcus, legionella, CMV, EBV, HIV, etc.; autoimmune SLE, sarcoidosis, cryoglobulinemia; idiopathic
  - Clinical manifestations: fever, maculopapular rash, arthralgias, eosinophilia
  - Urinalysis: WBC casts, urine eosinophils; increased serum IgE
  - Management: remove offending agent
- Glomerular (AGN)
- Vascular:
  - Microvascular: TTP (thrombotic thrombocytopenic purpura), HELLP syndrome in pregnant patients, DIC
  - Macrovascular: aortic aneurysm, renal artery dissection/thrombosis, renal vein thrombosis, atheroembolic (especially after catheterization, CABG, AAA repair)

Prerenal Injury

Characterized by decreased renal perfusion with nephrons still structurally intact; may lead to intrinsic injury (ATN) if not corrected

- Most common type of acute kidney injury (40–80%)
- Etiologies: reduced renal perfusion hallmark (hypovolemia, afferent arteriole vasoconstriction eg, NSAIDs, IV contrast) and efferent arteriole dilation (eg, ACE inhibitors, ARBs); hypovolemia from renal volume loss (diuretic therapy), GI loss (diarrhea or vomiting); blood loss
- Diagnosis: evidence of water and electrolyte conservation—increased BUN > increased creatinine (BUN:creatinine ratio >20:1), fractional excretion of sodium (FENA) <1% and urine sodium <20, high urine specific gravity (>1.020) and increased urine osmolarity (>500 mOsm/kg)
- Management: volume repletion (rapid response to treatment)

Postrenal Injury (Obstructive Uropathy)

Characterized by obstruction of the passage of urine

- Etiologies: kidney stones, tumors, bladder outlet obstruction (benign prostatic hypertrophy) and sloughed off renal papillae.
- Clinical manifestations: usually asymptomatic. May develop change in urine output, hypertension.
- Diagnosis: increased creatinine usually associated with bilateral kidney involvement. Ultrasound often the initial imaging test to look for signs of obstruction & hydronephrosis. Depending on the cause or site of obstruction, catheterization, CT scan, MRI or pyelography may be useful.
- Management: removal of the obstruction (readily reversible if corrected quickly).

HYPONATREMIA

Impaired kidney-free water excretion (increased ADH) preventing the kidney from making dilute urine in the setting of increased water intake

Etiology/Pathophysiology

- **MRS WHAT** eats so much **Tea and Toast** she pees until her **thyroid and adrenal levels are low**
    - **M**DMA (ecstasy)
    - **R**eset hypothalamic osmostat
    - **S**IADH

    - **W**ater intoxication
    - **H**ypothyroidism
    - **A**drenal insufficiency
    - **T**ea and toast syndrome

Clinical Manifestations/Physical Exam

- Asymptomatic
- CNS dysfunction due to cerebral edema: nonspecific neurologic symptoms (eg, headache, nausea/vomiting, decreased DTR)
- Neurologic complications: seizure, coma, permanent brain damage, respiratory arrest, death

Management/Prognosis

- Hypotonic hyponatremia
    - Isovolemic: H2O restriction; treat underlying cause
    - Hypervolemic: H2O, sodium restriction, diuretics
    - Hypovolemic: normal saline
- Severe (iso or hyper) volemic hyponatremia: hypertonic saline with furosemide
- Correct ≤0.5 mEq/L/h to prevent demyelination (central pontine myelinolysis) due to rapid shrinking of the brain cells

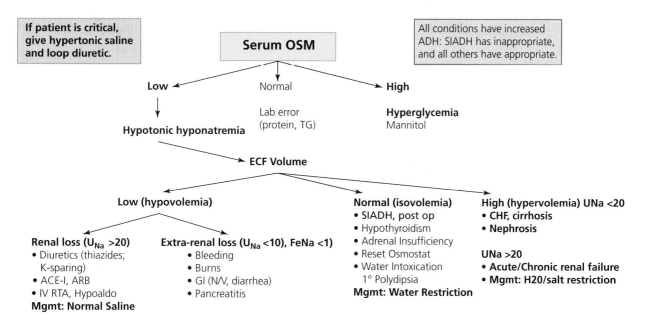

Figure 8.4 Hyponatremia

HYPERNATREMIA

Sustained hypernatremia seen when appropriate water intake not possible/impaired or impaired thirst mechanism

Etiology/Pathophysiology

- Most commonly caused by net water loss (free water loss or hypotonic fluid loss)
- Hypertonic sodium gain (iatrogenic)

Risk Factors

- Rare electrolyte disorder (eg, infants, elderly, debilitated patients)

Clinical Manifestations/Physical Exam

- Asymptomatic
- CNS dysfunction: confusion, lethargy, coma, muscle weakness, seizures

Management/Prognosis

- Hypotonic fluids:
  - Oral intake of water
  - D5W
  - 0.45% normal saline
  - 0.2% saline
- Correct ≤0.5 mEq/L/h to prevent cerebral edema

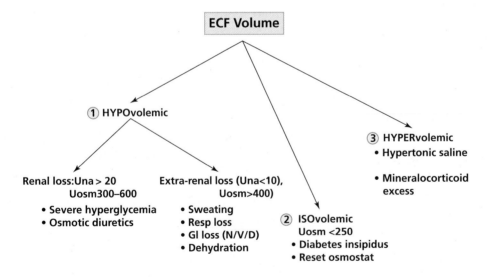

Figure 8.5 Hypernatremia

HYPOMAGNESEMIA

Low dietary intake or absorption or elevated excretion of magnesium

Etiology/Pathophysiology

- GI losses: malabsorption; alcoholism; celiac sprue; small bowel bypass; diarrhea; vomiting; laxatives
- Renal losses: diuretics (thiazide, loop); DM; renal tubular acidosis
- Medications: omeprazole, amphotericin B, cisplatin, cyclosporine, aminoglycosides

Clinical Manifestations/Physical Exam

- Neurovascular: altered mental status levels, lethargy, weakness, muscle cramps, vertigo, seizures, increased DTR, tetany
- Possible symptoms of hypocalcemia: Trousseau's/Chvostek's sign; possible symptoms of hypokalemia
- Cardiovascular: arrhythmias, palpitations

Diagnosis

- Serum magnesium <1.4 mEq/L (<0.70 mmol/L)
- Hypocalcemia and/or hypokalemia may be present
- ECG: ± prolonged QT interval, prolonged PR, QRS widening, atrial or ventricular fibrillation, ventricular tachycardia

Management/Prognosis

- IV magnesium sulfate: severe hypomagnesemia or patients with torsades de pointes
- Oral magnesium: milder cases
- Hypocalcemia and hypokalemia associated with hypomagnesemia is often refractory to correction until magnesium is repleted

When people lose too much magnesium they get <u>MAD</u> and have <u>wrist and cheek spasms</u> while yelling <u>DAMN.</u>

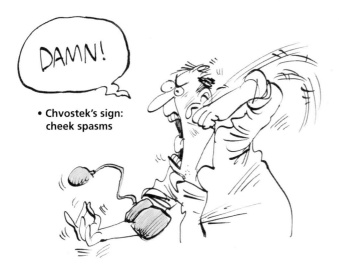

- Chvostek's sign: cheek spasms
- Trousseau's sign: wrist spasms

MAD (most common due to GI/renal losses) **=**
Malabsorption
Alcoholism
Diuretics

Signs and Symptoms: DAMN
- ↑ <u>D</u>TR
- <u>A</u>rrhythmias
- <u>M</u>ental status changes
- <u>N</u>eurovascular changes

Figure 8.6 Hypomagnesemia

HYPERMAGNESEMIA

Elevated levels of magnesium

Etiology/Pathophysiology

- Acute renal failure: iatrogenic excess IV magnesium administration (eg, in the management of asthma, eclampsia, torsades de pointes, arrhythmias); milk alkali syndrome
- Ingestion of magnesium-containing substances (eg, vitamins, antacids); lithium toxicity; adrenal sufficiency, milk alkali

Clinical Manifestations/Physical Exam

- Nausea, vomiting, skin flushing, weakness, lightheadedness, altered mental status, decreased DTR, palpitations

Diagnosis

- Serum magnesium >2.5 mEq/L
- ECG: may be similar to hypomagnesemia: prolonged QT and/or PR interval, wide QRS complex

Management/Prognosis

- IV fluids and furosemide (Lasix): enhances renal Mg excretion
- Calcium gluconate: antagonizes the toxic effects of magnesium by stabilizing the cardiac membrane if ECG changes are present
- Dialysis for severe or refractory cases

HYPERKALEMIA

Elevated levels of potassium

Etiology/Pathophysiology

- Increased renal excretion: acute or chronic renal failure (especially on dialysis), especially if coupled with increased K^+ intake (eg, bananas); hypoaldosteronism, adrenal insufficiency
- Medications: K^+ supplement, K^+ sparing diuretic, ACEI/ARB, digoxin, BB, NSAID, cyclosporine, succinylcholine
- Cell lysis: rhabdomyolysis, thrombocytosis, burns, leukocytosis
- K^+ Redistribution: metabolic acidosis (DKA), catabolic states
- Pseudohyperkalemia: venipuncture most common (lab error from hemolysis)

Clinical Manifestations/Physical Exam

- Serum levels and symptoms not consistent; rapidity in serum [K] change influences symptoms more than levels
- Neuromuscular: weakness (progressive ascending), areflexia, fatigue, paresthesias, paralysis
- Cardiovascular: palpitations, cardiac arrhythmias
- GI: abdominal distention, diarrhea, intestinal colic, nausea/vomiting

Diagnosis

- Serum potassium >5 mEq/L
- Workup may include CBC (hemolysis), creatinine kinase (rhabdomyolysis), glucose, bicarbonate
- ECG: ± tall peaked T waves lead to QR interval shortening, wide QRS, prolonged PR interval causing P wave flattening, sine wave, and arrhythmias

Management/Prognosis

- Repeat blood draw to verify not from hemolysis during venipuncture (may cause cell lysis)
- IV calcium gluconate: stabilizes the cardiac membrane used for severe symptoms, K^+ >6.5, ECG findings; given over 30–60 minutes
- Shift K^+ intracellularly: insulin (with glucose), albuterol
- Enhance K^+ excretion: sodium polystyrene sulfonate (Kayexalate), loop diuretics
- Bicarbonate: not usually given unless metabolic acidosis is also present
- Dialysis in severe cases and in some cases of renal failure

HYPOKALEMIA

Reduced levels of potassium

Etiology/Pathophysiology

- Increased urinary/GI losses most common causes include:
  - Vomiting
  - Diarrhea
  - Diuretic therapy
  - NG suction
  - Renal tubular acidosis: classic distal (Type I), proximal (II)
  - Increased mineralocorticoid activity
  - Hypomagnesemia
- Increased intracellular shifts:
  - Metabolic alkalosis
  - β2 agonists
  - Insulin
  - Chloroquine
  - Vitamin B12 treatment
  - Hypothermia
- Decreased potassium intake: (very rare unless superimposed with another cause)

Clinical Manifestations/Physical Exam

- Neuromuscular: severe muscle and weakness (including respiratory), cramps, nausea/vomiting, ileus, decreased DTR
- Nephrogenic diabetes insipidus: polyuria, rhabdomyolysis
- Myoglobinuria
- Cardiovascular: palpitations, arrhythmias

Diagnosis

- Serum potassium <3.5 mEq/L
- May also have hypomagnesemia
- ECG: T wave flattening (earliest change) leads to prominent U wave

Management/Prognosis

- Potassium replacement:
  - Oral potassium chloride (KCl) if possible
  - IV KCl given for rapid treatment/severe symptoms
  - High dose KCl given via central line
- Potassium sparing diuretics: spironolactone, amiloride
- Magnesium replacement if hypomagnesemia present (facilitates potassium repletion)
- Nondextrose IV solutions (because insulin shifts K^+ into cells)

Taking <u>diuretics</u> will cause so much <u>diarrhea, vomiting, and urination</u> that it will eventually <u>weaken and flatTen U.</u>

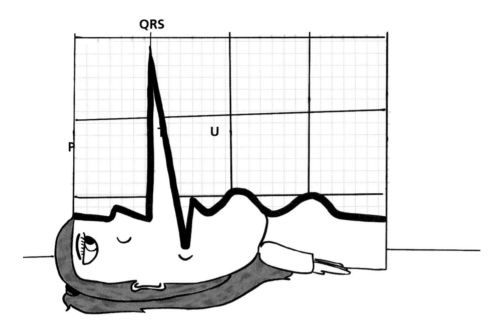

- MC due to increased urinary/GI K⁺ losses: **diarrhea, vomiting, diuretic therapy**
- **Clinical:** severe **muscle weakness, polyuria**
- **ECG: T wave flattening** → prominent **U waves**

Figure 8.7 Hypokalemia

PHIMOSIS

Foreskin (prepuce) is unable to retract over the glans; unlike paraphimosis, not a urologic emergency

- May result in pain during erection; otherwise not usually painful
- Maintain proper hygiene, stretch exercises (many spontaneously resolve).
- Topical therapy: 4–8 wks of topical corticosteroids to increase foreskin retractility
- Surgical: dorsal or ventral slits, preputioplasty, circumcision

Paraphimosis

Foreskin (prepuce) becomes trapped behind the corona of glans and cannot be reduced back to its normal anatomic position; a urologic emergency (can result in gangrene)

- Enlarged painful glans with irreducible prepuce
- Manual reduction: restore the foreskin to original position; cool compresses and/or dressing wraps to reduce the edema (usually not used if arterial compromise is suspected)
- Pharmacologic therapy: injection of hyaluronidase, granulated sugar (osmotic agent for the edema)
- Surgical: incision (dorsal slit incision) with circumcision performed at a later date

Just like **Para**chutes stay behind you when you go skydiving, in **Para**phimosis the **foreskin stays behind the corona of glans** penis due to entrapment.

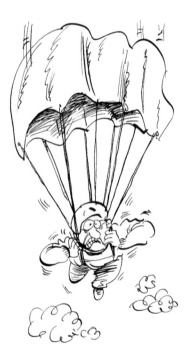

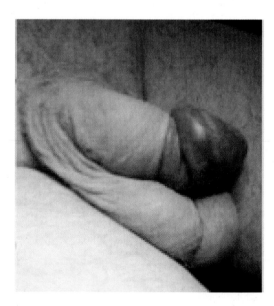

Figure 8.8 Differentiating Paraphimosis from Phimosis

ADULT POLYCYSTIC KIDNEY DISEASE

Autosomal dominant disorder due to mutations of gene PKD1 (85–90%) or PKD2 (10–15%), leading to formation of cysts primarily in the kidney and other organs (liver, spleen, pancreas)

Clinical Manifestations/Physical Exam

- Commonly age 20–40
- Flank/abdominal pain
- Hematuria, nephrolithiasis, progressive renal dysfunction
- Extrarenal: cerebral "berry" aneurysms in circle of Willis, hepatic cysts, MVP, and colonic diverticula
- HTN; palpable flank masses (often bilaterally), hepatomegaly

Diagnosis

- Renal U/S: bilateral masses
- CT scan/MRI: more sensitive than renal U/S
- Genetic testing

Management/Prognosis

- Control HTN
- ± need dialysis or renal transplant

After eating many <u>berries</u> from his <u>pouch,</u> the <u>MVP</u> developed <u>many cysts in his kidneys and liver</u>.

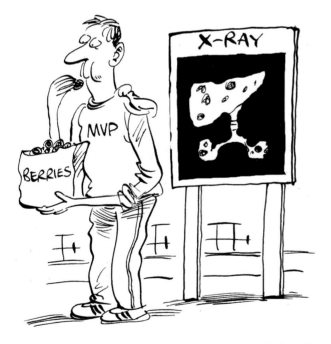

Clinical Manifestations:
- Cerebral **berry aneurysms**

- **Colonic diverticula** (outpouches)

- <u>M</u>itral <u>V</u>alve <u>P</u>rolapse

- **Hepatic and renal cysts**

Figure 8.9 Adult Polycystic Kidney Disease

NEPHROLITHIASIS AND UROLITHIASIS

Caliculi in the kidney or urinary tract, respectively

Etiology/Pathophysiology

- Calcium-containing stones: 80%; calcium oxalate (most common); calcium phosphate
  - Risk factors include decreased fluid intake, hypercalcemia, hypercalciuria, decreased urine citrate, increased oxalate absorption (eg, after bariatric surgery), increased protein and salt intake
- Uric acid: 5–8% increased acidity of the urine (eg, DM), gout (hyperuricemia)
- Cystine 1–3%: usually secondary to genetic disorders
- Struvite: (magnesium ammonium phosphate) due to urease producing organisms (eg, *Klebsiella* and *Proteus*); associated with alkaline urine pH >7.2

Clinical Manifestations/Physical Exam

- Renal colic: sudden onset of constant back/flank pain over the costovertebral angle radiating to the groin/anteriorly; patient often unable to find comfortable position
- ± hematuria, frequency, urgency, nausea, vomiting
- Physical Exam: costovertebral angle tenderness; usually afebrile

Diagnosis

- Urinalysis: hematuria (85%) either microscopic or gross, nitrites (if infection); urinary pH <5.0 (uric acid, cysteine); urinary pH >7.2 associated with calcium and struvite stones; urine strained for stone analysis
- Noncontrast CT of abdomen/pelvis: most common diagnostic test
- Renal U/S: rule out hydronephrosis and complications
- Abdominal x-ray: only calcium-containing stones can be seen on abdominal film so not as useful as other studies
- IV pyelography: done to rule out staghorn calculi

Management/Prognosis

- Stones ≤5 mm in diameter: fluids (IV or oral) 2.5–3 liters/day, analgesics (NSAIDs, opioids) and antiemetics (eg, metoclopramide), wait for spontaneous passage (most stones this size pass spontaneously); stones ≥10 mm and proximal ureter stones are unlikely to pass spontaneously
- Lithotripsy: may be used for larger stones to break them down to sizes that are more likely to pass spontaneously
- Alkalinization of the urine: used for uric acid, cystine, and oxalate stones
- Percutaneous nephrolithotomy: used for larger stones that fail other more conservative measures, struvite stones (especially staghorn calculi)
- Adjunctive medication to enhance stone passage: alpha blockers (eg, tamsulosin) which relaxes ureteral and urethral tone, facilitating stone passage; CCBs (eg, nifedipine)

Going out to the <u>CT (city)</u> after drinking <u>salty protein calcium shakes</u> instead of water makes you want to go back because of severe <u>FLANK</u> pain that makes you want to <u>CUS</u>s until you pee blood.

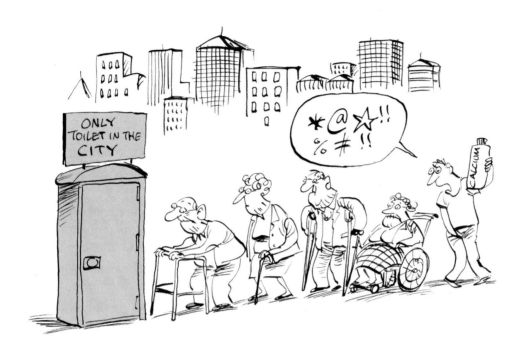

CT scan diagnostic test of choice

Risk Factors: increased salt for Ca stones Increased protein for uric acid Instead of water = **dehydration most important overall RF**

Stones Types:
Calcium oxalate (80%); calcium phosphate
Cystine
Uric acid
Struvite

Hallmarks:
- **Flank/back pain** may radiate to groin
- **CT:** costovertebral angle tenderness
- **Hematuria** (microscopic)

Management:
- **F**luids, analgesics
- **L**ithotripsy (stones >10 mm)
- **A**lpha 1a blocker (tamsulosin) to relax urethra/ureters
- **N**ephrolithotomy (stones large or refractory)
- **K**idney scope (ureteroscopy/pyeloscopy (at risk or obstructed kidneys)

Diagnosis:
Other: IVP, KUB
Ultrasound
Tomography (CT)

Figure 8.10 Nephrolithiasis (Kidney Stones)

INCONTINENCE

Stress Incontinence

Involuntary leakage of urine that occurs once increased abdominal pressure exceeds urethral pressure and resistance to urine flow

- Laxity of the pelvic floor muscles (childbirth, surgery, postmenopausal estrogen loss); post-prostatectomy in men (rare)
- Urethral hypermobility: insufficient support from the pelvic floor musculature and the vaginal connective tissue to the urethra and bladder neck
- Most common type of incontinence in younger women (mostly ages 45–49)
- Urine leakage during times of increased intra-abdominal pressure (coughing, laughing, sneezing); there is no urge to urinate prior to leakage
- Usually a clinical diagnosis
- Management: pelvic floor muscle (Kegel) exercises initial treatment of choice; Kegel supportive therapy includes supervised therapy, vaginal weighted cones or biofeedback; bladder training (eg, timed voidings), topical estrogen for postmenopausal women with vaginal atrophy
- Lifestyle modification used in conjunction with pelvic floor exercises—protective garments and pads, weight loss, smoking cessation, and drinking smaller amounts of water throughout the day
- Pessaries used if incomplete efficacy with lifestyle changes and muscle strengthening or situational stress incontinence
- Surgery midurethral sling (higher success rate than conservative therapy; more rapid/definitive treatment)
- Alpha-agonists: midodrine, pseudoephedrine (only mildly efficacious)

Overflow Incontinence

Urinary retention and incomplete bladder emptying leading to involuntary urine leakage once the bladder is full (it overflows)

- Neurological disorders/autonomic dysfunction: DM, MS, spinal injuries, spinal stenosis, peripheral neuropathy associated with B12 deficiency
- Bladder outlet obstruction: BPH, uterine fibroids, pelvic organ prolapse, overcorrection of the urethra from prior pelvic floor surgery
- Neurologic disorders or autonomic dysfunction
- Urine leakage with no warning (as in urge) or triggers (as in stress)
- Leakage or dribbling in the setting of incomplete bladder emptying
- Weak or intermittent urinary stream, hesitancy, frequency, and nocturia
- Leakage often occurs with changes in position
- Diagnosis: post-void residual >200 mL
- Management: intermittent/indwelling catheterization (first-line) for bladder atony; cholinergics eg, bethanechol to increase detrusor muscle activity; alpha-1 blockers improve urinary stream flow for BPH

Urge Incontinence

Involuntary urine leakage preceded by or accompanied by sudden urge to urinate

- Detrusor muscle overactivity: detrusor muscle is stimulated by muscarinic acetylcholine receptors; detrusor overactivity leads to uninhibited (involuntary) detrusor muscle contractions during bladder filling
- Most common in older women
- Increased urgency, frequency, small volume voids, nocturia
- Strong urge to void with an inability to make it to the bathroom in time
- Usually a clinical diagnosis
- Bladder training: 75% improvement; timed frequent voiding, using a voiding diary to identify the shortest voiding intervals, decreased fluid intake; diet: avoidance of spicy foods, citrus fruit, chocolate, alcohol, and caffeine; lifestyle modifications and Kegel exercises
- Anticholinergics: first-line medications; tolterodine, propantheline, oxybutynin (anticholinergic and antispasmodic); tricyclic antidepressants; mirabegron
- Surgery to increase bladder compliance: botulinum toxin injection, bladder augmentation

People with urge incontinence might have the urge to pee in their POT while cooking.

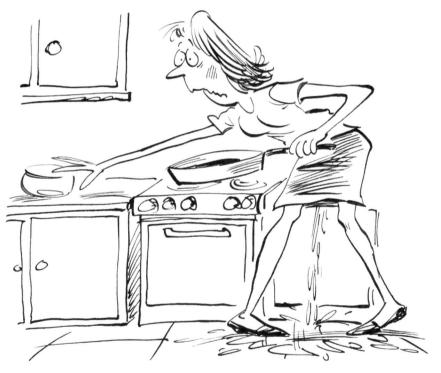

Anticholinergic drugs (first-line medications):
POT

Propantheline
Oxybutynin
Tolterodine

Figure 8.11 Urinary Incontinence

Chapter 9

Neurology

Neurology

ESSENTIAL FAMILIAL TREMOR (BENIGN)

Autosomal dominant inherited disorder of unknown etiology

Clinical Manifestations/Physical Exam

- Most commonly age 60–70
- Most common cause of action (intentional) tremor
- Postural, bilateral action (intentional) tremor
  - Commonly involves the hands, forearms, head, voice; upper extremities
  - Worsened with emotional stress and intentional movement (eg, finger-to-nose test where tremor increases as target approached)
  - Relieved with ETOH ingestion (short-term relief)
  - Not associated with a resting tremor
- No other physical or neurologic findings (except possible cogwheel phenomenon)

Management/Prognosis

- Treatment not usually warranted once secondary causes are excluded
- For severe symptoms (eg, disability): propranolol, primidone, alprazolam

The **pro auto** driver in his **prime** named **Dom** drank **alcohol** to calm down before the race but when he got closer to the **finish line, he had a tremor and crashed.**

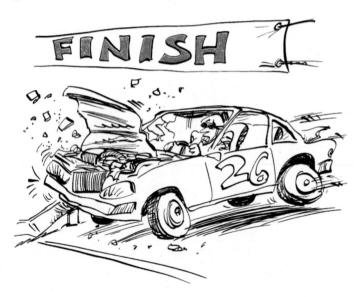

- **Autosomal dominant**

Clinical Manifestations:
- **Intentional tremor** (worse as finger gets closer to nose on exam) and **shortly relieved with alcohol**

Management:
- **Propranolol, primidone**

Figure 9.1 Essential Familial Tremor

Essential Familial Tremor (**EFT**)

- **E**TOH temporarily relieves tremor
- **F**amily history (autosomal dominant)
- **T**remor with intentional movement

PARKINSON'S DISEASE

Idiopathic dopamine depletion resulting in a failure to inhibit acetylcholine in basal ganglia

Etiology/Pathophysiology

- Characterized by cytoplasmic inclusions called Lewy bodies and loss of pigmented cells seen in the substantia nigra (which normally produces dopamine)

Risk Factors

- Most commonly age 45–65

Clinical Manifestations/Physical Exam

- Resting tremor: usually confined to one limb/one side for years before becoming generalized; often first symptom and manifests as "pill-rolling" if it involves the fingers; worse at rest/with emotional stress and better with sleep and voluntary activity/intention
- Bradykinesia: slowness of voluntary movement and decreased automatic movements: lack of swinging of arms while walking; akinesia (difficulty initiating movements); postural instability
- Rigidity: increased resistance to passive movement (flexed posture); often described as "cogwheel" in nature; festination (increasing speed while walking)
- Relatively immobile face (fixed facial expressions)
- Seborrhea of skin common; usually no muscle weakness
- Postural instability usually a late finding (stand behind patient and pull shoulders, leading patient to fall or step backward ["pull test"])
- Dementia is a late finding

Management/Prognosis

- Levodopa/carbidopa (most effective medication): increased dopamine
- Dopamine agonists: bromocriptine, pergolide, pramipexole
- Anticholinergics: benztropine, trihexyphenidyl
- Amantadine: increases of dopamine in mild disease
- MAO inhibitors (selegiline) and COMT inhibitors (entacapone)to prevent breakdown of dopamine

If you are unable to stop blinking, you cannot join the Myerson's TRIBE unless you shoot dope and rob the Benz with the MOB.

Tremors when you **Park** (at rest)

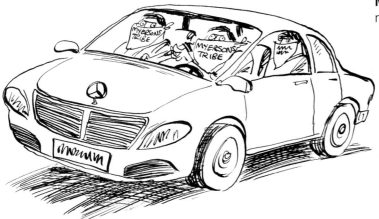

Myerson's sign: tapping the bridge of the nose repetitively causes a **sustained blink**

Treatment:
Levo**dopa**/Carbi**dopa**
Benztropine
Mao-B inhibitors

Tremor: worse at rest and with stress
Rigidity
Instability (postural)
Bradykinesia
Expression of face is fixed, leading
    to decreased blinking

Figure 9.2 Parkinson's Disease

HUNTINGTON'S DISEASE

Autosomal dominant neurodegenerative disorder

Etiology/Pathophysiology

- Trinucleotide (CAG) repeat expansion in huntingtin gene on chromosome 4p leads to neurotoxicity, especially of cerebrum, putamen, and caudate nucleus; leads to atrophy of these areas
- Symptoms usually appear age >30; often fatal within 15–20 yrs

Clinical Manifestations/Physical Exam

- Classic progression
  - **B**ehavioral changes (personality, cognitive intellectual, psychological) leads to chorea
  - **C**horea (rapid, involuntary, or arrhythmic; non-repetitive movement of face, neck, trunk, limbs initially); may have facial grimacing, ataxia leads to dementia
  - **D**ementia: executive and cognitive dysfunction
- Hypotonia, hyperreflexia, dystonia, nystagmus
- Cachexia and weight loss
- Restlessness; quick involuntary hand movements
- Fragility

Diagnosis

- CT scan shows cerebral and caudate nucleus atrophy
- Genetic testing

Management/Prognosis

- No cure (inevitable progression)
- Chorea-dominant: antidopaminergic agents (neuroleptics); benzodiazepines
- Bradykinesia and rigidity dominant: dopamine agonists

Huntington's disease will hunt down the caudate nucleus for a trophy, making you forget the A in the ABCDDs.

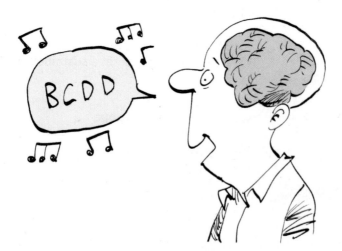

- **A**trophy of caudate nucleus
- **B**ehavioral changes
- **C**horea
- **D**ementia (late finding)
- **A**utosomal dominant

Figure 9.3 Huntington Disease

GUILLAIN-BARRÉ SYNDROME

Autoimmune condition targeting the peripheral nervous system

Etiology/Pathophysiology

- Acute/subacute inflammatory, immune-mediated demyelinating polyradiculopathy involving cranial & peripheral nerves (axonal variants may be seen)
- Often preceded by bacterial or viral infection (*Campylobacter jejuni* most common); respiratory or GI infection, CMV, EBV, immunization, surgery

Clinical Manifestations/Physical Exam

- Symmetrical ascending weakness: lower leads to upper extremity weakness
- Autonomic: tachycardia, hypotension/HTN, breathing difficulty, episodic diaphoresis, paresthesias
- Areflexia (decreased DTR), labile BP, decreased proprioception, cranial nerve palsies

Diagnosis

- CSF: high protein with normal WBCs (the high protein [>400 mg/L] often seen after 1–3 wks of symptoms)
- Nerve conduction evaluation: slow conduction velocity and reduced amplitude: conduction velocity may be preserved in axonal variant
- MRI may show enhancement with gadolinium

Management/Prognosis

- Plasmapheresis: best if within first 2 wks of symptoms (IVIG equally effective)
- Mechanical ventilation if respiratory failure occurs
- Corticosteroids are not indicated
- Most recover within 4 weeks

Rather than take <u>steroids,</u> Guillain went to <u>camp</u> where he learned to <u>SAW</u> trees and eat <u>lots of protein BARRS</u>.

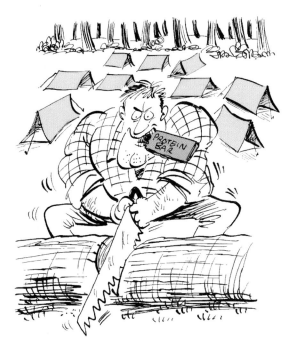

- **SAW: S**ymmetrical **A**scending **W**eakness

- Increased incidence with *Campylobacter jejuni*

- Steroids not recommended

Diagnosis:
CSF: high protein with normal WBCs

Figure 9.4 Guillain Barre Syndrome

LOWER MOTOR NEURON LESIONS

Damage to peripheral nerve cells

Etiology/Pathophysiology

- Normal physiology: lower motor neurons connect brainstem and anterior horn of spinal cord to muscle fibers; they terminate on an effector (muscle) at the neuromuscular junction and activate muscle by release of acetylcholine
- Pathophysiology: damage to the lower motor neurons leads to loss of acetylcholine release at the neuromuscular junction causing flaccid paralysis
- Etiologies: Guillain-Barré syndrome, botulism, cauda equina syndrome, poliomyelitis

Clinical Manifestations/Physical Exam

- Flaccid paralysis (hypertonia), decreased DTR
- Downward Babinski
- Fasciculations (due to end-stage muscle denervation)
- Loss of muscle tone, strength

Muscles are **FLABBY**

- **F**asciculations in advanced stage
- **F**laccid paralysis (flabby muscle)
- **L**oss of muscle tone and strength
- **A**reflexia (decreased DTR)
- **B**abinski toward the **B**asement (downward)
- **Y**oung (poliomyelitis known as infantile paralysis)

B conditions: Guillain-**B**arré Syndrome, **B**otulism, poliomyelitis (**B**aby), cauda equina Syndrome (**B**ack), **B**ell palsy

---

UPPER MOTOR NEURON LESIONS

Damage to nerve cells in the brain or spinal cord

Etiology/Pathophysiology

- Normal physiology: upper motor neurons originate in motor region of cerebral cortex or brain stem; they connect brain to appropriate level in spinal cord and also connect to lower motor neurons; the neurotransmitter glutamate transmits nerve impulse from upper motor to lower motor neurons
- Pathophysiology: damage to upper neuron causes loss of inhibitory influence of the cortex, causing spasticity
- Etiologies: stroke; MS; cerebral palsy; brain or spinal cord damage

Clinical Manifestations/Physical Exam

- Spastic paralysis (hypertonia), increased DTR
- Upward Babinski
- No fasciculations
- Little to no muscle atrophy

Muscles are **SPASTIC**

- **S**light muscle loss (no atrophy)
- **P**ositive Babinski (toe up)
- **P**osturing
- **A**bsence of fasciculations
- **S**trong tone (Spastic paralysis)
- **T**one increased (Spastic paralysis)
- **I**ncreased deep tendon reflexes
- **C**lonus

S conditions: **S**troke (CVA), multiple **S**clerosis, cerebral pal**S**y, **S**pinal cord or brain damage (eg, traumatic brain injury)

MYASTHENIA GRAVIS
Autoimmune disorder of the peripheral nerves

Etiology/Pathophysiology
- Pathophysiology: inefficient skeletal muscle neuromuscular transmission due to autoantibodies against acetylcholine (nicotinic) post synaptic receptor at the neuromuscular joints (decreased acetylcholine receptors)
- Leads to progressive weakness with repeated muscle use

Risk Factors
- Most commonly young women; associated with HLA-DR3
- 75% have thymic abnormality (hyperplasia or thymoma)

Clinical Manifestations/Physical Exam
- Ocular: extraocular muscle weakness leads to diplopia, eyelid weakness resulting in ptosis (more prominent with upward gaze); pupils usually spared
- Generalized muscle weakness: least in the morning and worsened with repeated muscle use throughout the day (relieved with rest), fluctuating; normal sensation/reflexes
  - Bulbar (aka oropharyngeal) muscle weakness (weakness with prolonged chewing, dysphagia)
  - Respiratory muscle weakness (possibly leading to respiratory failure, eg, myasthenic crisis)

Diagnosis
- Outpatient
  - Acetylcholine receptor antibodies initial test of choice.
  - Muscle specific tyrosine kinase (MuSK) antibodies
  - Electrophysiology: repetitive nerve stimulation or electromyography (most accurate test).
  - Chest CT or MRI done in all patients to detect abnormal thymus gland
- Suspected crisis
  - Edrophonium (Tensilon) test: rapid response to short-acting IV edrophonium with improvement of strength
  - Ice pack test (for ocular myasthenia gravis): improvement of ptosis after 10-min application of ice is positive

Management/Prognosis
- Long-term management with acetylcholinesterase inhibitors: pyridostigmine or neostigmine
- Myasthenic crisis: plasmapheresis or IVIG
- Thymectomy has been shown to improve disease
- Avoid exacerbating medications: fluoroquinolones, aminoglycoside, beta blockers, opioids

Without AC, <u>Thymama dug up so many graves</u> she got <u>so weak</u> and out of breath that she was unable to post up a sign to get help from <u>Edro during her crisis.</u>

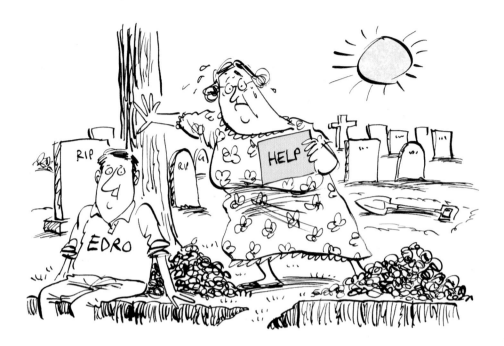

- Autoimmune disorder of the peripheral nerves

- 75% have a **thymic** abnormality (usually hyperplasia or **thymoma**)

- **Without AC = decreased Acetylcholine** due to antibodies against the **post**synaptic acetylcholine receptors
  <u>A</u>cetylcholine receptor <u>A</u>ntibody positive
  <u>C</u> "see"—ocular findings common

Weak after she dug up many graves = progressive weakness with repeated muscle use.

Figure 9.5 Myasthenia Gravis

Graves = Gravis

Respiratory failure = Myasthenia crisis

To distinguish myasthenia crisis from cholinergic crisis, administer **Edro**phonium (Tensilon).
- If **weakness resolves**, it indicates **myasthenia crisis**.
- If **weakness worsens**, it indicates **cholinergic crisis**.

MULTIPLE SCLEROSIS

Autoimmune, inflammatory demyelinating disease of the CNS; of idiopathic origin and associated with axon degeneration

Etiology/Pathophysiology

- Relapsing-remitting: episodic exacerbations (most common type)
- Progressive: decline without acute exacerbations
- Secondary progressive: relapsing-remitting that later becomes progressive

Risk Factors

- Most commonly 20–40
- Women 2x more common than men

Clinical Manifestations/Physical Exam

- Optic neuritis: unilateral eye pain worse with eye movements, diplopia, scotoma/vision loss (especially color); Marcus Gunn pupil (pupil dilation when light shined in affected eye)
- Sensory deficits: weakness, fatigue; Uhthoff's phenomenon: worsening of symptoms with heat (eg, exercise, fever, hot tubs); pain, numbness, paresthesias in a limb, muscle cramping (spasticity), trigeminal neuralgia (may be presenting symptom in young patients); Lhermitte's sign: lightning shock pain radiating from the spine down the leg with neck flexion
- Spinal cord symptoms: bladder, bowel, or sexual dysfunction; Charcot's neurologic triad: nystagmus, staccato speech, and intentional tremor; positive Babinski (upper motor neuron)

Diagnosis

- MRI with gadolinium: white matter hyperdensities (plaques); MRI is the test of choice in helping to confirm diagnosis; clinical diagnosis
- CSF analysis: increased IgG (oligoclonal bands) in CSF fluid

Management/Prognosis

- Acute exacerbations: corticosteroids (high dose), immune modulators (eg, cyclophosphamide); plasma exchange if not responsive to steroids
- Relapse-remitting/progressive disease: β-interferon or glatiramer acetate (Copaxone)—however teratogenic
- Amantadine is helpful for fatigue

Marcus and Amanda couldn't see and had extreme fatigue after getting muscle spasms while RACING UP multiple Mountain Ranges In the scorching heat during the triathlon.

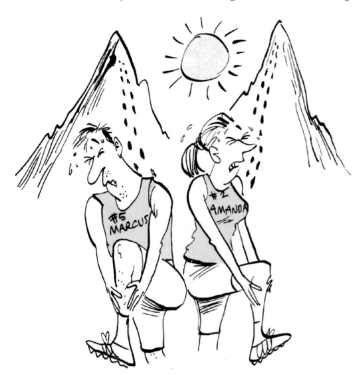

Clinical Manifestations:

- **Optic neuritis (CN II)** ocular pain worse movements, diplopia, scotomas, **vision loss**

- **Trigeminal neuralgia (CN V) may be presenting symptom (young patients)**

- **Marcus Gunn** pupil

- Uhthoff's phenomenon: **symptoms worsen with HEAT**

MRI test of choice to confirm diagnosis

- Weakness, paresthesias, **fatigue, and muscle spasms**

- **Upper** motor neuron involvement spasticity and **up**ward Babinski

Figure 9.6 Multiple Sclerosis

RACING

- **R**elief of **A**cute MS with **C**orticosteroids
- **IN**terferon (beta) and **G**latiramer for relapsing/remitting disease

Trigeminal neuralgia (CN V on Marcus' shirt) may be initial presenting symptom.

Neurology

DEMENTIA

Progressive, chronic deterioration of selective functions: memory loss and loss of impulse control, motor and cognitive functions

Alzheimer's Disease

- Most common type; loss of brain cells, amyloid deposition (senile plaques) in the brain, neurofibrillatory tangles (tau protein); cholinergic deficiency
- Short-term memory loss initially leads to long-term memory loss, language and visuospatial changes, disorientation and behavioral changes
- Diagnose with cerebral cortex atrophy on CT scan; clinical diagnosis
- Manage with ACh-esterase inhibitor (donepezil, rivastigmine, galantamine) and NMDA receptor antagonist (memantine, which slows calcium influx and nerve damage)

Vascular Disease

- Second most common type; brain disease due to chronic ischemia and multiple infarctions (eg, lacunar infarcts) seen on CT scan; increased incidence in patients with DM and HTN

Diffuse Lewy Body Disease

- Abnormal protein deposits (Lewy bodies) in nerve cells
- Visual hallucinations (visuospatial deficits), delusions
- Parkinsonism motor features with early-onset dementia

Creutzfeldt-Jakob Disease

- Spongiform encephalopathy; rapid onset of dementia due to prions producing neurotoxic beta sheets

Parkinson's Disease

- Dementia may occur later in disease

Frontotemporal Dementia (Pick's Disease)

- Localized frontotemporal brain degeneration (may progress globally)
- Marked personality changes (preserved visuospatial), aphasia initial symptom
- Dementia occurs later in disease
- Positive pick bodies (round aggregates of tau protein)

PICK couldn't get to the front of the Tau temple to take A PIC.

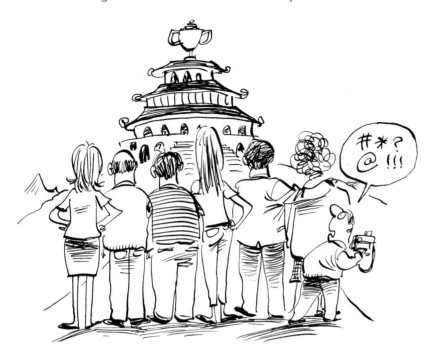

- **A**phasia and **a**trophy involving **frontotemporal** area

- **P**ersonality change seen early (a distinguishing factor from Parkinson's)

- **I**ntact visuospatial skills (a distinguishing factor from Alzheimer's, diffuse Lewy body, and Parkinson dementia)

- **C**ircular (round) intracellular aggregates of **Tau protein** (Pick bodies) (a distinguishing factor from Alzheimer's, where tau can be seen but in tangles)

Figure 9.7 Frontotemporal Dementia (Pick's Disease)

DEMENTIA:

- You must **CARE** for the elderly with Alzheimer's dementia
  - **C** = Cerebral cortex atrophy
- Treatment: acetylcholinesterase inhibitors:
  - **A**ricept (donepezil)
  - **R**azadyne (galantamine)
  - **E**xelon (rivastigmine)

Leads to **P**ersonality changes (**P**icks)

Diffuse **L**ewy Body Disease

- **L**ewy had ha**LL**ucinations/de**L**usions, and wandered off into the **Park in** the **sun** (Parkinsonism)

Neurology

CLUSTER HEADACHES

Sudden, painful headaches occurring at the same time

Etiology/Pathophysiology

- Etiology unknown but thought to be caused by activation of trigeminal-autonomic reflex via hypothalamus; leads to parasympathetic hyperactivity and sympathetic impairment

Risk Factors

- Predominantly young and middle-aged males
- Men 6x more common than women

Clinical Manifestations/Physical Exam

- Parasympathetic hyperactivity: severe unilateral periorbital or temporal pain (sharp, lancinating) headaches lasting <2 hours with spontaneous remission; bouts occur several times a day over 6–8 weeks
- Triggers: worse at night, ETOH, stress or ingestion of specific foods
- Physical exam: parasympathetic hyperactivity: ipsilateral Horner's syndrome: nasal congestion/rhinorrhea, conjunctivitis and lacrimation

Management/Prognosis

- Acute attacks
  - 100% oxygen (first-line treatment, 6–10 L) causes vasoconstriction of blood vessels
  - Anti-migraine medications: sumatriptan or dihydroergotamine
- Prophylaxis: verapamil (first-line treatment)
- Corticosteroids, ergotamine, valproic acid, lithium, methysergide

When middle-aged **men** who are not **"HORNE"** get headaches at <u>**night**</u>, <u>**100%**</u> <u>**of**</u> them will get a <u>**cluster**</u> of **sum symptoms** that are <u>**EVIL**</u> if they don't use **prophylaxis.**

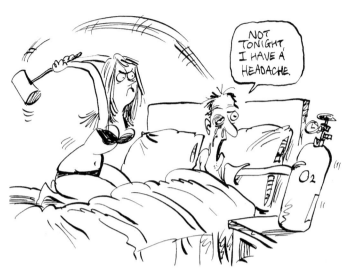

- Mostly young and middle-aged **men**

- Triggers are **worse at night** and with **ETOH**

- Ipsilateral Horner's syndrome **rhinorrhea, conjunctivitis, lacrimation, congestion**

- Acute management: **100% O$_2$**, anti-migraine med

Figure 9.8 Cluster Headache

Horner's syndrome: ipsilateral nasal congestion/rhinorrhea, conjunctivitis, lacrimation

Oxygen: **100% oxygen** first-line therapy for acute symptoms, then **sum**atriptan

Rapid headache (<2 hrs) **r**ecurrent (clusters)

Nighttime: increased incidence

Ergotamines for both acute and chronic

Conjunctivitis

Lacrimation

Unilateral

Sharp

Temporal headache

ETOH exacerbates symptoms

Rhinorrhea

Prophylaxis is EVIL

Ergotamines

Verapamil (first-line)

Indomethacin (long term use may benefit some patients)

Lithium

TOURETTE SYNDROME

Disorder marked by tics—uncontrollable, repetitive movements and vocalizations

Risk Factors

- Onset usually childhood (age 2–5) with onset of symptoms occurring age <18
- ± associated with OCD and ADHD

Clinical Manifestations/Physical Exam

- Tic-like movements of face, head, and neck
  - Motor: sudden, rapid recurrent tics (eg, blinking, shrugging, head thrusting, sniffling, jerking)
  - Verbal or phonetic: grunts, throat clearing, obscene words (coprolalia), repetitive phrases
  - Tics >1 year in duration (but may wax and wane; tic-free period usually <3 months)
  - Tics often diminish by adulthood

Management/Prognosis

- Dopamine-blocking agents: eg, haloperidol, olanzapine, risperidone, ziprasidone, tetrabenazine (presynaptic dopamine blocker)
- Alpha agonists: clonidine, guanfacine (fewer side effects compared to dopamine blocking agents)
- Behavioral habit reversal therapy

Tourette Syndrome: 3 Ts

- Motor **T**ics
- Verbal **T**ics
- Habit reversal **T**herapy

MIDDLE CEREBRAL ARTERY SYNDROMES

Conditions resulting from ischemia or infarction of the middle cerebral artery

Cerebral Blood Flow

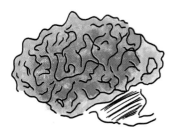

Middle cerebral artery
- Supplies 2/3 of lateral frontal of the hemisphere and temporal lobe

Anterior cerebral artery
- Supplies most of the medical surface of cerebral cortex (anterior 3/4) and anterior portions of corpus callosum

Posterior cerebral artery
- Supplies medulla, pons, cerebellum, occipital lobe, thalamus, subthalamus, midbrain, hippocampus, and medial portion of temporal lobe

- Normal physiology: right and left middle cerebral arteries arise from the internal carotid arteries into the lateral sulcus before branching into multiple areas of lateral cerebral cortex
- Left middle cerebral artery: left hemisphere is responsible for the learning/language of 95% of right-handed people and 70% of left-handed people
- Middle cerebral artery (left superficial division) is responsible for
  - Motor cortex: motor output; movement of the right head, arm, neck, and trunk
  - Sensory cortex: sensory input from the right head, arm, neck, and trunk
  - Broca's area: expressive speech (with input from other language areas)
  - Wernicke's area: receptive speech area (with input from other language areas)

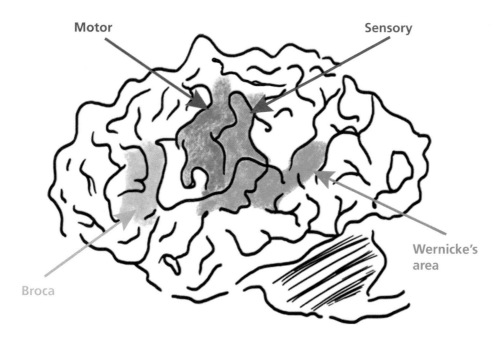

Figure 9.9 Left Middle Cerebral Artery

MIDDLE CEREBRAL ARTERY STROKE

Condition resulting from ischemia or infarction of the middle cerebral artery

Clinical Manifestations/Physical Exam

- Motor/sensory: contralateral face/arm hemiparesis (weakness), hemiplegia (paralysis); contralateral face/arm sensory loss; upper extremity involvement > lower extremity
- Visual
  - Contralateral homonymous hemianopsia (visual field loss on the same side of the vertical midline of both eyes) because the right half of the brain has visual pathways for the left hemifield of both eyes and vice versa
  - Gaze preference toward the side of the lesion (especially acutely)
- Dominant hemisphere involvement (usually left)
  - Aphasia: disorder of language
    - Broca: **o**utput problem (expressive), with understanding intact but nonfluent/hesitant/minimal speech
    - Wernicke: **i**nput problem (sensory), with severe comprehension deficits but fluent speech (especially when posterior section of superior 1st temporal gyrus is damaged)
  - Decreased math comprehension, agraphia (impaired writing ability), dysarthria (motor speech disorder)
- Nondominant hemisphere involvement (usually right)
  - Perceptual deficits: contralateral neglect syndrome: decreased awareness of left side (variable); spatial and time deficits, anosognosia: lack of awareness of the disability
  - Emotional: flat affect, impaired judgment, increased impulsivity, emotional lability

> Middle cerebral artery (MCA) is the **M**ost **C**ommon **A**rtery involved in stroke syndromes.

Neurology

MICA couldn't raise his right hand to answer the **math** question with a **graph**, so **he looked to the left** when he **couldn't express** that it **BROC** his heart and then **LEFT** out**SIDE** to **tell Wernicke,** who **couldn't understand what he was saying.**

MCA Stroke Symptoms
Motor and/or sensory deficit contralaterally (MICA can't raise his right hand)
Affects **face, upper > lower extremities**
Contralateral homonymous hemianopsia
Affected side of lesion is where the gaze goes (*he looked to the left*)

MCA on Dominant Side (Usually Left)
Motor speech disorder caused by impaired **M**ovement of the **M**uscles **(dysarthria)**
Can't calculate **math** problems (comprehension)
Agraphia (**writing** problems); **aphasia, eg, Broca** (can't express himself)
Wernicke (expressive and fluent) but doesn't always make sense (global aphasia [Paris image])

Left outside = Left side

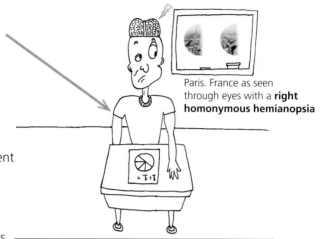

Paris. France as seen through eyes with a **right homonymous hemianopsia**

Note that **Mica can raise both eyebrows,** indicating it is a stroke; if it were CN VII palsy, raising the eyebrows wouldn't be possible

Figure 9.10 Left-Sided Middle Cerebral Artery Stroke

MICA's twin sister **ANA** couldn't raise her left hand because there was no space, so when she impulsively gazed **to the right,** she forgot to pay attention to her useless, flat, left hand.

MCA Stroke Symptoms
Motor and/or sensory deficit contralaterally (ANA can't raise her left hand)
Affects **face, upper > lower extremities**
Contralateral homonymous hemianopsia
Affected side of lesion is where the gaze goes (*she gazed to the right*)

MCA on Non-Dominant Side (Usually Right)
(MICA's **Twin Sister ANA**)
Memory Impairment
Contralateral neglect (gazed to the right side and forgot her left side)
Anosognosia (lack of insight/awareness) with increased impulsivity

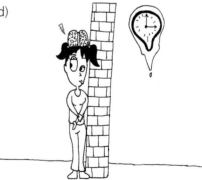

Twin **S**ister
Time and
Spatial deficits
ANA = Anosognosia

Figure 9.11 Right-Sided Middle Cerebral Artery Stroke

ANTERIOR CEREBRAL ARTERY STROKE

Condition resulting from ischemia or infarction of the ACA

Clinical Manifestations/Physical Exam

- Rare compared to MCA stroke because of the sufficient collateral circulation via the anterior communicating artery
- Supplies motor and sensory cortex of lower limb; supplemental motor area of dominant hemisphere; prefrontal cortex (involved in volition, planning, will, and organization of complex behavior)
- Motor/sensory deficits: contralateral leg/foot hemiparesis (weakness), hemiplegia (paralysis); contralateral leg/foot sensory loss
  - Lower extremity involvement (including the perineum and pelvic floor muscles) > upper
  - Facial and hand sparing: speech usually preserved (unless involving the prefrontal cortex and supplemental motor areas)
- Frontal lobe deficits:
  - Emotional: impaired judgment, confusion, personality changes (flat affect)
  - Reflexes: contralateral grasp, sucking reflex (medial surface of posterior frontal lobe)
- Urinary incontinence (sensorimotor section of paracentral lobule)
- Gait apraxia: loss of ability to have normal function of lower limbs (not due to loss of motor or sensory function)
- Abulia: lack of will with diminished motivation (medial inferior section of parietal, frontal, and temporal lobes, cingulate gyrus)

After **A BULL** stepped on a **FIRE ANT**, he **couldn't find the will to walk** to the **opposite side** of the **gate** so he **P'eed** on himself and said the **F word!**

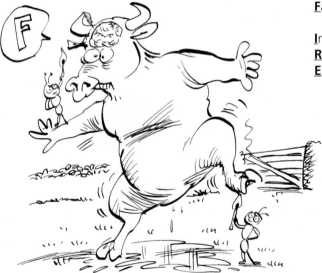

Face (speech) usually preserved, frontal lobe impairment, flat affect
Incontinence (urinary)
Reflex (grasp, sucking)
Emotional and personality changes

Abulia (A BULL): lack of will
Not on same side (contralateral weakness)
Toward side of the lesion (gaze)

Figure 9.12 Anterior Cerebral Artery Stroke

Gait ataxia: lower > upper involvement

P'eed: marked **P**ersonality changes and urinary incontinence, **p**aratonic rigidity

ANT: anterior

Gate: gait ataxia

Opposite side: contralateral weakness/sensory loss

POSTERIOR CEREBRAL ARTERY STROKE

Condition resulting from ischemia or infarction of the PCA

Clinical Manifestations/Physical Exam

- Posterior cerebellar artery (huge variety and combination of symptoms)
  - Larger infarcts (involving internal capsule and thalamus): contralateral hemisensory loss or hemiparesis
  - **P1 syndrome: thalamic, subthalamic, and midbrain signs**
    - CN III (oculomotor) palsy: diplopia (unable to focus), eye in outward and downward position (decreased ability to move eye inward or up), ptosis (malpositioning of the upper eyelid), enlarged pupil (unable to constrict the pupil)
    - Claude's syndrome: CN III palsy and contralateral ataxia (red nucleus involvement)
    - Weber's syndrome: CN III palsy and contralateral hemiplegia (cerebral peduncle)
    - Thalamic syndrome: contralateral hemisensory loss with subsequent burning pain in the areas associated with the loss (due to sensory impairment)
    - Subthalamus: contralateral hemiballismus
  - **P2 syndrome: medial temporal and occipital lobe involvement**
    - Occipital: contralateral homonymous hemianopsia with macular sparing
    - Medial temporal lobe: memory deficits ($\pm$ temporary)
    - Visual hallucinations
    - Dominant hemisphere involvement: alexia without agraphia
    - Anton syndrome: cortical blindness with patient unaware (bilateral occlusion in distal PCAs)
- Posterior inferior cerebellar artery
  - Vertigo, nystagmus, ataxia, dysphonia, dysarthria
  - Ipsilateral facial deficits, contralateral extremity deficits
- Vertebrobasilar artery
  - Can present with findings of a PCA or PICA
  - Crossed symptoms: ipsilateral cranial nerve deficits with contralateral sensory deficits
  - Syncope, diplopia, ataxia, nausea, vomiting, nystagmus, dysphagia, hiccups, coma

INTRACRANIAL HEMORRHAGE

Various forms of bleeding occurring within the skull

Epidural Hematoma

- Bleeding in the tough outer membrane covering the brain (dura mater) and the skull
- Most commonly due to rupture of the middle meningeal artery often associated with a temporal bone fracture; may lead to hemorrhagic stroke and brain herniation
- Risk factors: head trauma
- Three classic phases: (1) brief loss of consciousness, (2) followed by a lucid interval (patient regains consciousness and seems fine) and subsequent neurologic deterioration, (3) mental status changes to coma as a result of increased intracranial pressure; during the deterioration phase, headache, vomiting, aphasia, hemiparesis, and seizure may occur
- Uncal herniation: CN III palsy–dilated "blown" pupil can be seen on ipsilateral side of injury (tentorial herniation compressing CN III); Cushing reflex: triad of HTN, bradycardia with respiratory irregularity
- Diagnose with head CT without contrast (initial test of choice): convex (lens-shaped) hyperdensity usually in the temporal area that does not cross suture lines
- In most cases, hematoma evacuation or craniotomy is the treatment of choice to prevent irreversible brain injury and death; may be observed closely with serial imaging if small and the patient is in good condition

Shooting <u>Epi</u> through the <u>skull temp</u>orarily constricts the lens of the eye and the <u>middle meningeal artery</u> (MMA).

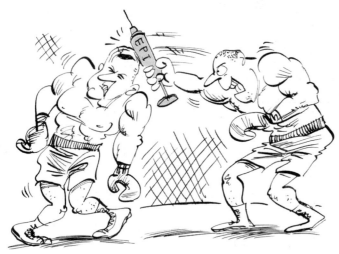

- **Arterial** bleed (MMA most common)

- Often post-skull fracture, especially temporal bone

- **Diagnosis:** head CT will show **convex (lens**-shaped) bleed that **does not cross suture line**, usually in **temp**oral area (constricts = does not cross suture line)

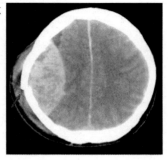

Figure 9.13 Epidural Hemorrhage (CT scan)

Subdural Hematoma

- Bleeding between the dura and arachnoid membranes
- Most commonly due to rupture of the cortical bridging veins after blunt trauma
- Because the bleeding is venous, can develop over a longer period compared to epidural hematoma
- Risk factors: elderly age; alcoholism (brain atrophy puts tension on bridging veins); anticoagulant use; shaken baby syndrome (child abuse)
- Clinical manifestations vary but usually a gradual increase in generalized neurologic symptoms (eg, headache, dizziness, nausea, vomiting) or focal neurologic symptoms
- Head CT without contrast will show concave (crescent-shaped) bleed that may cross suture lines (if severe, midline shift may occur as a result of increased intracranial pressure); CT scan may be negative immediately post-injury so serial imaging may be needed)
- Nonoperative management: if clinically stable with a small hematoma or no CT signs of brain herniation (eg, midline shift <5 mm) or increased intracranial pressure
- Surgical management: surgical evacuation may be indicated if ≥5 mm midline shift or severe; options include: burr hole trephination, craniotomy and decompressive craniectomy

Venus drove across the bridge and into the tunnel cave on the other side to catch the subway.

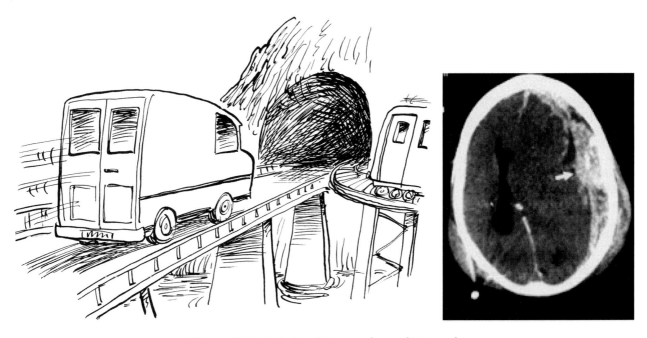

Figure 9.14 Subdural Hemorrhage (CT scan)

- **Venous** bleed most common between dura and arachnoid due to tearing of **bridging veins**
- Most common due to blunt trauma
- May cause bleeding **on other side (contre-coup)**
- Diagnosis: CT head con**cave** (crescent-shaped bleed)
- **Can cross suture lines**

Subarachnoid Hemorrhage

Bleeding between the arachnoid membranes and pia mater

- Most commonly due to a ruptured berry aneurysm at the anterior communicating artery (circle of Willis); AVM stroke or trauma
- Risk factors: PCOS, atherosclerotic disease, smoking, excessive alcohol intake, Ehlers-Danlos, and Marfan syndrome
- Clinical manifestions include sudden, intense thunderclap headache often unilateral in occipital area; often described as "worst headache of my life"; may be associated with delirium, seizures, nausea/vomiting; meningeal symptoms (photophobia, neck stiffness, fever)
  - May have initial loss of consciousness
  - Possible meningeal signs: nuchal rigidity, positive Brudzinski and Kernig signs
  - Not usually associated with focal neurologic deficits, Terson syndrome, retinal hemorrhage, or CN III palsy
- Head CT without contrast (initial test of choice) will show subarachnoid bleeding
  - Lumbar puncture performed if CT is negative and no papilledema or focal signs: xanthochromia (yellow to pink color of CSF fluid due to breakdown of RBCs in CSF; increased CSF protein from bilirubin; increased CSF pressure)
  - Four-vessel angiography usually performed after confirmed SAH to identify source of bleeding and other aneurysms
- Manage with bed rest, stool softeners, lower intracranial pressure; nimodipine to cerebral vasospasms, improving neurologic outcomes
  - Endovascular coiling or surgical clipping of aneurysm or AVM used to prevent rebleeding (coiling often preferred over clipping)
  - Lowering BP may decrease the risk of rebleeding but may also increase the risk of infarction; if needed, labetalol, nicardipine, and enalapril are preferred antihypertensives
  - Ventriculostomy may be needed if SAH is associated with hydrocephalus

During the <u>thunderstorm, Avum</u> had a <u>severe headache and stiff neck</u> after she vomited <u>UP yellow blood</u>.

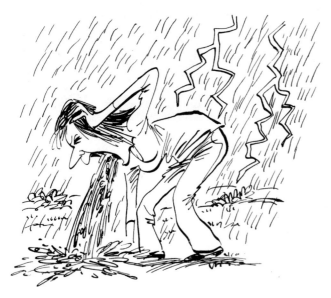

- Most common due to **AVM/aneurysm**

- **Thunderclap severe headache (worst headache of my life) and stiff neck**

- CT first; if negative, must do lumbar puncture

- On lumbar puncture, look for **Xanthochromia yellow CSF fluid due to blood (RBCs) and Increased** CSF pressure

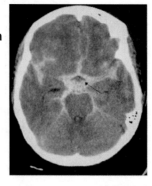

Figure 9.15 Subarachnoid Hemorrhage (CT scan)

Intracerebral Hemorrhage

Bleeding within the brain parenchyma; may compress the brain, ventricles, and sulci

- Etiologies:
  - HTN most common overall cause of spontaneous ICH
  - Cerebral amyloid angiopathy most common cause of nontraumatic ICH in the elderly, but AVM most common cause in children
- HTN most important risk factor; AVM; amyloidosis; trauma; older age; high alcohol intake; and coagulopathy
- Neurologic symptoms usually increase gradually (minutes to hours): headache, nausea/vomiting, syncope, focal neurologic symptoms (hemiplegia, hemiparesis, seizures), altered mental status (lethargy, obtundation, etc.); not usually associated with a lucid interval; CN III palsy; possible focal motor and sensory deficits
- Head CT without contrast will show parenchymal bleeding
- Supportive management: gradually reduce BP; reduce intracranial pressure (raise head 30° off bed, limit IV fluids, manage BP, analgesia, and sedation); IV mannitol, temporary hyperventilation
  - BP reduction: IV labetalol, nicardipine, esmolol, hydralazine, nitroprusside, and nitroglycerin
  - Aggressive reduction only if systolic BP >200 mm Hg or mean arterial pressure >150 mm Hg

Neurology

BACTERIAL MENINGITIS

Life-threatening infection of the meninges

Etiology/Pathophysiology

- Neonates: Group B Streptococcus (most common), *E. coli, L. monocytogenes, S. pneumoniae*
- Children age 1 month–18 years: *N. meningitidis, S. pneumoniae, Haemophilus influenza*
- Age 18–50: *Streptococcus pneumoniae* (most common), *N. meningitidis, H. influenzae, L. monocytogenes*, gram-negative rods
- Age >50: *S. pneumoniae, L. monocytogenes* (increased risk), gram-negative rods

Clinical Manifestations/Physical Exam

- Fever, photophobia, headache, altered mental status, seizures
- Neck stiffness (meningismus)
- Positive Kernig and Brudzinski signs

Diagnosis

- Blood cultures, CBC
- CSF: **increased WBCs, markedly decreased glucose, and elevated protein** (the bacteria need to eat and bulk up on their protein in order to live, so they will eat up the glucose and increase their protein)
- Lumbar puncture: do CT scan first to rule out mass (contraindicated with papilledema or focal neurological deficits)

	Bacterial Meningitis	Viral Meningitis	TB/Fungal Meningitis
Protein	Increased	Normal to increased	Increased
Glucose	Decreased	Normal	Decreased
Cells	Increased neutrophils	Increased lymphocytes	Increased lymphocytes
Pressure	Increased	Normal	Increased

Management/Prognosis

- Antibiotics
  - Neonates: ampicillin + cefotaxime (may add gentamicin for synergy)
  - Empiric treatment age 3 mos–50 yrs: vancomycin + ceftriaxone (or cefotaxime)
  - Empiric treatment age >50 yrs: vancomycin + ceftriaxone + ampicillin (added for *Listeria monocytogenes*)
- Dexamethasone: shown to reduce mortality and sequelae of *S. pneumoniae, H. influenzae,* and *N. meningitidis* in adults; also recommended in children if *H. influenzae* type B is suspected (reduces incidence of CN VIII-related hearing loss)
- Seizures: benzodiazepines, phenytoin
- Cerebral edema: IV mannitol
- Prophylaxis for close contacts: rifampin, ciprofloxacin

Bacterial Meningitis

Treatment: age <1 month and >50 yrs

- You must turn on the **AC** for **infants** and the **elderly** with fevers and disinfect with **Listerine**
- **A**mpicillin and **C**efotaxime/**c**eftriaxone
- Increased risk for *Listeria monocytogenes*

Treatment: all others

- You must submit your **CV** in order to be treated for meningitis
- **C**eftriaxone and **V**ancomycin

- In bacterial meningitis, the CSF will show **increased WBCs**: the bacteria need to eat and bulk up on their protein in order to live, so they will eat the glucose and increase their protein.
- Therefore, **CSF glucose will be markedly decreased and protein will be elevated.**

INCOMPLETE SPINAL CORD INJURY

Spinal cord injury in which there is some retention of sensory or motor ability below the point of injury

Anterior Cord Syndrome

- Motor deficit: lower extremity > upper extremity (corticospinal)
- Sensory deficit: pain, temperature (spinothalamic tract), light touch
- Possible bladder dysfunction (retention, incontinence)
- Preservation of proprioception, vibration, pressure (dorsal column spared)

Central Cord Syndrome

- Motor deficit: upper extremity > lower extremity; distal portion of the upper extremity more severe involvement (eg, hands) from corticospinal involvement
- Sensory deficit: pain, temperature (spinothalamic tract) deficit in upper extremity > lower extremity (a "shawl" distribution)
- Preservation of proprioception, vibration

> **CENT**
>
> - **C**audal (upper > lower)
> - **E**xtension injuries, **e**lderly after a fall (common mechanisms)
> - **N**umb to pain
> - **T**emperature

Brown Sequard Syndrome

- Rare; may be seen with penetrating trauma
- Ipsilateral deficit: motor (lateral corticospinal tract); vibration and proprioception (dorsal column)
- Contralateral deficit: pain and temperature (lateral spinothalamic tract) usually 2 levels below the injury (where spinothalamic tract crosses at spinal cord level)

Posterior Cord Syndrome

- Very rare; loss of proprioception and vibration only
- Spares both temperature and pain

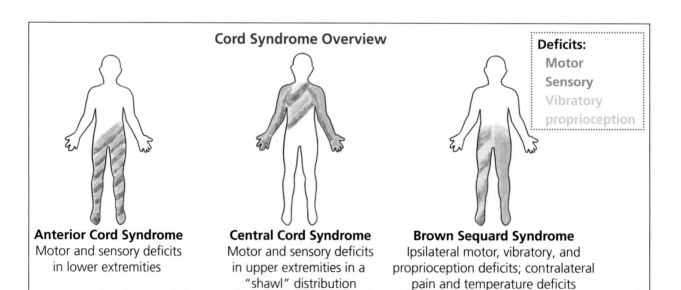

Cord Syndrome Overview

Deficits:
Motor
Sensory
Vibratory
proprioception

Anterior Cord Syndrome
Motor and sensory deficits in lower extremities

Central Cord Syndrome
Motor and sensory deficits in upper extremities in a "shawl" distribution

Brown Sequard Syndrome
Ipsilateral motor, vibratory, and proprioception deficits; contralateral pain and temperature deficits

Because ANT couldn't walk to the bathroom in the TeePee, he peed in his pants when his bladder busted into flecks.

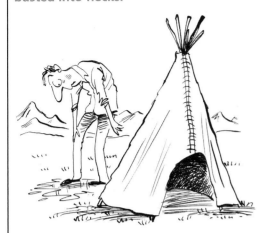

- **Couldn't walk: lower extremity motor deficit**

- **TeePee:** loss of **T**emperature and **P**ain sensation

- **Peed in his pants:** bladder dysfunction, lower extremity involvement

- **Flex:** flexion compression injury (common mechanism)

Figure 9.16 Anterior Cord Syndrome (ACS)

Because Malefi**cent** developed frostbite when she **extend**ed her hand to touch the cold window pane, she couldn't put on her **shawl** with her **weak hands**.

- **Extension** injuries

- Loss of pain and temperature sensation

- **Upper extremity** > **lower** (esp. hands)

- **Shawl distribution**

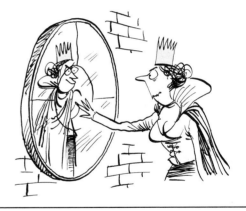

Figure 9.17 Central Cord Syndrome

The MVP on the winning side was oblivious 2(to) the stabbing heat of the pain of defeat from the losing side.

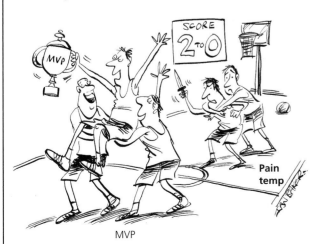

Ipsilateral Deficits:
- **M**otor, **V**ibratory, and **P**roprioception deficits

Contralateral Deficits:
- **Pain and temperature deficits, usually seen 2 levels below level of injury**

Mechanism:
Stabbing: penetration injuries

Figure 9.18 Brown-Sequard Syndrome

Canadian Head CT Rules

CANADA IS Anti Skull Fractures!

- **C**oma scale (<15 points 2 hours after head injury)
- **A**ny sign of basilar skull fracture (raccoon eyes, battle sign)
- **N**eurologic deficits
- **A**ge (>65)
- **D**angerous mechanism of injury
- **A**mnesia

- **I**ncreased vomiting
- **S**eizures

- **Anti**coagulant use
- **Skull Fractures**: suspected open/depressed

Chapter 10

Dermatology

ATOPIC DERMATITIS (ECZEMA)

Chronic, inflammatory pruritic skin condition

Etiology/Pathophysiology

- Closely related to other atopic diseases (**atopic triad: asthma, allergic rhinitis, eczema**)
- Triggers: heat, perspiration, allergens, contact irritants (eg, wool, nickel, foods)
- Associated with increased IgE and altered immune reaction
- Types: eczema, contact dermatitis

Risk Factors

- Often starts in childhood

Clinical Manifestations/Physical Exam

- Pruritus is a hallmark, "itch-scratch cycle"
  - Acute lesions: tiny erythematous, edematous blisters (ill-defined); later, dries/crusts over and scales (looks similar to psoriasis); most common in flexor creases (eg, antecubital and popliteal folds)
  - Nummular eczema: sharply defined coin-shaped lesions especially on dorsal hand, feet, extensor surfaces (knees, elbows)

Management/Prognosis

- Acute management
  - High-strength topical corticosteroids first-line therapy; antihistamines for itching; wet dressings (eg, Burrow's solution); antibiotics if secondary infection develops
  - Topical calcineurin inhibitors (eg, tacrolimus, pimecrolimus) are alternatives to steroids (they do not cause skin atrophy).
  - Systemic treatment: phototherapy (UVA, UVB and narrow-band UVB), cyclosporine, azathioprine, mycophenolate mofetil, methotrexate, dupilumab
- Chronic management
  - Daily hydration and emollients; oral antihistamines for pruritus
  - Avoid exacerbating factors/irritants (soap, detergent, frequent baths) and maintain skin hydration (skin emollient 2x daily and within 3 min after a lukewarm shower/bath)

LICHEN PLANUS

Inflammatory condition that develops on flexor surfaces of extremities, mucous membranes on skin, mouth, scalp, genitals, and nails

Etiology/Pathophysiology

- Cell-mediated immune response of idiopathic origin
- Increased incidence with hepatitis C, drug reactions, graft vs host and malignant lymphoma; adults > children and women > men

Clinical Manifestations/Physical Exam

- Skin rash
  - Pruritic rash most common on the extremities, especially the volar surfaces of wrist and ankles; may involve the mouth, scalp, genitals, nails, and mucous membranes
  - 5 Ps: purple, polygonal, planar, pruritic papules/plaques
  - Fine scales and irregular borders with possible Wickham striae (fine white lines on skin lesions or oral mucosa)
  - Koebner's phenomenon (new lesions at sites of trauma)
- Nail dystrophy
- Scarring alopecia

Management/Prognosis

- Topical corticosteroids first-line with occlusive dressings; antihistamines for pruritus
- Second-line: PO or intralesional corticosteroids, topical tretinoin, or photosensitizing psoralen and ultraviolet light therapy (generalized eruptions)
- Rash usually resolves spontaneously in 8–12 mos

> Wickham the snake caught hepatitis C and developed a purple, polygonal, pruritic, planar rash on his scales.

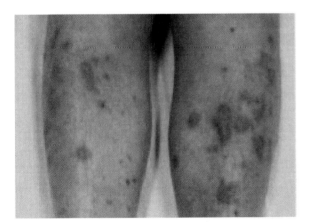

Figure 10.1 Lichen Planus

PITYRIASIS ROSEA

Idiopathic, self-limiting skin outbreak

Etiology

- Uncertain etiology; may be associated with viral infections (eg, human herpesvirus 6 or 7)

Risk Factors

- Increased incidence in spring/fall
- Commonly older children/young adults

Clinical Manifestations/Physical Exam

- Early: herald patch (solitary salmon-colored macule) on trunk (2–6 cm diameter) leads to general exanthem 1–2 weeks later
- Later: smaller, very pruritic 1 cm round or oval salmon-colored papules with white circular (collarette) scaling in a Christmas tree pattern (oriented along skin cleavage lines); confined to trunk and proximal extremities (face usually spared); may be preceded by a viral prodrome

Diagnosis

- Primary a clinical diagnosis
- Can mimic syphilis so do RPR if patient is sexually active

Management/Prognosis

- No treatment needed for most
- If pruritis present, educate, reassure, and treat: oral antihistamines; topical corticosteroids; oatmeal baths; lotion for scaling; UVB phototherapy if severe (start week 1 of eruption); oral acyclovir or erythromycin may speed up healing but not routinely used

> **Rosea** developed an itchy rash in **Herald** square after touching a **Christmas tree** so her boyfriend had **pity** and took her out to eat a **salmon** dinner.

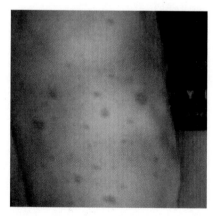

Figure 10.2 Pityriasis (Tinea) Versicolor)

PSORIASIS

Chronic, multisystemic, inflammatory immune disorder

Etiology/Pathophysiology

- Keratin hyperplasia (proliferating cells in the *stratum basale* and *stratum spinosum* due to T-cell activation)

Clinical Manifestations/Physical Exam

- **Plaque psoriasis** (most common): raised, dark-red plaques/papules with thick silver/white scales most common on extensor surfaces, scalp
    - Nail pitting (25%); yellow-brown discoloration under nailbed (oil spot) pathognomonic
    - Auspitz's sign: punctuate bleeding with removal of plaque
    - Koebner's phenomenon: skin lesions at lines of trauma
- **Pustular psoriasis**: deep, sterile yellow pustules evolve into red macules on palms/soles
- **Guttate psoriasis**: small, erythematous papules with fine scales; discrete lesions and confluent plaques; often appears after streptococcal pharyngitis
- **Inverse psoriasis**: lacks scale; erythrodermic—generalized, involving most of the skin (worst type)
- **Psoriatic arthritis**: inflammatory arthritis (10% of those with psoriasis and higher in those with HLA-B27 positivity); patients with stiffness >30 min and relieved with activity; swelling of an entire finger or toe ("sausage digits"); x-ray shows "pencil in cup" deformities

Management/Prognosis

- Topical: corticosteroids (high strength), tar-based, anthralin; vitamin D analogs (calcipotriene) and retinoids (vitamin A analogs)
- UVB light therapy; immune agents: methotrexate, cyclosporine A, alefacept

Koebner placed **thick, silver-white** blocks on a scale **To sell** to **Auspitz**, and they were so heavy that they caused **pitting of her nails**.

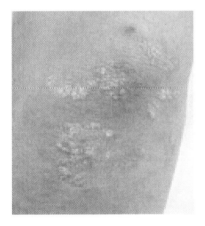

Figure 10.3 Psoriasis

Psoriasis
- Thick silver/white scales
- Koebner
- T cells
- Auspitz's sign
- Nail pitting

Dermatology

PITYRIASIS (TINEA) VERSICOLOR

Overgrowth of the yeast *Malassezia furfur* (formerly called *Pityrosporum ovale*) that is part of the normal skin flora

Clinical Manifestations/Physical Exam

- Well-demarcated round/oval macules with fine scaling may be hyper/hypopigmented
- Often associated with pruritus
- Affected skin does not tan with sun exposure

Diagnosis

- Primarily a clinical diagnosis
  - Potassium hydroxide preparation: short, hyphae "spaghetti and meatball" appearance of the scales
  - Wood's lamp: yellow-green fluorescence (enhanced color variation)

Management/Prognosis

- Topical: selenium sulfide shampoo; sodium sulfacetamide; zinc pyrithione; *"azoles"*
- Systemic therapy: itraconazole in adults if widespread or if topical treatment failed; ketoconazole can be used but associated with hepatotoxicity (patients must not shower for 8–12 hrs post oral intake because it is delivered to skin via sweat)

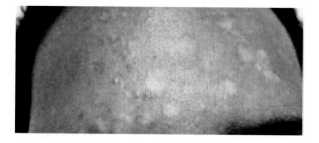

Figure 10.4 Pityriasis (Tinea) Versicolor

SEBORRHEIC DERMATITIS

Hypersensitivity to the fungus *Malassezia furfur* (formerly called *Pityrosporum ovale*) that is part of the normal skin flora

Etiology/Pathophysiology

- Etiology not clearly defined
- Occurs in areas of high sebaceous gland oversecretion (scalp, face, eyebrows, body folds)

Risk Factors

- Neonatal; adult men
- Immunocompromised state (eg, AIDS)
- Parkinson's disease

Clinical Manifestations/Physical Exam

- Infants: "cradle cap": erythematous plaques with fine white scales
- Adults: erythematous plaques with fine white scales common in scalp (dandruff), eyelids, beard mustache, nasolabial folds, trunk (chest), intertriginous regions of the groin

Management/Prognosis

- Topical: selenium sulfide, sodium sulfacetamide, ketoconazole (shampoo or cream), topical corticosteroids; zinc pyrithione
- Systemic: corticosteroids for severe disease

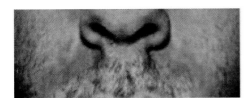

Figure 10.5 Seborrheic Dermatitis

ERYTHEMA MULTIFORME

Acute self-limiting type IV hypersensitivity reaction

Risk Factors

- Most commonly age 20–40
- Infections: HSV (most common), *Mycoplasma* (especially in children), *S. pneumoniae*
- Medications: sulfa drugs, beta-lactams, phenytoin, phenobarbital
- Malignancies, autoimmune

Clinical Manifestations/Physical Exam

- Skin lesions usually evolve over 3–5 days and last approximately 2 weeks
- Target (iris) lesions: pathognomonic (dull "dusty-violet" red, purpuric macule/vesicle or bullae in center surrounded by pale edematous rim and peripheral red halo); often febrile
    - **EM minor:** target lesions distributed acrally; no mucosal membrane lesions
    - **EM major:** target lesions with involvement of ≥1 mucous membrane(s) (oral, genital, ocular mucosa); <10% body surface area acrally end up centrally; no epidermal detachment

Management/Prognosis

- Symptomatic: discontinue drug causing rash, antihistamines, analgesics, skin care
- For oral lesions: steroid/lidocaine/diphenhydramine mouthwash

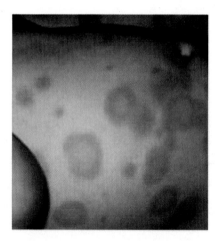

Figure 10.6 Erythema Multiforme

STEVENS-JOHNSON SYNDROME AND TOXIC EPIDERMAL NECROLYSIS

Life-threatening skin conditions associated with peeling skin, sores, and blisters

Risk Factors

- Most commonly after drug eruptions (especially sulfa and anticonvulsants) and infections (mycoplasma, HIV, HSV, malignancy, idiopathic)

Clinical Manifestations/Physical Exam

- Fever and URI symptoms lead to widespread blisters (begin on trunk/face), erythematous/pruritic macules ≥1 mucous membrane with epidermal detachment
- Sloughing <10% body surface area suggests **SJS**
- Sloughing >30% body surface area suggests **TEN**
- Positive Nikolsky sign seen in both (sloughing of epidermis with gentle pressure)

Diagnosis

- Based on clinical history and symptoms
- Skin biopsy may distinguish staphylococcal scalded skin syndrome from TEN

Management/Prognosis

- Treat like severe burns (admit to burn unit)

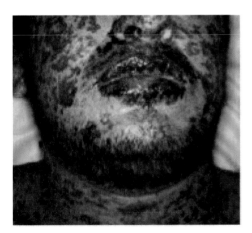

Figure 10.7 Toxic Epidermal Necrolysis

Dermatology

ROSACEA

Persistent vasomotor instability with lesion formation (adult acne)

Etiology/Pathophysiology

- Unclear etiology

Risk Factors

- Alcohol; temperature: hot drinks, hot/cold weather, hot baths, spicy foods, emotional stress

Clinical Manifestations/Physical Exam

- Acneiform lesion with erythema, facial flushing, telangiectasia, skin coarsening, papulopustules with burning, stinging
- Red eyes
- Absence of comedones (blackheads) in rosacea distinguishes it from acne

Management/Prognosis

- Topical metronidazole first-line; azelaic acid, ivermectin cream. sulfacetamide, anti-acne topical antibiotics
- Moderate–severe: oral antibiotics (eg, tetracyclines); laser therapy; oral isotretinoin for refractory cases
- Facial erythema: topical brimonidine, laser or intense pulsed light
- Lifestyle modification: sunscreen, avoid toners/astringents, menthol/camphor, triggers

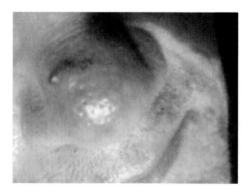

Figure 10.8 Rosacea

After **eating hot and spicy food and drinking alcohol, Rosacea** had a **burning stinging rash on her face** and had to run and take the **metro.**

ACTINIC KERATOSIS

Premalignant condition to SCC (most common premalignant skin condition)

Etiology/Pathophysiology

- Proliferation of atypical epidermal keratinocytes

Risk Factors

- Lighter skin, increasing age, prolonged sun exposure
- Male gender

Clinical Manifestations/Physical Exam

- **Dry, rough, scaly macules/papules that feel like "sandpaper" with transparent or yellow scaling**
- May be **erythematous** or **hyperkeratotic (hyperpigmented) plaques**
- May have a projection on the skin (cutaneous horn)

Diagnosis

- Clinical diagnosis based on inspection and palpation
- Punch or shave biopsy to distinguish actinic keratosis from SCC; classic findings include atypical epidermal keratinocytes and cells with large hyperchromatic pleomorphic nuclei from the basal layer upward (no invasion into dermis)
- Consider biopsy for lesions >1 cm in diameter, indurated, ulcerated, rapidly growing, or that fail to respond to appropriate therapy

Management/Prognosis

- Surgical: liquid nitrogen cryotherapy (most common); dermabrasion; electrodesiccation; curettage
- Medical (most commonly used if multiple lesions): topical 5-fluorouracil, imiquimod
- Observation is an option for low-risk patients

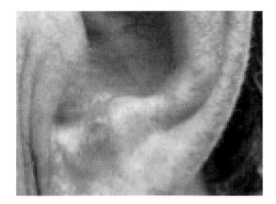

Figure 10.9 Actinic Keratosis

SEBORRHEIC KERATOSIS

Most common benign epidermal skin tumor

Etiology/Pathophysiology

- Benign proliferation of immature keratinocytes

Risk Factors

- Most common in fair-skinned elderly patients who have had prolonged sun exposure

Clinical Manifestations/Physical Exam

- Well-demarcated round/oval velvety warty lesions with a greasy or "stuck on" appearance; color varies (flesh-colored, grey, brown, black)

Diagnosis

- Usually a clinical diagnosis
- Biopsy if diagnosis is uncertain; biopsy reveals well-demarcated proliferation of keratinocytes with characteristic small keratin-filled cysts

Management/Prognosis

- **No treatment needed (benign)**
- Cosmetic or symptomatic management includes cryotherapy (most common treatment); curettage; electrodessication; laser therapy

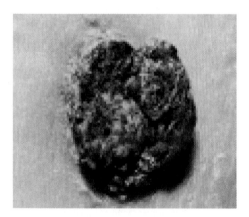

Figure 10.10 Seborrheic Keratosis

SQUAMOUS CELL CARCINOMA

Second most common skin cancer

Etiology/Pathophysiology

- Malignancy of keratinocytes that invade the dermis or beyond characterized by hyperkeratosis & ulceration.
- **Bowen's disease = SCC in situ** (has not invaded the dermis)

Risk Factors

- Sun exposure major risk factor (often preceded by actinic keratosis)
- HPV infection
- Lighter-skin, xeroderma pigmentosum
- Chronic wounds, old scars, burns
- Chronic immunosuppression (eg, post transplant).

Clinical Manifestations/Physical Examination

- Erythematous, elevated thickened nodule with adherent white scaly or crusted, bloody margins; may present as a nonhealing ulceration or erosion evolving slowly
- Most commonly lips, hands, neck, head

Diagnosis

- Biopsy: atypical keratinocytes and malignant cells with large, pleomorphic, hyperchromatic nuclei in epidermis, extending into dermis; may form nodules with laminated centers ("epithelial/keratinous pearls")

Management/Prognosis

- Surgical excision with clear margins (most frequently done)
- Electrodessication & curettage for small, well-defined superficial lesions in low risk noncritical sites; also cryotherapy for small, well-defined, low risk lesions and Bowen's disease
- Mohs micrographic surgery for recurrent/aggressive tumors and cosmetically sensitive areas
- Radiation therapy: nonsurgical choice in select patients or as adjuvant therapy
- Slow growing (rarely metastasizes)

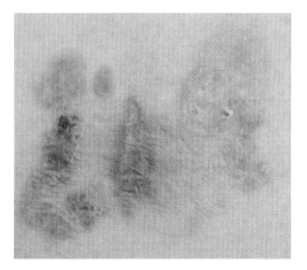

Figure 10.11 Squamous Cell Carcinoma

BASAL CELL CARCINOMA
Most common skin cancer in the United States; most common cancer in humans

Risk Factors
- Lighter-skinned individuals; prolonged sun exposure; xeroderma pigmentosum (genetic disorder with inability to repair damage caused by UV light exposure)

Clinical Manifestations/Physical Exam
- Flat, firm area with small, raised, translucent, pearly/waxy papule with raised, rolled borders and central ulceration with overlying telangiectatic vessels; often friable (bleeds easily)
- Most commonly face, nose, neck, trunk

Diagnosis
- **Punch or shave biopsy**: clusters of basaloid cells with a palisade arrangement of the nuclei at periphery of the clusters
- Excisional biopsy may also be performed

Management/Prognosis
- Mohs micrographic surgery for facial involvement, difficult and high-risk cases, or cases that recur (best long-term cure rates and tissue-sparing benefit)
- Electrodesiccation and curettage most common for nonfacial tumors with low risk of recurrence
- Surgical excision for tumors with either low or high risk of recurrence (cryosurgery)
- Small superficial: imiquimod & 5-FU for superficial non-facial lesions (cryosurgery)

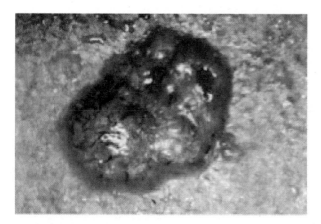

Figure 10.12 Basal Cell Carcinoma

Basil slowly **punched** the **base** of a **friable, waxy, pearly** piece of pottery, causing a **central crater** with **raised borders.**

MALIGNANT MELANOMA

Most common cause of skin cancer-related death; aggressive with high malignant potential (3% of all skin cancer but 65% of all skin cancer-related deaths)

Etiology/Pathophysiology

- Type of cancer developing from the melanocytes most commonly affecting the skin
- Most commonly metastasizes to regional lymph nodes, skin, liver, lungs, brain

Risk Factors

- **UV radiation** associated with 80% of cases, blistering sunburns, family history, >3 burns before age 20, tanning booth use, large number of nevi, Caucasian, light hair/eye color, xeroderma pigmentosum
- Most commonly on sun-exposed areas but it can occur anywhere on the body

Clinical Manifestations/Physical Examination

- Change to an existing mole in size, color, and symmetry; band of darker skin around a fingernail/toenail; slow-growing patch of thick skin that looks like a scar
- Lesions on upper back, upper arm, neck, and scalp decrease the likelihood of survival

Diagnosis

- **Full-thickness wide excisional biopsy** + lymph node biopsy
- Shave biopsy discouraged
- Major subtypes:
  - **Superficial spreading** (most common, 70%); may arise de novo or from pre-existing nevus; in men commonly trunk; in women commonly legs
  - **Nodular** second most common; may be associated with rapid vertical growth phase
  - **Lentigo maligna**: most common on face
  - **Acral lentiginous**: most commonly darker-skinned individuals; seen on palms, soles, nail beds
  - **Desmoplastic**: most aggressive

Management/Prognosis

- Complete wide surgical excision with sentinel lymph node biopsy
- Adjuvant therapy in some high risk: interferon-alfa, immune therapy, or radiotherapy. This includes talimogene (modified HSV injected into lesion)
- Thickness most important prognostic indicator for metastasis

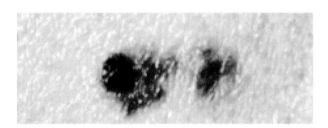

Figure 10.13 Malignant Melanoma

ABCDEs of Malignant Melanoma

Asymmetric

Borders irregular

Color varied

Diameter usually ≥6 mm

Evolution (rapid change in appearance)

MOLLUSCUM CONTAGIOSUM

Benign viral infection (*Poxviridae* family)

Etiology/Pathophysiology

- Highly contagious (skin to skin and fomites)

Risk Factors

- Most common in children, sexually active adults, patients with HIV

Clinical Manifestations/Physical Exam

- Single or multiple dome-shaped, flesh-colored to pearly-white, waxy papules with central umbilication
- Curd-like material expressed from the center if squeezed

Management/Prognosis

- No treatment needed in most cases; usually spontaneously resolves in 3–6 months
- Curettage (rapid resolution) first-line when therapy is indicated; cryotherapy, podophyllotoxin electrodessication; imiquimod
- Topical retinoids may be needed in severe cases

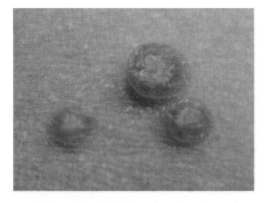

Figure 10.14 Molluscum Contagiosum

ROSEOLA (SIXTH'S DISEASE) HHV 6

Transmitted via respiratory droplets

Etiology/Pathophysiology

- Caused by human herpesvirus (HHV) 6 (and 7)
- 10-day incubation period

Risk Factors

- Most commonly age <5

Clinical Manifestations/Physical Exam

- High fever over 3–5 days leads to defervescence and coincides with rose pink maculopapular blanchable rash trunk/back and eventually the face
- Only childhood viral exanthem that starts on trunk and spreads to face
- Child appears well during febrile phase

Management/Prognosis

- Supportive, anti-inflammatories

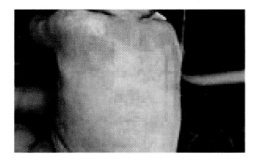

Figure 10.15 Roseola (Sixth's Disease) HHV 6

Dermatology

MUMPS

Paramyxovirus

Etiology/Pathophysiology

- Transmission via respiratory droplets
- 12–14-day incubation period

Clinical Manifestations/Physical Exam

- Low grade fever, myalgias, headache leads to painful parotid gland swelling
- Complications: older patients: orchitis in males (usually unilateral), deafness, encephalitis; mumps are the most common cause of acute pancreatitis in children

Diagnosis

- Serologies; often clinical diagnosis

Management/Prognosis

- Supportive, anti-inflammatories
- Symptoms usually last 7–10 days
- Patients are contagious for up to 9 days after initial onset
- MMR vaccine: give at 12–15 months, then again age 4–6

Remember the **Ps** of mum**Ps**:

- **P**arotid swelling
- **P**ancreatitis
- **P**aramyxovirus
- **P**enis-orchitis (males)

RUBEOLA (MEASLES)

Paramyxovirus

Etiology/Pathophysiology

- Transmission via respiratory droplets
- 10–12-day incubation period

Clinical Manifestations/Physical Exam

- **Prodrome**: high fever and "3 Cs" (**c**ough, **c**oryza, **c**onjunctivitis) followed by the enanthem
- **Enanthem**: approximately 48 hours prior to onset of the exanthem, possible Koplik spots (1–3 mm grayish, whitish or bluish elevations with an erythematous base) usually seen on the buccal mucosa opposite first and second molars
- **Exanthem**: maculopapular, erythematous rash beginning on the face and hairline followed by involvement of the neck, trunk and extremities rash usually lasts 7 days
- Fever usually concurrent with rash

Management/Prognosis

- Supportive, anti-inflammatories; isolate for 1 week after onset of rash
- Complications: otitis media, pneumonia, diarrhea, encephalitis

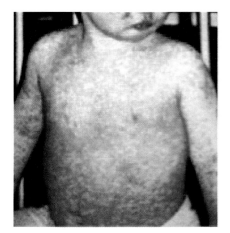

Figure 10.16 Rubeola (Measles)

Koplik developed **3 Cs** after throwing **red bricks** off the roof for **7 days**.

RUBELLA (GERMAN MEASLES)

Togavirus

Etiology/Pathophysiology

- Transmission via respiratory droplets
- "3-day rash"

Clinical Manifestations/Physical Exam

- Fever, cough, anorexia, lymphadenopathy (posterior cervical, posterior auricular) leads to pink, light-red spotted rash on face and extremities (3 days); transient photosensitivity and joint pains may be seen (especially in young women); may develop posterior cervical lymphadenopathy
- Teratogenic, especially first trimester: congenital syndrome: sensorineural deafness, cataracts, TTP "blueberry muffin rash," mental retardation

Management/Prognosis

- Anti-inflammatories, supportive
- Generally no complications in children compared to rubeola

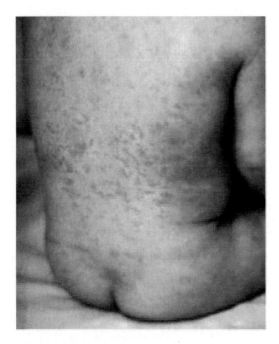

Figure 10.17 Rubella (German Measles)

Infectious diseases associated with arthropathy:

- **Bella** got **slapped on the cheek for the 5th time** with a **lime** and fell down a **valley** causing diffuse body pains!
- Rubella, 5th disease, Lyme disease, Coccidioidomycosis (Valley Fever)

Chapter 11

Infectious Disease

COMMONLY USED ANTIBIOTICS FOR INFECTIOUS DISEASE

Penicillins

- **Natural penicillins:**
  - Penicillin VK oral; penicillin G benzathine IM
  - Penicillin G aqueous IM, IV; penicillin G potassium IM, IV
- **Antistaphylococcal penicillins:**
  - Oxacillin IV, dicloxacillin PO, nafcillin IV, methicillin
- **Aminopenicillins:**
  - Amoxicillin PO; ampicillin PO, IM, IV
- **Aminopenicillins with beta-lactamase inhibitor:**
  - Amoxicillin/clavulanate PO
  - Ampicillin/sulbactam IV
- **Antipseudomonal penicillins:**
  - Piperacillin/tazobactam IV
  - Ticarcillin/clavulanate IV
  - Carbenicillin PO
- MOA: betalactam ring inhibits last step of cell wall synthesis, leading to osmotic rupture of bacterial cells; destruction of existing cell wall by bacterial autolysins (bactericidal)
- Distribution: broad distribution in body; penicillins have the ability to cross the placental barrier but are not teratogenic; are least toxic drugs known
- Penicillins are only active against bacteria with peptidoglycan cell walls (not active against viruses, mycobacteria, protozoa, and fungi)
- Penicillins and aminoglycosides have synergistic effects when used together; the penicillins break down the cell walls, allowing for easier entry of the aminoglycosides
- Hypersensitivity: drug class most commonly associated with hypersensitivity reactions
- **GI:** nausea, vomiting, diarrhea
- Neurotoxicity: may cause seizures at higher doses
- Acute interstitial nephritis
- Hematologic: thrombocytopenia, neutropenia, methemoglobinemia; IV penicillin G benzathine or penicillin procaine is associated with cardiopulmonary arrest and death; should be given IM in the buttocks (upper outer quadrant) or thigh (anterolateral)

After eating a plate of lettuce and bad penicillin, Piper developed a rash, seizures, and diarrhea, causing her to break down the bathroom wall to leave a beta-lactam ring IN the toilet bowl.

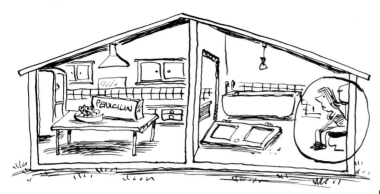

Side Effects:
- **Thrombocytopenia** (Plate of lettuce = platelets)
- **Rash, seizures, diarrhea**

Mechanism of Action:
- **Beta-lactam ring which breaks down the cell wall of bacteria**

Piper = piperacillin

Figure 11.1 Penicillin

- Peni**cillin** can **kill** by causing **I**nterstitial **N**ephritis
- **Amp**icillin will **amp**lify the rash when given to people infected with infectious mononucleosis

GLYCOPEPTIDE VANCOMYCIN

MOA/Pharmacokinetics

- Cell wall inhibition (by inhibition of phospholipids and peptidoglycans)

Indications

- Restricted use by CDC
  - Oral: *Clostridium difficile* colitis; oral vancomycin otherwise has poor tissue penetration
  - IV: MRSA; MRSE infections; adverse reactions
- Spectrum of activity
  - Mainly gram positive only: *S. aureus* (including MRSA, MRSE, *S. pneumonia*, enterococcal infections)
  - Synergistic use with aminoglycosides

Contraindications/Cautions/Side Effects

- **Red man syndrome:** flushing and pruritus due to histamine release if given too rapidly via IV; prevented by giving the infusion slowly over 1–2 hours and antihistamine administration; severe histamine release may lead to anaphylaxis in some patients
- Fevers/chills
- Thrombophlebitis at the IV site
- Ototoxicity: tinnitus or hearing loss; may be reversible in some cases
- Nephrotoxicity, especially if given with other antibiotics having similar adverse effects (eg, aminoglycosides); increased risk with longer duration of treatment
- Monitoring: trough levels may be needed in those with renal impairment for renal dosing, in those taking other nephrotoxic medications, or in those with severe infection

While on his cell phone, the red man drove too fast, causing HIS VAN to CRASH into a POST, only to leave him lying in a trough deaf with a busted kidney and a crushed license plate at the site.

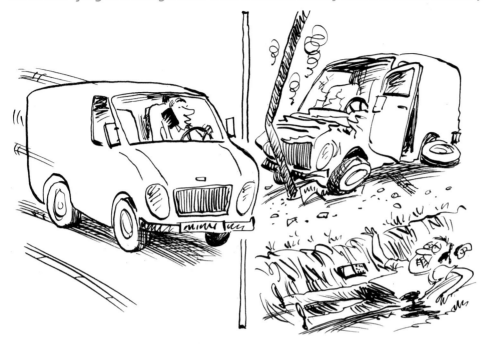

Figure 11.2 Vancomycin

C. *difficile* infection treatment in some patients (second-line treatment in most but first line with severe *C. difficile*)

Red man syndrome, to treat **R**esistant organisms (MRSA, MRSE), **R**estricted use by CDC

Antihistamines to premedicate if infusion has to be given rapidly to prevent red man syndrome

Slower infusion reduces the incidence of red man syndrome

Histamine release from rapid infusion causes flushing (red man syndrome)

- Cell wall inhibitor
- Red man syndrome when infusion is too fast
- HIS = red man syndrome due to histamine release
- Deaf busted kidney = ototoxicity, nephrotoxicity
- Post only = gram positive only
- Crushed license plate at the site = thrombophlebitis (platelets) at IV site
- Trough levels may be needed in some patients receiving other nephrotoxic drugs (eg, aminoglycosides, amphotericin B, cyclosporine), or some patients with severe life-threatening infections

CEPHALOSPORINS

- **First generation: cephalexin (PO), cefazolin (IV), cefadroxil (PO)**
  - Spectrum: gram-positive cocci, anaerobes, gram-negatives rods (*E. coli, H. influenzae, P. mirabilis, K. pneumoniae*)
  - Indications include skin and soft tissue infection (staph, strep); surgical prophylaxis
- **Second generation: cefaclor (PO), cefuroxime (IV, IM, PO), cefoxitin (IV), cefotetan (IM, IV)**
  - Spectrum: broader gram-negative coverage (*Neisseria spp, M. catarrhalis*) with weaker gram-positive coverage
  - Indications include skin, respiratory/ENT, UTI
  - Cefoxitin has excellent coverage against *Bacteroides fragilis*
  - Cefotetan and cefoxitin used for anaerobic infections (abdominal infection); inpatient PID treated with IV doxycycline + cefoxitin or cefotetan
- **Third generation: ceftriaxone (IM/IV), ceftazidime (IM, IV), ceftibuten, cefotaxime, cefixime**
  - Spectrum: broader gram-negative coverage (including *Serratia* and enteric organisms)
  - Good CNS penetration (especially ceftriaxone)
  - Indications include bacterial meningitis, gonorrhea, CAP (hospitalized) (combined with macrolides), Lyme disease involving the heart or brain
  - Ceftazidime has coverage vs. *Pseudomonas aeruginosa*
- **Fourth generation: cefepime (IV)**
  - Spectrum: gram-negative coverage including *P. aeruginosa*; gram positive only for methicillin-susceptible organisms
- **Fifth generation: ceftaroline (IV)**
  - Spectrum: gram-positives (including **MRSA**) and gram-negatives; does not cover *P. aeruginosa* or anaerobes

MOA/Pharmacokinetics

- Structurally and functionally similar to penicillin family with a beta-lactam ring but are effective against beta-lactamase producing bacteria

Indications

- Categorized by generations based on their spectrum of activity
- Increasing level of gram-negative activity and loss of gram-positive activity as you go, from first to fourth generation
- Cephalosporins are not typically effective against *Enterococci*, MRSA, *L. monocytogenes*, or *Clostridium difficile*

Contraindications/Cautions/Side Effects

- Allergic reaction: 5–15% cross-reactivity with penicillin (thus, do not use in those with an anaphylactic reaction to penicillin); 1–2% occurrence in those without a penicillin allergy
- Disulfiram-like reaction (due to blockage of the second step in alcohol oxidation), especially with cefotetan
- Increase the risk of bleeding with cefotetan and cefoxitin can (hypoprothrombinemia due to effect on vitamin K-dependent clotting factors)
- Inadequate biliary metabolism with ceftriaxone especially in neonates. Cefotaxime is preferred over ceftriaxone in neonates (eg, neonatal meningitis)

AMINOGLYCOSIDES

- Antibiotics that are derived from the *Streptomyces* bacteria end in **-mycin** (neomycin, streptomycin), while those antibiotics derived from Micromonospora bacteria end in **-micin** (gentamicin, amikacin)

MOA/Pharmacokinetics

- Binds to 30S ribosomal subunit, inhibiting bacterial protein synthesis (bactericidal)
- Concentration-dependent bacterial killing

Indications

- Distribution: varied tissue penetration; aminoglycosides not as good for CNS penetration in adults; needs to be "renally dosed" in patients with renal impairment; reduced activity in sites with acidic pH
- Gentamicin: HAP gram-negative bacteremia, GU infections, septic shock, neonatal meningitis (used with ampicillin), yersiniosis, tularemia, septic shock
- Tobramycin: slightly increased activity against *Pseudomonas;* topical use for keratitis
- Neomycin: similar to tobramycin; used as bowel prep; topically (a component of neomycin/polymyxin B/bacitracin + corticosporin); topical for otitis externa (must be able to visualize the tympanic membrane)
- Amikacin: reserved for serious infections
- Streptomycin: TB, tularemia, yersinia

Contraindications/Cautions/Side Effects

- Nephrotoxicity: acute tubular necrosis
- Ototoxicity: (vestibular and cochlear): cautious use of gentamicin with other ototoxic drugs, such as cisplatin, furosemide, bumetanide, ethacrynic acid, high-dose NSAIDs
- Neuromuscular paralysis: increased muscular weakness in patients with myasthenia gravis.
- Monitor serum drug levels in patients with renal impairment; peak level is typically evaluated 30 min post-infusion. Trough levels should be drawn immediately before next dose is administered.
- Contact dermatitis with topical neomycin

The gentleman drove his 1930's mu**STANG** into a NO_2 Noise zone, so he took the tube off his cute but bad kid's knee and put it in the muffler but still got sued by MONA.

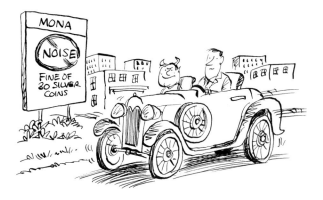

- Binds to **30S** ribosomal unit

N O
- **Gram Negatives Only** not used solo for positives

- **Nephrotoxic and Ototoxic (Acute Tubular Necrosis)**

- **NOt good if No O$_2$xygen** (used for aerobic infections)

- **Good activity against pseudomonas**

MOA: binds to 30S ribosomal unit
Streptomycin, **T**obramycin, **A**mikacin, **N**eomycin, **G**entamicin
Tube, cute = acute tubular necrosis
Bad kid's knee = bad kidneys (nephrotoxic)
Sued MONA = good activity against pseudomonas

Figure 11.3 Aminoglycosides

TETRACYCLINES

Doxycycline, tetracycline, minocycline, demeclocycline

MOA/Pharmacokinetics

- Binds to **30S ribosomal** subunit, inhibiting bacterial protein synthesis (bacteriostatic)

Indications

- Distribution: broad tissue penetration (both orally and IV); doxycycline is ideal tetracycline for IV administration and is safest in the group for those with renal impairment
- Spectrum of activity: broad (good against gram-positive, gram-negative, atypical, and organisms other than bacteria)
  - Doxycycline drug of choice: *Chlamydia spp*, including *C. trachomatis* STIs, PID, lymphogranuloma venereum; *C. pneumophila* pneumonia, *C. psittaci*), *M. pneumoniae*, Lyme disease, Rocky Mountain spotted fever, *Vibrio cholerae*, Q fever, bubonic plague, cat scratch fever, acne
  - Tetracycline, minocycline: acne
  - Demeclocycline: SIADH

Contraindications/Cautions/Side Effects

- Poor GI tolerance: may cause diarrhea and gastritis
- Deposition in calcified tissue: deposition in teeth causes tooth discoloration and may affect growth (not given to children age <8 except with Rocky Mountain spotted fever)
- Hepatotoxic (especially in pregnancy); contraindicated in pregnancy
- Photosensitivity; vestibular side effects, pseudotumor cerebri
- Impaired absorption if given at same time with dairy products, calcium, aluminum, magnesium, iron
- Contraindicated in patients with renal impairment (except doxycycline)

After playing **Tetras** all day **and avoiding drinking his pregnant mother's breast milk**, the 7-year-old had **difficulty looking at light** and had **very bad teeth.**

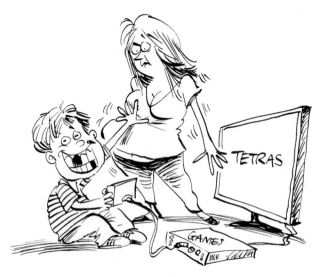

Side Effects and Contraindications:

<u>**Deposition in calcified tissue**</u> causes tooth discoloration (not given age <8)

Contraindicated in pregnancy

Photosensitivity; vestibular side effects, GI side effects

Impaired absorption if given simultaneously with dairy, calcium, aluminum, magnesium, iron

Figure 11.4 Tetracycline

Infectious Disease

MACROLIDES

Erythromycin, azithromycin, and clarithromycin

MOA/Pharmacokinetics

- Protein synthesis inhibitor: binds to 50S ribosomal subunit (bacteriostatic at low doses)

Indications

- Spectrum of activity: broad (good against gram-positive, gram-negative, atypical, and organisms other than bacteria (eg, *Babesia microti*)
- Erythromycin: Strep pharyngitis (if penicillin allergy), pneumonia, *C. diphtheriae*, acne (topical use); less gram-negative activity compared with others in class; safe in pregnancy
- Azithromycin: pneumonia
  - Best macrolide atypical coverage (*Mycoplasma, Chlamydia & Legionella*), *Chlamydia trachomatis*; acute bacterial exacerbations of chronic bronchitis (ABECB); anti-inflammatory in lung
  - Compared with erythromycin, increased activity vs. *H. influenzae & M. catarrhalis* but less activity vs. *Staph* and *Strep*
- Clarithromycin: CAP, *legionella, H. pylori*, sinusitis, bronchitis ABECB
- Clarithromycin and azithromycin are drugs of choice for *Mycobacterium avium complex*

Contraindications/Cautions/Side Effects

- GI upset (increases peristalsis): diarrhea and abdominal cramps (especially erythromycin)
- Ototoxicity: may cause deafness (usually reversible)
- Prolonged QT interval
- Acute cholestatic hepatitis (especially erythromycin estolate)
- Many drug-drug interactions so use caution (macrolides inhibit the CP450 system); increased levels of warfarin, digoxin, theophylline, carbamazepine, statins; increased muscle toxicity if used with niacin or statins
- In pregnancy, avoid the macrolides (exception is erythromycin); clarithromycin is embryotoxic

ACE got butterflies in his stomach and became so nervous that he couldn't hear the cutie (QT) that he had been pining over for 50 days calling him until she increased her voice, causing his liver to quiver and his muscles to get weak.

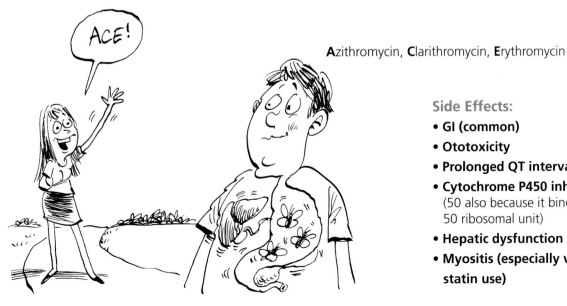

Azithromycin, **C**larithromycin, **E**rythromycin

Side Effects:
- **GI (common)**
- **Ototoxicity**
- **Prolonged QT interval**
- **Cytochrome P450 inhibition** (50 also because it binds to 50 ribosomal unit)
- **Hepatic dysfunction**
- **Myositis (especially with statin use)**

Figure 11.5 Macrolides

Infectious Disease

FLUOROQUINOLONES

Antibiotics with a broad spectrum of activity, excellent bioavailability, tissue penetration, prolonged half-life

MOA/Pharmacokinetics

- DNA gyrase inhibition removes excess positive supercoiling in the DNA helix (primary target in gram-negative bacteria); primary target in gram-negative bacteria
- Topoisomerase IV inhibition (affects separation of interlinked daughter DNA molecules); primary target for many gram-positive bacteria

Indications

- **Second generation:** increased activity vs. aerobic gram-negative bacteria
  - Ciprofloxacin: best gram-negative coverage in this class, including *Pseudomonas*, enteric organisms, *H. influenzae, Neisseria*
    - Indications: UTI, pyelonephritis, gastroenteritis, PID, malignant otitis externa, sinusitis, gonococcal arthritis, anthrax
  - Ofloxacin and lomefloxacin: enhanced coverage of *Staph* and *Strep* spp
    - Indications: same as above + acute bacterial exacerbation of chronic bronchitis and CAP
- **Third generation:** increased activity vs. gram-positive and atypical
  - Levofloxacin: better activity vs. *S. pneumoniae*
    - Indications: CAP, pyelonephritis, prostatitis, acute cystitis, gastroenteritis
  - Moxifloxacin: best gram-positive, anaerobic, and atypical coverage of the 3 generations. Poor *Pseudomonas* coverage
    - Indications: intra-abdominal infection (can be used as monotherapy), respiratory infection, sinusitis, ophthalmic infection, skin infection
  - Gatifloxacin: ophthalmic infections

Contraindications/Cautions/Side Effects

- GI (most common): possible nausea/vomiting, diarrhea
- CNS dysfunction: headache, memory impairment, agitation, delirium, seizures, peripheral neuropathy; may exacerbate myasthenia gravis
- Arthropathy: may be associated with tendinitis or tendon rupture in adults
- Contraindicated in pregnancy and age <18 (articular cartilage derangements)
- Photosensitivity
- QT prolongation
- Increased risk of hyperglycemia or hypoglycemia
- Renal or hepatic dysfunction
- Avoid for the treatment of uncomplicated infection (eg, acute sinusitis, simple cystitis), when risks outweigh the benefits

Infectious Disease

Although it is okay for **Quinn alone** to **gyrate** topless at club **DNA**, it would be a **grave sin** to do if she were **pregnant** or **under age 18.** She would have to get on her knees to pray to **Achilles** for a **prolonged time** for forgiveness.

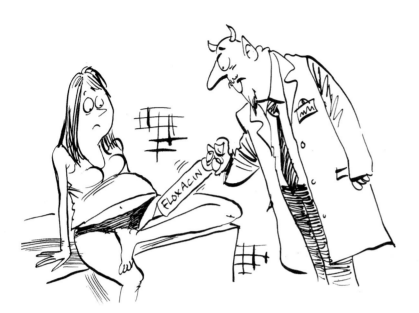

Figure 11.6 Fluoroquinolones

Mechanism of Action:
DNA gyrase (gram negative) and **topoisomerase** (gram positive)

- <u>**Grave**</u> = may exacerbate myasthenia gravis
- Sin: floxaCIN

Side Effects/Contraindications:
- Achilles tendon rupture and cartilage formation problems
- Prolonged QT interval

- Pregnancy, age <18

METRONIDAZOLE

Inhibits DNA synthesis

MOA/Pharmacokinetics

- Forms metabolites which inhibit bacterial DNA synthesis; in anaerobic bacteria, it is activated by ferredoxin (present in anaerobic parasites) to form reactive cytotoxic products
- Available in oral, IV, and topical forms

Indications

- Spectrum of activity: effective against protozoa and anaerobes
  - Anaerobes "below the diaphragm" (drug of choice)
  - Anaerobes including *B. fragilis, C. difficile,* and *Gardnerella vaginalis*
  - Protozoa including *Entamoeba histolytica, Giardia lamblia, Trichomonas spp*
  - *H. pylori*
- Intra-abdominal infection, vaginitis, vaginosis, pseudomembranous colitis, and amoebic liver abscess

Contraindications/Cautions/Side Effects

- Disulfiram-like reaction if used with alcohol (acetaldehyde accumulation)
- Neurotoxicity: peripheral neuropathy, headache, dizziness, nausea
- Metallic taste

You cannot take the underground metro to Anazoa while drinking alcohol with a metallic taste or you will die suffering a reaction from neurotoxicity!

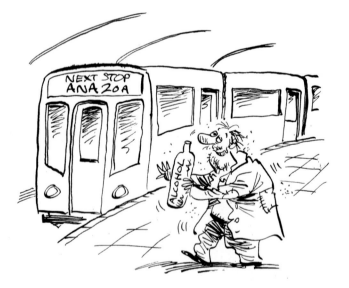

Mechanism of Action:
- **Great against anaerobes and protozoans (especially anaerobes below the diaphragm)**

- **Disulfiram reaction if used with alcohol**

- **Metallic taste**

- **Neurotoxicity**

Figure 11.7 Metronidazole

TRIMETHOPRIM-SULFAMETHOXAZOLE

Antimetabolite

MOA/Pharmacokinetics

- Folic **acid antagonist** and **inhibitor of folic acid synthesis;** bactericidal
- Available in oral and IV forms

Indications

- Spectrum of activity: broad (excellent against gram-negative and gram-positive)
  - Second best oral coverage vs. MRSA (linezolid is first but is used less frequently than TMP-SMX)
  - Not active vs. *Group A streptococcus* (thus often added with cephalexin for empiric oral treatment of MRSA cellulitis where the cephalexin covers the Strep)
- Soft tissue infections with MRSA, UTI, PCP treatment and prophylaxis, acute bacterial exacerbation of chronic bronchitis, toxoplasmosis, shigellosis, otitis media in children only, traveler's diarrhea

Contraindications/Cautions/Side Effects

- Side effects: rash, photosensitivity, and folate deficiency are most common; appetite loss; nausea/vomiting; dizziness; tinnitus; fatigue; hyperkalemia
- Hematologic abnormalities (due to folic acid inhibition); may cause hemolytic anemia in those with G6PD deficiency
- May increase levels of warfarin and digoxin
- **Contraindications:** those requiring increased folic acid (pregnancy, nursing mothers, neonates <6 wks [causes kernicterus]; sulfa allergy

Bac**trim** will **Trim** your folic acid levels if you are pregnant with a **son that has G6PD** but it will help you get closer to take a **selfie** with your **PCP and your Murse.**

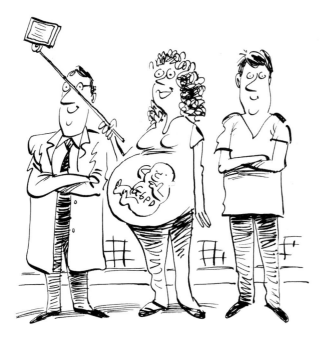

Mechanism of Action:

- Inhibitor of folic acid

- Broad coverage: gram positives/negatives, PCP, MRSA

- Not active against group A Strep

Caution:

- Sulfa allergy, G6PD deficiency

Figure 11.8 Trimethoprim-Sulfamethoxazole

Infectious Disease

AMPHENICOL CHLORAMPHENICOL

MOA/Pharmacokinetics

Binds to 50S ribosomal subunit, inhibiting bacterial protein synthesis

Indications

- Broad tissue penetration (both orally and IV); good CNS penetration
- Spectrum of activity:
  - Broad spectrum of activity: good against gram positive, gram negative, anaerobes, and other organisms (eg, *Rickettsiae*)
  - Because of high incidence of toxicity, it is usually reserved for severe anaerobic infections or other life-threatening infections that are not responsive to other antibacterials

Contraindications/Cautions/Side Effects

- Bone marrow suppression: aplastic anemia, reversible anemia, hemolytic anemia (especially if GPD deficient), aplastic anemia
- Overgrowth of *Candida albicans* (common)
- Grey baby syndrome (due to abnormal mitochondrial activity in neonates because of the drug) leading to cyanosis and hemodynamic collapse (may be fatal)
- Drug interactions: may increase levels of phenytoin, warfarin, and chlorpropamide

> Chlorampheni**COL** = **Call** the doctor if baby turns grey or if you have anemia!

STREPTOCOCCAL PHARYNGITIS

Group A beta-hemolytic *Streptococcus* (GABHS/*Strep pyogenes*)

Risk Factors

- 20–40% of all cases of exudative pharyngitis occur in children

Clinical Manifestations/Physical Exam

- Sore throat
- Centor criteria

Diagnosis

- Rapid antigen detection test: 95% specific but only 55–90% sensitive (most useful if positive, but if negative obtain throat culture (especially in children age 5–15)
- Throat culture: definitive diagnosis (gold standard)

Management/Prognosis

- Normal course of illness is 3–5 days; treatment shortens by 48 hrs so is given mostly to prevent complications and rheumatic fever
  - Penicillin G or penicillin VK; amoxicillin/clavulanic acid (Augmentin)
  - Macrolides if penicillin-allergic
  - Other alternatives include clindamycin, cephalosporins
- Complications:
  - Rheumatic fever (preventable with antibiotics)
  - Glomerulonephritis (not preventable with antibiotics)
  - Peritonsillar abscess, cellulitis

Children who miss school due to strep throat will "FALE" instead of getting an A.

Fever
Absence of cough
Lymphadenopathy (tender, anterior)
Exudate on tonsils

Age (modified Centor)
3–14: add 1 point
15–44: add 0 points
$\geq$45: subtract 1 point

Centor criteria help to identify patients in whom neither antibiotic or throat culture is necessary; **criteria <3 means strep pharyngitis is unlikely**

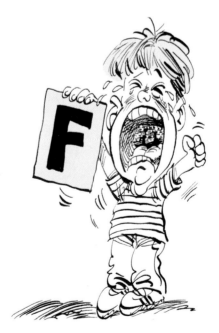

Figure 11.9 Centor Criteria 4 Strep Throat

RASHES THAT AFFECT THE PALMS AND SOLES

- **Kawasaki Syndrome:** commonly children (especially age <5), boys (Asians at highest risk); thought to occur after respiratory pathogen or viral syndrome
  - **W**arm + **CREAM** – fever + **c**onjunctivitis; **r**ash (polymorphous); **e**xtremity changes (rash on hands and feet, induration); **a**denopathy (cervical, erythematous, no pus); **m**ucous membrane involvement (strawberry tongue, lip swelling); treatment: IVIG + aspirin
- **Janeway Lesions:** seen in infective endocarditis: embolic/immune response, painless erythematous macules on palms and soles
- **Coxsackie A virus**
  - Fever, URI symptoms lead to oral vesicular, erythematous lesions resulting in vesicular lesions on distal extremities, palms and soles
- **Syphilis:** secondary syphilis associated with maculopapular rash
- **Toxic Shock Syndrome:** red, diffuse, maculopapular rash with desquamation of palms and soles
- **Reactive Arthritis (Reiter's syndrome):** keratoderma blennorrhagica refers to hyperkeratotic lesions on palms and soles

King James of Switzerland Climbed Rocky Mountain and Spotted Many Toxic Reactive Measly Markings on His hands and Feet

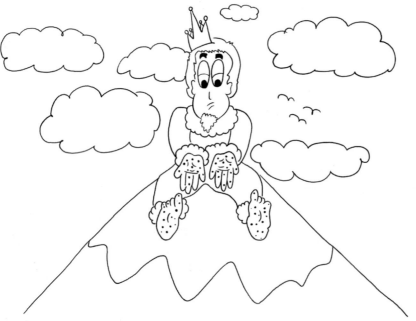

Kawasaki syndrome
Janeway lesions (painless)
Osler's nodes (painful)
Secondary syphilis
Coxsackie virus
Rocky mountain spotted fever

Figure 11.10 Palm & Sole Rashes

ROCKY MOUNTAIN SPOTTED FEVER

Potentially fatal but curable tick-borne disease: *Rickettsia rickettsii* (spread by ticks)

Etiology/Pathophysiology

- *R. rickettsii* (gram negative, obligate intracellular bacterium)
- Vector: *Dermacentor andersoni/variabilis* (wood/dog tick) is especially in south central and southeastern states (especially in the spring/summer)

Clinical Manifestations/Physical Exam

- 2–14 days after tick bite; fevers/chills, myalgias, arthralgias, headache, nausea/vomiting, lethargy, seizures; leads to blanching; erythematous macular rash first on wrists/ankles and palms/soles (characteristic) and spreading centrally over 2–3 days (10% of those affected don't get rash)
- ± faint macules lead to papules, petechiae; patient may develop encephalitis, ARDS, cardiac or bleeding disorders

Diagnosis

- Clinical diagnosis (don't wait for serologies)
- Serologies: indirect fluorescent antibody test for IgM and IgG antibodies; four-fold rise in titers indicates acute disease; an infected patient may have negative serology tests in the first few days
- Skin biopsy, thrombocytopenia, hyponatremia
- CSF: low glucose and pleocytosis (increased cell count)

Management/Prognosis

- Doxycycline (even in children) for 5–14 days (dental staining not as likely with short course)
- Chloramphenicol (second-line treatment) (treatment of choice in pregnancy); keep in mind that third trimester usage of chloramphenicol is also associated with grey baby syndrome

After climbing a **Rocky mountain in the South, Rick** developed **fevers, headaches, and a rash that spread to his Palms and Soles** so he couldn't wait and was rushed to his **Doc's** office on his **cycle** before he developed **multi-organ failure.**

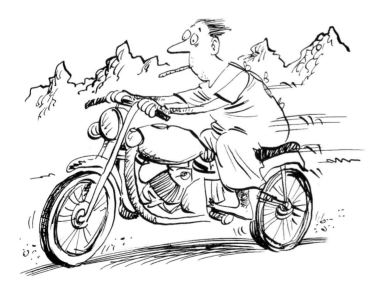

- *Rickettsia rickettsii* **cause**

- *Dermacentor* **spp. Vector (wood/ dog tick)**

Clinical Manifestations:
- **Fevers, rash, multi-organ involvement**

Diagnosis:
- **Clinical, serologies**

Management:
- **Doxycycline, chloramphenicol**

Figure 11.11 Rocky Mountain Spotted Fever

Infectious Disease

OSTEOMYELITIS

Rare but serious bone infection

Etiology/Pathophysiology

- Notable pathogens
  - *S. aureus* most common organism overall; Group *A beta hemolytic Strep (S. pyogenes)*
  - *S. epidermis* (coagulase-negative): increased incidence after recent prosthetic joint placement
  - *Salmonella* pathognomonic for sickle cell disease
  - *Group B streptococcus* increased incidence in neonates
  - *P. aeruginosa:* calcaneal osteomyelitis associated with puncture wound through tennis shoe
- Pathogenesis
  - Hematogenous spread is most common source in children; commonly affects tibia, femur, or humerus in children and in adults and IV drug users, commonly affects vertebral bodies
  - Contiguous infection close to bone (most common overall source in adults); occurs with local trauma, breaks in the skin, etc
  - Chronic osteomyelitis: often includes the development of sinus tracts

Clinical Manifestations/Physical Exam

- Local pain or signs of inflammation/infection over site of the involved bone
- Possible systemic signs such as fever
- Chronic cases usually can have a subacute presentation

Diagnosis

- Labs: increased ESR and CRP; positive blood cultures in 50%
- Plain x-ray: periosteal reaction leads to bony destruction, sequestra (segments of necrotic bone separated from living bone by granuloma [sequestra = chronic]; may take weeks to develop radiologic evidence of osteomyelitis
- MRI: most sensitive test in early disease
- Radionuclide or gallium scan: sensitive in early disease
- Bone biopsy (gold standard); percutaneous needle aspiration of the bone for chronic osteomyelitis

Management/Prognosis

- Age birth to 3 months: third-generation cephalosporin (cefotaxime preferred) or ceftazidime + an antistaphylococcal agent (vancomycin, nafcillin, oxacillin)
- Age >3 months
  - MSSA suspected: nafcillin, oxacillin, cefazolin
  - MRSA suspected: vancomycin, clindamycin, or linezolid
- Puncture wound to foot (*Pseudomonas*): ceftazidime or cefepime; ciprofloxacin (adults only)

Miles walked with a **stuff** until he developed **sickle cell disease.** After his diagnosis he went fishing for **salmon** and couldn't because the **MRI** machine made a magnetic field around his body.

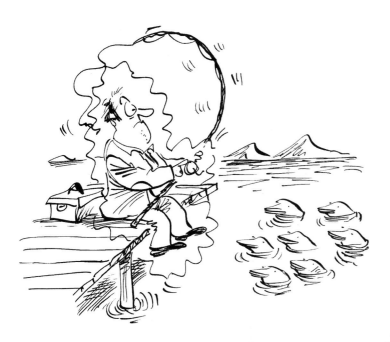

Figure 11.12 Osteomyelitis

- *Staph aureus* most common cause (salmonella often seen with sickle cell disease)

- **Diagnostic MRI** to detect early disease

SYPHILIS

Chronic infection caused by spirochete *Treponema pallidum*

Etiology/Pathophysiology

- Transmission: direct contact of an infected lesion during sexual activity and contact with lesions (including mucous membranes); may also be transmitted to the fetus via the placenta

Clinical Manifestations/Physical Exam

- Early syphilis: clinical syndrome that occurs within first year of infection: includes primary, secondary, and early latent
- Latent syphilis: asymptomatic infection with a normal exam but positive testing; late latent (>1 year) is associated with a lower transmission rate (except in fetal transmission)
- Clinical Manifestations (incubation period is 3 days–3 months):
  - Primary:
    - Chancre: painless ulcer at inoculation site with raised indurated edges (usually begins as a papule that ulcerates); on average heals spontaneously within 3–4 weeks (even without treatment)
    - Nontender regional lymphadenopathy near the chancre site lasting 3–4 weeks
  - Secondary:
    - Maculopapular rash, diffuse bilateral maculopapular lesions (involvement of the palms/soles common); lesions may be pustular in some patients
    - Condyloma lata: wart-like lesions involving mucous membranes and other moist areas
    - Systemic symptoms: fever, lymphadenopathy (may be tender), arthritis, meningitis, hepatitis (elevated alkaline phosphatase); secondary symptoms may occur a few weeks to 6 months after initial symptoms
  - Tertiary (late): may occur 1–20 years after initial infection
    - Gumma: noncancerous granulomas on skin and body tissues (eg, bones)
    - Neurosyphilis: headache, meningitis, dementia, vision/hearing loss, incontinence; tabes dorsalis (demyelination of posterior columns leads to ataxia, areflexia burning pain, weakness)
    - Argyll Robertson pupil: small, irregular pupil that constricts normally to near accommodation but not to light
    - Cardiovascular: aortitis, aortic regurgitation, aortic aneurysms
  - Congenital syphilis:
    - Hutchinson teeth (notches on teeth), sensorineural hearing loss
    - Saddle nose deformity
    - ToRCH syndrome

Diagnosis

- Screening (nontreponemal) tests
  - RPR: look at titers (eg, a positive test indicates titer ≥1:32); usually positive 4–6 weeks post-infection; changes in titer also help determine therapeutic response
  - VDRL
  - Because they are nonspecific, a positive RPR or VDRL must be confirmed by specific treponemal testing (eg, FTA-ABS)
  - False-positives can be seen with antiphospholipid syndrome, pregnancy, TB, rickettsial infections (eg, Rocky Mountain spotted fever)
- Confirmatory (treponemal) testing via FTA-ABS and micro-hemagglutination test for *T. pallidum* antibodies
- Darkfield microscopy allows for direct visualization of *T. pallidum* from clinical specimens (chancre or condyloma lata)

Management/Prognosis

Penicillin is treatment of choice for all stages of syphilis:

- **Early syphilis:** (primary, secondary, and early latent): penicillin G benzathine 2.4 million units IM × 1 dose; doxycycline for 14 days if penicillin-allergic
- **Late syphilis:** (tertiary or late latent): penicillin G benzathine 2.4 million units IM once weekly × 3 weeks
- **Neurosyphilis:** IV penicillin G preferred (3–4 million units every 4 hrs for 10–14 days)
- For penicillin allergy, pregnancy, neurosyphilis, CV manifestation of late syphilis, or prior treatment failure, test for true penicillin allergy and desensitize (if immediate-type reaction) or rechallenge (if delayed reaction) with penicillin
- **Jarisch-Herxheimer** reaction is an acute, self-limited febrile reaction seen within 24 hrs post-therapy of a spirochetal infection (eg, syphilis, Lyme); thought to be caused by release of cytokines and immune complexed from killed organisms; classically presents with fever, headache, myalgia, hypotension, and may worsen the rash; is self-limited and usually resolves in 12–24 hrs but NSAIDs and antipyretics may help
- Monitoring
  - All patients with syphilis should be tested for HIV and other STIs
  - All patients should be reexamined clinically and serologically at 6 months and 12 months post-treatment; those with HIV may be monitored more frequently
  - A nontreponemal titer should be obtained prior to initiating therapy; a fourfold decline in the nontreponemal titer within 6 months is considered an acceptable response

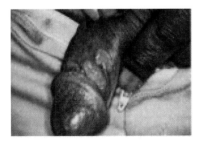
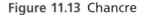

Figure 11.13 Chancre

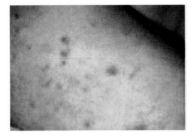

Figure 11.14 Maculopapular Rash

When **Trep** and his **pal imitated Argyll Robertson** the First, he **accommodated** them by taking them out to a **dark-field** and gave them a **chancre**. After that, he used his **palms and soles** to beat them until they developed **visual/hearing loss, notches on their teeth, and saddle nose deformities**.

Infectious Disease

LYME DISEASE

Borrelia burgdorferi (gram-negative spirochete) spread by vector *Ixodes* (deer) tick, especially in Northeast, Midwest, and Mid-Atlantic regions of the United States

Etiology/Pathophysiology

- Transmitted by an *Ixodes* species tick in nymphal phase, especially in spring and summer when nymphs feed
- Highest likelihood of transmission if tick is engorged and/or has been attached for $\geq$72 hours

Clinical Manifestations/Physical Exam

- Early localized: erythema migrans (90%); expanding warm annular erythematous rash (classically seen with central clearing or "bull's eye" appearance usually within a month of the tick bite, often near the site of the bite) expanding slowly over days to weeks; may be accompanied with viral-like syndrome (headaches, fevers, malaise, or lymphadenopathy)
- Early disseminated: (1–12 weeks) rheumatologic arthritis (especially large joints); neurologic (headache, meningitis, weakness, CN VII palsy, neuropathy); cardiac (AV block); multiple erythema migrans lesions
- Late disease: persistent synovitis, persistent neurological symptoms

Diagnosis

- Clinical: especially with early localized Lyme disease (eg, erythema migrans rash); at this early stage patients are often seronegative so treat those who have the rash and who reside in/have traveled to an endemic area for Lyme
- Serologic testing: ELISA, followed by Western Blot if ELISA is positive or equivocal; serologic testing is used in patients who fit **all** of the following criteria:
  - **Reside in or travel to an endemic area**
  - **Risk factor for exposure to ticks**
  - **Symptoms consistent with early disseminated or late Lyme disease (arthritis, meningitis, CN palsy, carditis, radiculopathy, mononeuritis)**
- Because serologic testing takes weeks to become positive and does not distinguish acute from past infection, serologic testing is **not used in** patients with an erythema migrans; for screening of asymptomatic patients living in an endemic area; or in patients with non-specific symptoms only
- If ELISA is false-positive, consider other spirochetal diseases: syphilis, yaws; viral/bacterial illnesses; or another *Borrelial* species

Management/Prognosis

- **Early disease:** doxycycline bid over 10–21 days (early disseminated duration 14–28 days) (if doxycycline contraindicated or if penicillin-allergic, azithromycin and erythromycin are alternatives); amoxicillin over 14–21 days for children age <8 or for pregnancy (cefuroxime is an alternative)
- **Late or severe:** IV ceftriaxone if second/third AV heart block, syncope, dyspnea, chest pain, CNS disease other than CN VII palsy such as meningitis; prophylaxis is doxycycline (200 mg) $\times$ 1 dose within 72 hours of removal of an *Ixodes* tick that has been latched on for $\geq$36 hrs from an area with $\geq$20% tick infection rate

After eating **Lime, shopping at Burgdorf's,** and **migrating** in the spring and summer, **Ixodes** developed **arthritis** and rang the **Bell** on his **cycle** to try to get **Elisa's** attention who lived up the **Av**e on the **second block next to Moxy.**

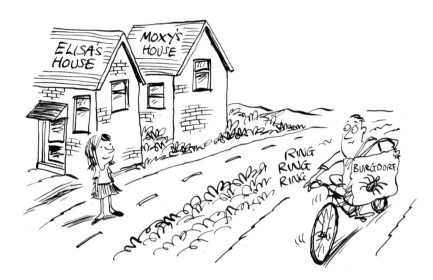

Figure 11.15 Lyme Disease

- *Borrelia **burgdorferi*** causative agent
- ***Ixodes*** (deer) tick vector

Clinical Manifestations
- Erythema migrans, arthritis, CNS symptoms, atrioventricular heart **blocks**

Diagnosis
- **ELISA**, clinical, titers

Management
- Doxy**cycl**ine; A**mox**icillin (if age <8)

MALARIA

RBC disease caused by *Plasmodium* (falciparum, vivax, ovale, malariae, knowlesi) transmitted by female *Anopheles* mosquito (especially at dusk and dawn)

Etiology/Pathophysiology

- Found throughout most of the tropics, especially in Sub-Saharan Africa
- *Plasmodium* species infect RBCs and lead to RBC lysis, resulting in cyclical fevers; **falciparum** is most dangerous type
- Sickle cell trait and thalassemia trait are protective against the disease

Clinical Manifestations

- Febrile illness (cold stage/chills)
  - Cyclical fever every 48 hrs (*P. vivax & P. ovale*) and 72 hrs (*P. malariae*)
  - With *P. falciparum*, irregular fever plus possible cerebral malaria (altered mental status, delirium, seizures, coma) or Blackwater fever (severe hemolysis, hemoglobinuria [dark urine], and renal failure)
- Cold stage is followed by hot stage/fever which is followed by diaphoretic stage every 2–3 days)
- Headache; myalgia; GI symptoms; splenomegaly

Diagnosis

- Clinical diagnosis: suspect in patients with fever who have traveled to endemic area + laboratory evidence of parasitic infection
- Giemsa-stained blood smear: (thin and thick): parasites (trophozoites and schizonts) in RBCs with light microscopy; Schüffner's dots (small brick-red granules throughout erythrocyte cytoplasm) seen with *P. vivax & ovale*
- Rapid diagnostic tests: antigen or antibody (can pick up very low parasitemia)
- Thrombocytopenia, hemolytic anemia, increased LDH, leukopenia

Management/Prognosis

Check with CDC for resistance patterns and pharmacologic recommendations

- Chloroquine-sensitive regions
  - **Chloroquine: first-line treatment for uncomplicated *P. falciparum*** (hydroxychloroquine is an alternative)
  - Primaquine: add-on to kill latent hypnozoites in *P. vivax* and *P. ovale* infection and prevent recurrence
- Chloroquine-resistant *P. falciparum*
  - Artemisinin combination therapy (eg, artemether–lumefantrine) or atovaquone–proguanil
  - Second-line: quinine sulfate + doxycycline, tetracycline, or clindamycin
- Chloroquine-resistant *P. vivax*
  - Quinine sulfate + doxycycline or tetracycline + primaquine
  - Atovaquone–proguanil + primaquine
  - Mefloquine + primaquine

Anopheles traveled to Africa and got multiple **mosquito** bites and developed **cyclic fevers, hemolytic anemia, and Malaria,** so he started to stain his pants and had to use **chlorox** to **qleen** up the mess.

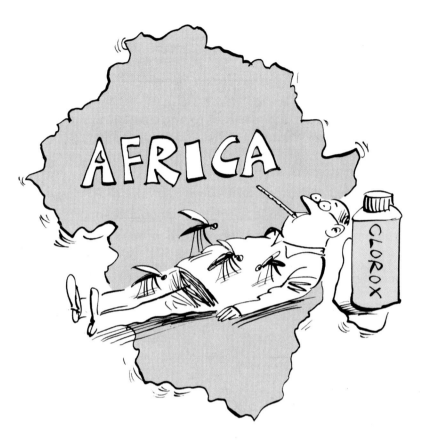

- Plasmodium spp **(falciparum, ovale, malariae, vivax)**

- **Female anopheles mosquito is the vector**

Clinical Manifestations:
- **Cyclical fevers, hemolytic anemia**

Diagnosis:
- **Thin/thick smear (Giemsa stain)**

Management:
- **Chloroquine if sensitive; check with CDC for resistant areas**

Figure 11.16 Malaria

Infectious Disease

TULAREMIA
Francisella tularensis, gram-negative coccobacillus

Etiology/Pathophysiology

- Incubation period: 2–15 days
- Transmission: tick/insect bite or handling animal tissues; rabbits are important reservoir hosts

Clinical Manifestations/Physical Exam

- Most are asymptomatic
- Ulceroglandular (most common): fever, headache, nausea; leads to single papule at site of inoculation, results in ulceration of papule with central eschar and tender regional lymphadenopathy; ulcers of the hand /arm are most common after animal exposure; ulcers of the head/trunk/legs are most common after tick exposure
- Glandular (most common type in children): tender regional LAD with absence of skin lesions
- Oculoglandular: if splashed in eye with infected material: pain, photophobia, tearing
- Pharyngeal: due to ingestion of contaminated food/water; fevers, sore throat
- Typhoidal: febrile illness
- Possible pneumonia after ingestion of meat (eg, undercooked rabbit meat); GI symptoms; stupor or delirium if severe

Diagnosis

- Serologies, blood cultures

Management/Prognosis

- Streptomycin (drug of choice), gentamicin, doxycycline

Silly Easter **Rabbit with "TULips and TRICKS"** are for **LADs.**

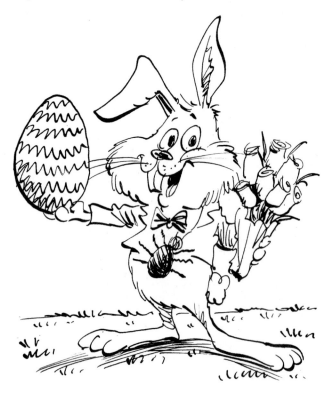

- **T**ick or animal tissue most common mode of transmission

- **R**egional **LAD (lymphadenopathy)**

- **I**noculation site-papule

- **C**entral Eschar

- **K**ids develop glandular type most often

- **S**treptomycin drug of choice

Figure 11.17 Tularemia

BABESIOSIS

Infectious disease caused by malaria-like protozoa of the *Babesia spp* (eg, *Babesia microti*)

Etiology/Pathophysiology

- Tick vectors (eg, *Ixodes scapularis,* same tick for Lyme disease); blood transfusion, transplantation, or congenital condition (rare)
- Similar to malaria, the *Babesia* protozoa infect and lyse RBCs

Risk Factors

- Endemic to upper Midwest & Northeastern United States (eg, Long Island, Massachusetts)
- Elderly age, history of asplenia, and immunocompromised status

Clinical manifestations/Physical exam

- Fever, chills, fatigue, sweats, headache, myalgia, jaundice, arthralgia, anorexia

Diagnosis

- Peripheral blood smear with Giemsa or Wright stain; parasites within RBCs especially in pathognomonic tetrads (Maltese cross appearance); intraerythrocytic ring forms with central pallor
- CBC: mild to severe hemolytic anemia (decreased haptoglobin, increased reticulocytes), lymphopenia, thrombocytopenia; increased transaminases
- Polymerase chain reaction (PCR) for detection of *Babesia* DNA
- Serologies

Management

- Atovaquone + azithromycin or quinine + clindamycin
- Tick *Ixodes scapularis* is the vector for Lyme disease, Babesiosis, and Ehrlichiosis; as many as 2/3 of patients with Babesiosis also have concurrent Lyme, and as many as 1/3 also experience concurrent human granulocytic anaplasmosis (Ehrlichiosis)

When the **Malta** knights conquered **the babies** of **Long Island and Massachusetts in tetrads,** they placed their **Maltese cross** banners **on the blood** they spilled during the war.

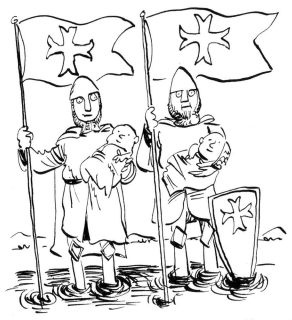

- **Common in Long Island, Massachusetts (northeast United States)**

Peripheral Smear:
- **Tetrads within the RBCs (Maltese cross-shaped)**

Diseases Transmitted by Ixodes Tick:

You can get a CN VII (BEL) palsy with a bite from an Ixodes tick.

- **Babesiosis**
- **Ehrlichiosis**
- **Lyme disease**

Figure 11.18 Babesiosis

Infectious Disease

EHRLICHIOSIS

Tick-transmitted bacterial infection

Etiology/Pathophysiology

- Human granulocytic *Anaplasma phagocytophilum* (HGA): transmitted by *Ixodes* tick (same tick of Lyme disease)
- Human monocytic ehrlichia (HME): *Ehrlichia chaffeensis* and *canis* transmitted by lone star tick (*Amblyomma americanum*); both organisms infect and destroy WBCs

Clinical Manifestations/Physical Exam

- Prodrome of rigors, malaise, and nausea leads to high fever, toxicity, myalgia, headache
- Usually no rash; ± splenomegaly; symptoms begin 7–10 days after tick bite

Diagnosis

- Serologies (titers)
- Leukopenia, thrombocytopenia, increased LFTs
- Peripheral smear/buffy coat: morulae in WBCs (*Ehrlichia* clusters in cell vacuoles forming large mulberry shaped aggregates) especially HGA

Management/Prognosis

- Doxycycline, rifampin, chloramphenicol

Ana and Ixodes always wear a lone star over their **mono**gram on their **mulberry-colored puffy coats** when they visit **Earl, Morris,** and **Little Luke.**

- Human granulocytic **anaplasma (HGA) phagocytophilum** transmitted by Ixodes

- Human monocytic ehrlichia (HME): Ehrlichia chaffeensis and canis lone star tick (*Amblyomma americanum*)

Diagnosis:
- **Leukopenia**

- Peripheral smear/puffy coat: **morulae** in WBCs (mulberry-shaped aggregates)

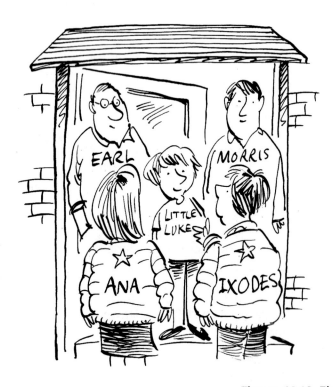

Figure 11.19 Ehrlichiosis

CYTOMEGALOVIRUS (HHV 5)

Common viral infection affecting people of all ages

Risk Factors

- Present in most people (70% of U.S. population)
- Clinical disease in immunocompromised patients

Clinical Manifestations/Physical Exam

- Primary disease: mononucleosis-like illness (most have no symptoms)
- Congenital CMV: sensorineural hearing loss common and "blueberry muffin rash" (TTP). ToRCH syndrome occurs with Toxoplasmosis, Other (Syphilis), Rubella, CMV & HSV
- Reactivation: seen in immunocompromised patients: HIV, steroid use, patients on chemotherapy, post transplant
- Retinitis: scrambled eggs/ketchup appearance (pizza pie) on fundoscopy (hemorrhage with soft exudates); retinitis seen if CD4 <50; pneumonitis, encephalitis; colitis (CD4 <100)
- Esophagitis: odynophagia; large superficial ulcers on EGD

Diagnosis

- Serologies (antigen tests, IgM, IgG titers)
- Owl's eye appearance on biopsy of tissues

Management/Prognosis

- Ganciclovir (first-line treatment); foscarnet, cidofovir

A gang of sick owls whose eyes were bigger than their colons developed esophagitis after swallowing too many blueberries, scrambled eggs with ketchup, and pizza pies.

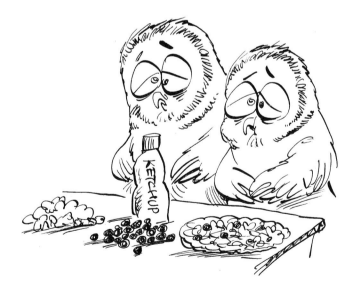

- **Owl's eye appearance on biopsy**

- **Esophagitis, colitis, retinitis**

- **Retinitis on fundoscopic exam: scrambled eggs/ketchup aka pizza pie sign**

- **Blueberry rash in infants with ToRCH syndrome**

- **Ganciclovir treatment of choice (gang sick)**

Figure 11.20 Cytomegalovirus

Infectious Disease

WOUND MANAGEMENT

Workup/Management for General Wounds:
- **W**hen/Where did wound occur?
- **O**paque/lucent (x-ray needed)?
- **U**nder water (irrigation)/**U**pdate tetanus
- **N**euro exam
- **D**irect pressure (if active bleeding)
- **S**top infection (Antibiotics)/**S**uture

Workup/Management for Bites:
- **B**roken bones (get x-ray)
- **I**rrigate
- **T**etanus up to date?
- **E**xplore for foreign body, tendon injury
- **S**top infection (antibiotics)

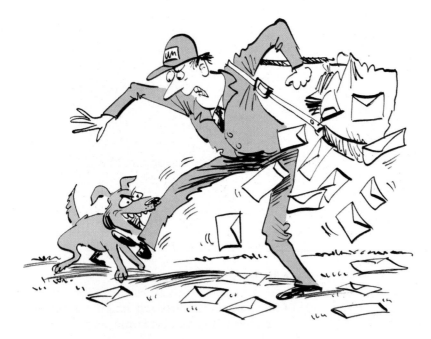

Figure 11.21 Wound Management

Chapter 12

Hematology

ANEMIA

Decrease in hemoglobin and hematocrit

Etiology/Pathophysiology

- Microcytic anemia: iron deficiency anemia (most common), thalassemias, lead poisoning, early anemia of chronic disease
- Macrocytic anemia: B12 deficiency, folate deficiency, liver disease, alcoholism, hypothyroidism
- Normocytic anemia: early iron deficiency anemia, mixed anemia, endocrine, dilutional, G6PD deficiency, sickle cell anemia, hemolytic anemia

Risk Factors

- Blood loss, nutritional deficiency, alcohol use, and genetics

Clinical Manifestations/Physical Exam

- Palpitations, tachycardia, high-output heart failure, orthostatic hypotension, dizziness, syncope
- Skin pallor, purpura, petechiae, jaundice
- Fatigue and weakness
- Headache

Diagnosis

- Complete blood count with peripheral smear
- Coombs testing for autoimmune hemolytic anemia
- Hemolytic anemia: increased reticulocyte, increased lactate dehydrogenase, increased indirect bilirubin, decreased haptoglobin; peripheral smear is positive for schistocytes

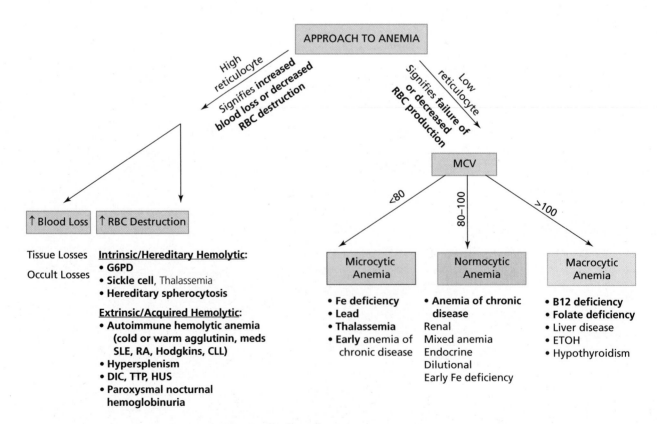

Figure 12.1 Approach to Anemia

Management/Prognosis

- Treat underlying cause

Iron Deficiency Anemia

- Most common cause of low RBCs caused by insufficient amounts of iron in body
- Caused by blood loss (excessive menstruation, occult blood loss eg, colon cancer, parasitic hook worm infection) or decreased dietary intake (in children, eg, diet high in cow's milk)
- Classic symptoms include pagophagia (craving for ice); pica (appetite for non-food substances, eg, clay); Plummer–Vinson syndrome (dysphagia + esophageal webs + atrophic glossitis + iron deficiency); and angular cheilitis (inflammation of ≥1 corner(s) of mouth), koilonychia (spooning of the nails), tachycardia, glossitis (smooth, enlarged tongue)
- Diagnose with CBC: classically microcytic, hypochromic anemia (may be normocytic early on or if a mixed disorder occurs, such as B12 deficiency)
  - Decreased reticulocyte count
  - Iron studies: low serum iron and ferritin, increased TIBC, decreased reticulocyte count in chronic cases, decreased transferrin saturation
  - Increased RDW
- Management is iron replacement (vitamin C may increase absorption); GI side effects may result so gradually increase dose

---

Microcytic Anemia (Etiologies):

Singing the **ABCDs** while bleeding can **lead** to a microcytic anemia.

- **A**lpha thalassemia
- **B**eta thalassemia
- **C**hronic disease (early on)
- **D**eficiency of iron

- **L**ead poisoning

THALASSEMIA

Inherited blood disorder which lowers the production of functional hemoglobin

Alpha Thalassemia

- Decreased production of alpha globin chains
- Most commonly Southeast Asians (68%), Africans (30%), and those of Mediterranean descent (5–10%)
- **Abnormal alleles:** carrier state 1/4; alpha thalassemia minor (trait) 2/4; hemoglobin H disease 3/4; hydrops fetalis 4/4
- Carrier state is usually asymptomatic
- Alpha thalassemia minor presents with mild microcytic anemia
- Hemoglobin H disease presents with chronic anemia, hepatosplenomegaly, frontal and maxilla bone overgrowth, pigmented stones
- Hydrops fetalis is associated with stillbirth or death shortly after birth
- Diagnose with **CBC** (hypochromic, microcytic anemia [usually decreased] with normal or increased RBCs and normal or increased serum iron stores; **peripheral smear** shows target cells, tear drop cells, basophilic stippling; Heinz bodies (hemoglobin H disease) (beta-chain tetramers); **Hgb electrophoresis** shows normal hemoglobin ratios in adults
- Manage as follows: no treatment needed for **mild disease** (alpha-trait); folate (if reticulocyte count is high) and avoid oxidative stress (eg, sulfa drugs) for **moderate disease**; weekly blood transfusion, iron-chelating agents (deferoxamine, deferasirox), and vitamin C and folate supplementation for **severe disease** (bone marrow transplantation definitive treatment in major cases)

Beta Thalassemia

- Decreased production of beta-globin chains leading to excess alpha chains
- Most commonly those of Mediterranean descent (eg, Greek, Italian), Africans, Indians
- **Abnormal alleles:** beta thalassemia trait (minor) 1/2; beta thalassemia major (Cooley's anemia) 2/2; beta thalassemia intermedia: mild homozygous form
- Beta thalassemia trait (minor) is usually asymptomatic but may have mild/moderate anemia
- Beta thalassemia intermedia presents with milder symptoms compared to major
- Beta thalassemia major (Cooley's anemia) usually become symptomatic at age 6 months: severe hemolytic anemia (jaundice, dyspnea, pallor, splenomegaly), frontal bossing, iron overload, pigmented gallstones
- Diagnose with **CBC**: hypochromic, microcytic anemia (decreased most common) with normal or increased RBCs, normal or increased serum iron; **peripheral smear** shows target cells, tear drop cells, basophilic stippling
- **Hgb electrophoresis** shows:

	Hgb F	Hgb A$_2$	Hgb A
β-thal trait (minor)	Increased	Increased	Decreased
β-thal major (Cooley's)	Increased up to 90%	Increased	Little to none

- Manage as follows: genetic counseling for **beta thalassemia trait (minor)**; periodic transfusions, deferoxamine/other chelating agent, possible bone marrow transplantation; vitamin C, folate, splenectomy for **beta thalassemia major/severe anemia**

LEAD POISONING (PLUMBISM)

Lead poisoning causing cell death and poisoning of enzymes needed for heme synthesis; leads to acquired sideroblastic anemia

Risk Factors

- Most commonly children (age <6)

Clinical Manifestations/Physical Exam

- May be asymptomatic or nonspecific symptoms (eg, anorexia)
- Neurologic symptoms: ataxia, fatigue, learning or developmental delays, hearing loss
- Peripheral neuropathy may be seen with sickle cell anemia and lead poisoning
  - Encephalopathy: mental status changes, vomiting
- GI symptoms: Lead colic leads to intermittent abdominal pain, vomiting, anorexia, and constipation
- Anemia: pallor, shock, coma; renal: chronic interstitial nephritis and metabolic acidosis

Diagnosis

- Peripheral smear: microcytic hypochromic anemia with basophilic stippling (dots of denatured RNA seen in RBCs) and ringed sideroblasts in bone marrow (iron accumulation in mitochondria due to failure of incorporation of iron into Hgb)
- Increased serum lead >97.5th percentile for pediatric population (5 mcg/dL or 0.24 mmol/L), increased serum iron; decreased TIBC
- Increased erythrocyte protoporphyrin: elevations can be seen in both iron deficiency and lead poisoning (usually worse in lead poisoning)
- X-ray: "lead lines" linear hyperdensities at metaphyseal plates; lead lines in gums (adults)

Management/Prognosis

- Remove source of lead
- Chelation therapy: may be needed if severe or >45 mcg/dL; 2-,3-dimercaptosuccinic acid, calcium disodium EDTA, dimercaprol, and penicillamine

Hematology

B12 (COBALAMIN) DEFICIENCY

Deficiency in the water-soluble vitamin B12

Etiology/Pathophysiology

- Natural sources derived from food of mainly animal origin; B12 is released by the acidity of the stomach and combines with intrinsic factor, where it is absorbed mainly by the distal ileum
- B12 deficiency causes abnormal synthesis of DNA, nucleic acids, and metabolism of erythroid precursors; B12 is needed to convert homocysteine into methionine and for DNA synthesis
- On average, it takes about 3–4 years to develop deficiency once B12 intake/absorption is impaired
- Malabsorption:
  - Pernicious anemia is the most common cause (lack of intrinsic factor due to parietal cell antibodies, leading to gastric atrophy)
  - Crohn's disease (affects the terminal ileum); ileal resection, gastrectomy, tropical sprue, Zollinger–Ellison syndrome
  - Meds: H2 receptor antagonists, PPIs, decreased nucleic acid synthesis (zidovudine, hydroxyurea), anticonvulsants
- Decreased intake (eg, vegans, who do not eat animal products and are therefore low in B12)

Clinical Manifestations/Physical Exam

- Anemia symptoms, pallor, glossitis, stomatitis, GI symptoms, psychological symptoms, hyperhomocysteinemia, hyperpigmentation
- Neurologic symptoms: B12 deficiency causes spinal cord demyelination, degeneration and peripheral neuropathy (especially in lower extremities), leads to ataxia, weakness, vibratory, sensory, and proprioception deficits, decreased DTR; abnormal Babinski, seizures, hypotonia

Diagnosis

- Peripheral smear:
  - Increased MCV >115 almost exclusively seen in B12 or folate deficiency especially if hypersegmented neutrophils seen (>5 lobes); oval macrocytes
- Increased homocysteine and methylmalonic acid levels
- Pernicious anemia: positive intrinsic factor antibodies, parietal cell antibodies, increased gastrin levels; positive Schilling test

Management/Prognosis

- B12 replacement: start with IM B12 hydroxycobalamin injections (6) at 3–7-day intervals and provide maintenance therapy of IV B12 every 3 months; watch for signs of hypokalemia

PAM the **vegan** wore the **crown** for drinking **alcohol**.

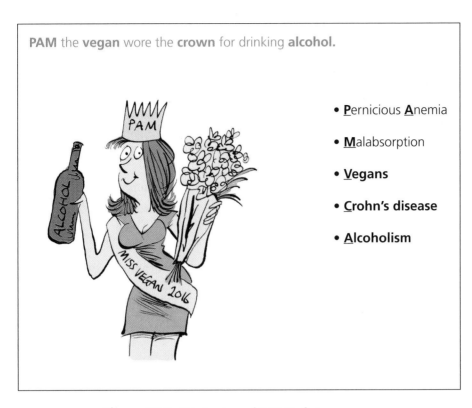

- **P**ernicious **A**nemia
- **M**alabsorption
- **V**egans
- **C**rohn's disease
- **A**lcoholism

Figure 12.2 Etiologies of B12 Deficiency

After **1:00** AM, Pam couldn't type **SMH** on her phone because of **paresthesias in her fingertips.**

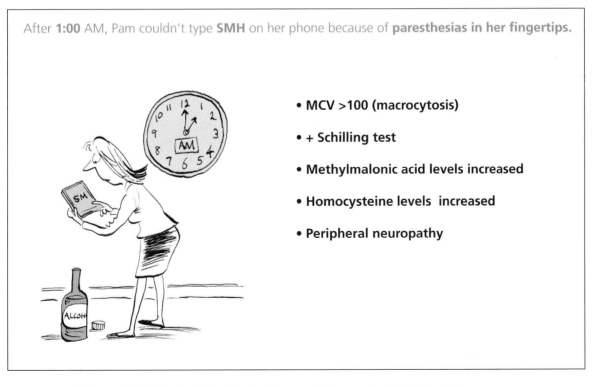

- **MCV >100 (macrocytosis)**
- **+ Schilling test**
- **Methylmalonic acid levels increased**
- **Homocysteine levels increased**
- **Peripheral neuropathy**

Figure 12.3 Clinical Manifestation and Diagnosis of B12 Deficiency

FOLATE DEFICIENCY

Deficiency in folate, a water-soluble B vitamin found in animal organs (eg, liver, kidney), green vegetables, and fruits to name a few; folate absorption occurs in the jejunum

Etiology/Pathophysiology

- Etiology
  - Inadequate folic acid intake usually occurs in the setting of increased vitamin requirements (eg, growth in infancy, chronic hemolysis)
  - Malabsorption: chronic diarrhea or chronic inflammation (eg, celiac or inflammatory bowel disease); some anticonvulsants (eg, phenytoin, phenobarbital)
  - Folic acid inhibition: methotrexate, pyrimethamine, trimethoprim
- Pathophysiology
  - Folate deficiency causes abnormal synthesis of DNA, nucleic acids and metabolism of erythroid precursor cells
  - Folate stores last only for 2–4 months; peak incidence in children occurs age 4–7 months

Clinical Manifestations/Physical Exam

- Anemia symptoms similar to B12 but without significant neurologic abnormalities

Diagnosis

- Peripheral smear: increased, most commonly >115 (macrocytic anemia), hypersegmented neutrophils, low reticulocyte count
- Decreased serum folate levels; increased LDH
- Increased homocysteine; methylmalonic acids are not elevated

Management/Prognosis

- Oral folic acid: 1 mg PO daily until hematologic correction
- IV folic acid (for severe folic acid deficiency and folate deficiency in pregnancy associated with neural tube defects); replacing folic acid in those with B12 deficiency will correct anemia but will worsen neurological symptoms

ANEMIA OF CHRONIC DISEASE

Multifactorial anemia due to the presence of a chronic inflammatory condition, such as infection, autoimmune disease, or cancer

Etiology/Pathophysiology

- Etiology: chronic inflammatory conditions (e.g., chronic infection, inflammation, autoimmune disorders, malignancy)
- Pathophysiology
  - Increased hepcidin (an acute phase reactant) blocks release of iron from macrophages and GI absorption
  - Increased ferritin (as an acute phase reactant) sequesters iron into storage
  - Erythropoietin inhibition: via cytokines

Diagnosis

- CBC: mild normochromic normocytic anemia (± present with hypochromic microcytic anemia early on)
- Increased ferritin and decreased TIBC, decreased serum Fe (serum ferritin and TIBC may be in normal limits)

Management/Prognosis

- Treat underlying disease
- Erythropoietin alpha if renal disease

In anemia of chronic disease, iron goes from the serum and hides in the stores!

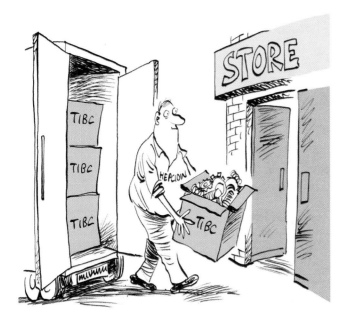

- **Decreased serum Fe** (hepcidin decreases Fe absorption and availability)

- **Increased ferritIN** (storage protein, ie, puts iron IN storage)

- **Decreased TIBC** (similar to transferrin)

Figure 12.4 Anemia of Chronic Disease

HEREDITARY SPHEROCYTOSIS

Autosomal dominant intrinsic hemolytic anemia

Etiology/Pathophysiology

- Most commonly Northern Europeans
- Pathophysiology: deficiency in RBC membrane/cytoskeleton (lack of spectrin protein) leads to increased protein fragility and sphere-shaped RBCs, resulting in RBC hemolysis in spleen by splenic macrophages

Clinical Manifestations/Physical Exam

- Anemia, jaundice, splenomegaly, pigmented gallstones

Diagnosis

- CBC with peripheral smear
  - 80% spherocytes (round RBC)
  - Microcytosis with **hyperchromia** (lack of RBC central pallor)
  - Increased MCHC, increased RDW
  - Possible evidence of hemolysis (eg, schistocytes)
- Coombs test negative; helps distinguish hereditary spherocytosis from autoimmune hemolytic anemia
- Confirmatory tests: **osmotic fragility test** (RBC lysis occurs more easily than normal when placed in hypotonic solution indicative of hereditary spherocytosis) and **eosin-5'-maleimide (EMA) binding** (preferred)

Management

- Folic acid supplementation to sustain RBC production and DNA synthesis (not curative but helpful)
- Splenectomy (severe disease) stops splenic RBC destruction; if possible, delay in children until age ≥ 4 after risk of severe sepsis from encapsulated organisms has peaked; give anti-pneumococcal vaccine prior to splenectomy
- Complications of hereditary spherocytosis include aplastic crisis, hemolytic crisis, folate deficiency, and pigmented gallstones

---

Autoimmune hemolytic anemia

With enough effort, you **can Comb** away acquired diseases.

- **Coombs positive**
- Also associated with spherocytosis with Coombs testing positivity

---

SICKLE CELL DISEASE

Autosomal recessive genetic disorder of Hgb SS leading to valine substitutes for glutamic acid on β-chain

Etiology/Pathophysiology

- Sickle cell trait: heterozygous hemoglobin S (8% of African Americans); confers some resistance to *Plasmodium falciparum* (malaria); usually asymptomatic unless exposed to severe hypoxia; 25–45% of their hemoglobin is hemoglobin S
- Pathophysiology: decreased solubility of Hgb S under stressful conditions (hypoxemia, infection, dehydration, cold weather, pregnancy) leads to RBC sickling and causes microthrombosis (± organ damage) and hemolytic anemia; sickled cells are destroyed by spleen

Risk Factors

- 0.15% of African Americans

Clinical Manifestations/Physical Exam

- Signs of microthrombosis (infarctions):
  - Skeletal: avascular (ischemic) necrosis of bones (eg, femoral or humeral head), "H"-shaped vertebrae
  - Painful occlusive crises: acute chest syndrome, back, abdominal, bone pain; renal or hepatic dysfunction; priapism common
  - Splenic sequestration crisis: acute splenomegaly and rapid drop in decreased hemoglobin (± fatal)
  - Skin ulcers: especially on the tibia
  - Dactylitis (painful swelling of hands and feet), most common in infants
- Infections due to widespread microthrombosis and early functional asplenia in childhood (increased risk of infection with encapsulated organisms like *S. pneumo, H. flu, N. meningitidis*, GBS)
- Aplastic crisis associated with parvovirus B-19 infection
- Patients with sickle cell trait may have painless hematuria

Diagnosis

- CBC with peripheral smear
  - Decreased hemoglobin (5–9 g/dL), decreased hematocrit (17–29%)
  - Target cells, sickled erythrocytes; ± Howell–Jolly bodies (indicates functional asplenia)
- Hemoglobin electrophoresis
  - Sickle cell disease: Hgb S, no Hgb A, increased Hgb F
  - Sickle cell trait: Hgb S, decreased Hgb A

Management/Prognosis

- Crisis management: IV hydration, oxygen, analgesia (high dose meperidine may lead to seizures and renal failure)
- Supportive medications for those with severe or frequent crisis episodes: hydroxyurea; folic acid
- Childhood immunizations:
  - *S. pneumococcus: Haemophilus influenzae* type B and N. *meningitidis* ("**SHiN**")
  - Children should receive prophylactic penicillin until age 5–6
- Allogeneic stem cell transplant: only potentially curative treatment but has significant side effects
- RBC transfusion for severe anemia (eg, acute chest syndrome, splenic sequestration)

IMMUNE (IDIOPATHIC) THROMBOCYTOPENIC PURPURA

Bleeding disorder in which the immune system destroys platelets

Etiology/Pathophysiology

- Primary ITP: idiopathic; most common in children/boys often after a viral infection (usually self-limiting)
- Secondary ITP: immune-mediated but often associated with underlying disorders (eg, systemic lupus erythematosus, HIV, hepatitis C virus, Hodgkins, non-Hodgkins, etc.); most common type in adults and is usually recurrent
- Pathophysiology
  - Autoimmune antibody reaction against glycoprotein IIb/IIIa receptors on platelets leads to splenic-mediated platelet destruction
  - Evans syndrome: ITP and autoimmune hemolytic anemia

Clinical Manifestations/Physical Exam

- Often asymptomatic; not associated with splenomegaly
- Mucocutaneous bleeding: petechiae, purpura, bruises, bullae, ecchymosis, menorrhagia, GI, bleeding of gums, epistaxis

Diagnosis

- Isolated thrombocytopenia with normal PTT, PT/INR
- Peripheral smear: usually normal but ± megakaryocytes
- Bone marrow: normal; marrow testing usually reserved for older patients or non-responsive patients

Management/Prognosis

- Children: observation (approximately 80% of cases are resolved without treatment within 6 months) leads to ± IV immunoglobulin (IVIG)
- Adults: corticosteroids first; if unresolved, consider IVIG or additional immunosuppressants (rituximab, anti-CD20/B-cell monoclonal antibody) for those needing splenectomy; platelet transfusion may be required if count <20,000/μL to prevent spontaneous intracranial hemorrhage

THROMBOTIC THROMBOCYTOPENIC PURPURA

Bleeding disorder in which clots form in small blood vessels leading to low platelet count

Etiology/Pathophysiology

- Primary TTP: idiopathic (autoimmune); Ab versus ADAMTS13 leads to decreased ADAMTS13 (a von Willebrand factor cleaving protease) resulting in large vWF multimers which stick to platelets and cause endothelial platelet adhesion and eventual small vessel thrombosis
- Secondary TTP: secondary to malignancy, bone marrow transplantation, estrogen, pregnancy, HIV1, ticlopidine, clopidogrel

Clinical Manifestations/Physical Exam

- Pentad (rare for patients to present with all five simultaneously since plasma exchange therapy has been developed)
  - Thrombocytopenia
  - Microangiopathic hemolytic anemia
  - Kidney failure/uremia (less common)
  - Neurologic symptoms (headache, CVA, altered sensorium)
  - Fever (rare)
- Splenomegaly (common)

Diagnosis

- CBC with peripheral smear: thrombocytopenia, hemolytic anemia (schistocytes, increased reticulocytes)
- Hemolysis: increased LDH, decreased haptoglobin, increased indirect bilirubin
- Normal PT/INR and PTT. Coombs negative

Management/Prognosis

- Plasmapheresis is treatment of choice
- Immunosuppression: corticosteroids, cyclophosphamides, etc.; no platelet transfusions (may cause thrombi formation)
- ± splenomegaly if refractory to plasmapheresis and corticosteroids

On his 13th birthday, Adam von Willebrand went FAR away to TAN and watch his new splendid big screen Plasma TV.

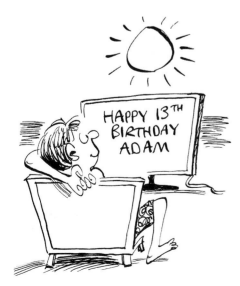

Pathophysiology:
- Antibodies against **ADAMTS13** lead to **decreased cleavage of vWF**

Clinical Manifestations:
Pentad:
- **F**ever, **A**cute **R**enal failure
- **T**hrombocytopenia, **A**nemia, and **N**eurological symptoms
- Splenomegaly (splendid big)

Management:
Plasmapheresis

Figure 12.5 Thrombotic Thrombocytopenic Purpura (TTP)

Hematology

HEPARIN-INDUCED THROMBOCYTOPENIA (HIT)

Acquired thrombocytopenia due to heparin; commonly seen within the initial 5–10 days of heparin administration

Etiology/Pathophysiology

- Antibody formation to the hapten of heparin and platelet factor 4, causing platelet activation, leading to simultaneous thrombocytopenia and thrombosis
- Differs from other types of thrombocytopenia in that HIT patients don't usually develop severe thrombocytopenia
- Not associated with bleeding
- Usually associated with increased risk of thrombosis
- Can occur with low molecular weight heparin but is 10 times more common with unfractionated heparin

Diagnosis

- 4 Ts: thrombocytopenia; timing of platelet count drop; thrombosis; other sequelae

Management/Prognosis

- Direct thrombin inhibitor: argatroban, bivalirudin
- Fondaparinux: a synthetic factor Xa inhibitor
- Long-term anticoagulation with warfarin only after other non-heparin anticoagulation has been started and the thrombosis has decreased because of the initial prothrombotic state normally associated with the first 5 days of the initiation of warfarin therapy

HIT with **other anticoagulants** but **don't start a WAR!!**

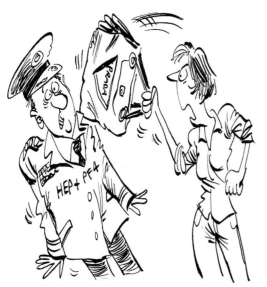

- **Due to hapten formation between heparin + platelet factor 4 leads to Ab formation**

HIT

- **HIT antibody testing (platelet factor 4 antibodies)**
- **Immediate discontinuation of heparin**
- **Thrombin inhibitors: bivalirudin, argatroban. Fondaparinux (a Factor Xa inhibitor can also be used)**

Management:
DO not use warfarin as INITIAL therapy (may cause thrombosis).

Figure 12.6 Heparin-Induced Thrombocytopenia (HIT)

Hematology

HEMOLYTIC UREMIC SYNDROME

Triad of thrombocytopenia, microangiopathic hemolytic anemia, and kidney failure (uremia), which is more common in HUS than TTP

Etiology/Pathophysiology

- D$^+$ HUS (classic): associated with diarrhea; platelet activation by exotoxins (eg, *Shigella* toxin and Shiga-like toxin in *E. coli* 0157:H7) enters the blood where it damages vascular endothelium, activating platelets (microthrombi formation), eventually depleting platelets (causing thrombocytopenia); the toxins preferentially damage the kidney (causing uremia and HTN); these micro-clots damage circulating RBCs, leads to hemolytic anemia
- D-HUS (atypical): not associated with diarrhea
- P-HUS: *Streptococcus pneumoniae* releases neuraminidase, which initiates an inflammatory reaction

Diagnosis

- Same labs/peripheral smear as TTP (hemolytic anemia, normal PT/INR, PTT); increased BUN/creatinine

Management/Prognosis

- Observation in most children (usually self-limiting); may need supportive dialysis
- Plasmapheresis ($\pm$ FFP) if severe, neurologic complications and non-renal complications
- Antibiotics may actually worsen condition (due to increased verotoxin release)

DISSEMINATED INTRAVASCULAR COAGULATION

Overactivity of blood clotting proteins

Etiology/Pathophysiology

- Etiology
  - Infections (eg, gram-negative sepsis endotoxins)
  - Malignancies: acute myelogenous leukemia; lung, GI, or prostate malignancies
  - Obstetric: preeclampsia; abruptio placentae, septic abortion, amniotic embolus
  - Massive tissue injury and trauma: burns, liver disease, aortic aneurysm, adult respiratory distress syndrome
- Pathophysiology
  - Pathological activation of coagulation system leads to widespread microthrombi, which consumes coagulation proteins (V, VIII, fibrinogen) and platelets causing severe thrombocytopenia

Clinical Manifestations/Physical Exam

- Acute illness with widespread hemorrhage (oozing from venipuncture sites, mouth, nose; extensive bruising) and thrombosis (renal failure, gangrene [as clots block circulation], hepatic/respiratory dysfunction)

Diagnosis

- Increased thrombin formation: decreased fibrinogen, increased PTT/PT/INR; severe thrombocytopenia
- Increased fibrinolysis: increased D-dimer (most sensitive test)
- Peripheral smear: fragmented RBCs (schistocytes)

Management/Prognosis

- Treat underlying cause
- Platelet transfusion if platelets <20,000/μL
- Fresh frozen plasma if severe bleeding (replaces all the coagulation factors)
- Cryoprecipitate (replaces fibrinogen in patients with severely low levels)
- ± heparin for thrombosis

Hematology

VON WILLEBRAND DISEASE

Autosomal dominant disorder and most common hereditary bleeding disorder (1% of population); may also be acquired

Etiology/Pathophysiology

- Von Willebrand factor (vWF) has two roles: serves as an adhesion molecule for the platelet to adhere to exposed endothelium and serves to prevent factor VIII degradation
- Deficiency in vWF leads to prolonged bleeding (eg, after minor lacerations)

Clinical Manifestations/Physical Exam

- Mucocutaneous bleeding: easy bruising, epistaxis, gums, GI bleeding, menorrhagia; varying degrees of bleeding
- Petechiae: common in vWF

Diagnosis

- Screening tests
  - Plasma vWF antigen: decreased vWF antigen or vWF activity ≤30 IU is diagnostic
  - Plasma vWF activity (ristocetin cofactor activity and vWF collagen binding): no platelet aggregation with ristocetin
  - Factor VIII activity: possibly decreased
- Specialized assays help to determine the type
  - vWF multimer distribution using gel electrophoresis
  - Ristocetin-induced platelet aggregation (gold standard)
- Coagulation studies: prolonged PTT
  - PTT corrects with mixing study
  - PTT and bleeding time prolongation worse with aspirin
  - Platelet count usually normal except in type 2B, which is associated with mild thrombocytopenia

Management/Prognosis

- **Type I:** quantitative deficiency (most common, 75%)
  - Mild disease: no treatment needed
  - Mild to moderate bleeding: DDAVP (desmopressin)
  - Severe bleeding: vWF-containing product (eg, factor VIII concentrates, purified vWF concentrates, recombinant vWF)
- **Type II** (qualitative deficiency): DDAVP for most; vWF or DDAVP prior to procedures
- **Type III** (severe, absent VWF): vWF-containing product (eg, human-derived factor VIII concentrates, purified vWF concentrates, recombinant vWF)

ACUTE LYMPHOCYTIC LEUKEMIA

Malignancy arising from immature lymphoid cells in bone marrow, lymph nodes, spleen, liver, other organs

Etiology/Pathophysiology

- B cell most common type, T cell, null type (non-B/T cell)
- TdT positive is a common marker of lymphoblasts
- B precursor cell surface markers: CD10+, CD 19+, CD 20+
- Mature B cell surface markers: CD10± 19, 20, 22, 25
- T precursor cell surface markers: CD2 through CD8 (no CD10)
- Cytogenetics in B cell all:
  - Translocation t(12;21) associated with a better prognosis
  - t(9;22) Philadelphia chromosome; positively associated with poorer prognosis (seen only in approximately 4% of children, usually older age)

Risk Factors

- Most common childhood leukemia (peak age 3–7)
- High incidence with Down syndrome (age ≥5)

Clinical Manifestations/Physical Exam

- Pancytopenia symptoms, fatigue, lethargy, bone pain
- CNS symptoms: headache, stiff neck, visual changes, vomiting
- **T** cell variant: **t**hymus gland mass, most common in **t**eenagers, **TdT** positive
- Physical exam: lymphadenopathy (50%); hepatosplenomegaly; anemia (pallor, fatigue; thrombocytopenia: petechiae, bruising)

Diagnosis

- Bone marrow: hypercellular with >20% blasts
- Increased WBCs: 5,000–100,000 (despite increased WBCs, these immature cells are incapable of fighting off infection)
- Anemia, thrombocytopenia, peripheral smear may show cytoplasmic aggregates with periodic acid-Schiff (PAS) positivity

Management/Prognosis

- Highly responsive to combination chemotherapy; remission >90%
- Treatment regimens may include oral chemotherapy (eg, imatinib in Philadelphia positive types)
- Methotrexate for CNS disease
- Stem cell transplant for certain cases of relapse

Of ALL the children with ALL, some have a BALL and a blast DOWN in Philadelphia, PA.

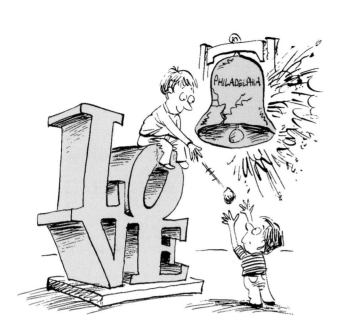

- ALL most common in children

- **B** cell precursor most common type

- **A**spiration of bone marrow to look for:
  - **L**ymphoblasts (>20%)
  - **L**ymphadenopathy (50%)

- **DOWN** syndrome: increased risk for ALL after age 5

- Philadelphia chromosome positive in some patients with ALL (usually older children)

- **PA:** lymphoblasts in ALL often have coarse clumps of PAS-positive material in their cytoplasm

Figure 12.7 Acute Lymphocytic Leukemia

Hematology

CHRONIC LYMPHOCYTIC LEUKEMIA (B Cell)

Clonal malignancy of mature (but incompetent) B lymphocytes

Etiology/Pathophysiology

- Small lymphocytic lymphoma: variant associated with predominant lymph node involvement with little peripheral blood involvement

Risk Factors

- Most commonly Caucasian men, age ≥50
- Most common form of leukemia in adults

Clinical Manifestations/Physical Exam

- Usually asymptomatic (often incidental lab finding)
- Pancytopenia: anemia symptoms, increased infections (due to neutropenia)
- Lymphadenopathy, splenomegaly

Diagnosis

- Peripheral smear: well-differentiated lymphocytes with scattered "smudge cells" (fragile B cells that become smudged during slide preparation)
- Peripheral blood flow cell cytometry: looks for cloning
  - CD19 and CD20 positivity; CD5 positivity (normally CD5 is a T-cell surface marker but can be seen on B cells in CLL)
- Prognostic markers:
  - Prognostic markers: include ZAP-70, CD38, IGHV gene mutation
  - Cytogenetics: del(13q), trisomy 12 have a favorable prognosis; del(17p), del(11q) have a poorer prognosis

Management/Prognosis

- Varied treatment but includes oral chemotherapy if in chronic phase (acute blastic crisis may be treated like AML in some cases)

The old, fragile lab tech born Before 1920 slowly ZAPped the slide, smudging the CeLL until only a small lymphocyte remained.

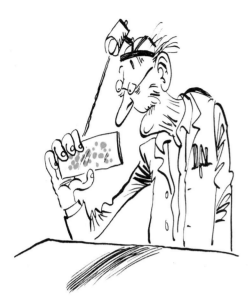

- **B cells are mature**
- **B cell most common type**
- **B cell surface marker positivity CD 19, CD 20**
- **Smudge cells: fragile B cells that smudge when preparing slides**

Figure 12.8 Chronic Lymphocytic Leukemia

- Old: most common leukemia in adults (usually presents age >50)
- B cell most common type (~95%) are mature
- 1920 B cell surface marker positivity for CD19 and CD 20 but may also contain CD5 marker (normally present on T cells)
- Slowly: most indolent form; slow onset of symptoms; doesn't commonly progress to acute form
- ZAP: biomarker positivity associated with a poorer prognosis
- Smudge cells: fragile B cells that smudge when preparing the slides
- Small lymphocytic lymphoma: identical cells to CLL (but seen primarily only in lymph node)

Hematology

CHRONIC MYELOGENOUS LEUKEMIA (CML)

Overproduction of WBCs (granulocytes)

Etiology/Pathophysiology

- Chromosome translocation 9;22 (Philadelphia chromosome) leads to fusion gene BCR-ABL1 leads to inhibition of apoptosis and increased cell division (proliferation) of well-differentiated granulocytes, especially neutrophils (but often have peripheral basophilia and eosinophilia)

Clinical Manifestations/Physical Exam

- 70% asymptomatic
- Patients usually age >50
- Splenomegaly (especially if converting to acute leukemia)

Diagnosis

- Translocation 9;22 (Philadelphia chromosome) oncogene positive
- Increased WBC counts: strikingly elevated (eg, 100,000); increased LDH
- Decreased LAP (leukocyte alkaline phosphatase) score (LAP only found in functioning non-leukemic WBCs, eg, leukemoid reaction)
- Chronic <5% blasts; accelerated >5% to 30% blasts; acute blast crisis: >20%

Management/Prognosis

- Imatinib: oral chemotherapy in Philadelphia positive CML (inhibits tyrosine kinase activity of the BCR-ABL protein); other tyrosine kinase inhibitors include dasatinib, ponatinib
- Other agents may be used in resistant cases

Imatinib put a breakable bottle of Philadelphia CreaM cheese down on his LAP with glee and ate so much of the white cream his spleen popped BEfore the clock struck 9:22.

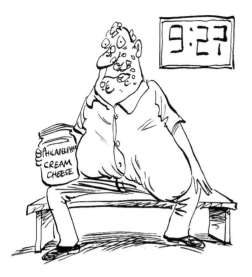

- **Imatinib (Gleevec): oral treatment used in Philadelphia positive leukemia**

- **Philadelphia chromosome** translocation between chromosome **9 and 22** giving rise to a fusion gene **BCR-ABL1** (breakable)

- **Markedly elevated WBC count with** low leukocyte alkaline phosphatase (LAP) score

Figure 12.9 Chronic Myelogenous Leukemia

- **Imatinib (Gleevec)** oral treatment used in Philadelphia positive leukemia
- **Philadelphia chromosome** translocation between chromosome **9 and 22** giving rise to a fusion gene
- **BCR-ABL1** (breakable) most commonly associated with CML
- **Down on LAP:** low leukocyte alkaline phosphatase score helps distinguish CML from leukemoid reaction
- So much white cream, struck: associated with a **strikingly elevated WBC count**
- **BE: B**asophilia, **E**osinophilia
- **Splenomegaly**

ACUTE MYELOID LEUKEMIA (AML)

Most common acute leukemia in adults (80% of cases) due to myeloblast proliferation in the bone marrow

Etiology/Pathophysiology

- Major subtypes:
  - Acute promyelocytic leukemia (APL): associated with t(15;17), leading to disruption in retinoic acid receptor that normally promotes maturation of the myeloblast; myeloperoxidase positive compared to the other two; increased risk of DIC
  - Acute megakaryoblastic leukemia: associated with Down syndrome in children age <5 (ALL seen if age >5)
  - Acute monocytic leukemia: gingival infiltration and hyperplasia

Risk Factors

- Majority of patients are older than 50
- May be a complication of myelodysplastic syndrome

Clinical Manifestations/Physical Exam

- Symptoms of anemia, thrombocytopenia and/or neutropenia
- Splenomegaly, hepatomegaly, bone pain
- Leukostasis (WBC >100,000) leads to CNS deficits: headaches, confusion, transient ischemic attacks, CVA (stroke)

Diagnosis

- Bone marrow:
  - >20% blasts
  - Auer rods: crystalized myeloperoxidase aggregate in APL
  - Myeloperoxidase staining negative in monocytic and megakaryoblastic variants

Management/Prognosis

- Induction:
  - Combination chemotherapy: eg, cytarabine and anthracycline (doxorubicin) chemotherapy usually given until <5% blasts and <20% cellularity
  - All-trans-retinoic acid: used in APL
  - Stem cell bone marrow transplant if age <70 and normal organ function
- Postremission therapy:
  - Given to eradicate residual leukemic cells; intensive chemotherapy and stem cell transplantation
- Supportive:
  - Granulocyte-macrophage stimulating colony factor: improves neutrophil recovery; may be given in elderly patients or patients with complicated courses
- Complications of treatment:
  - Tumor lysis syndrome: potentially lethal complication occurring 48–72 hours after initiation of chemotherapy (due to large number of cells being destroyed) leads to hyperuricemia, hyperkalemia, hypocalcemia, hyperphosphatemia, acute renal failure; management: allopurinol, IV fluids
  - DIC: either prior to treatment or with treatment (release of Auer rods into circulation may promote prothrombotic state)

While **FISH**ing in the **CRIST**al clear water, **AMIL** casted his **AUER rod down** and it got **stuck** on some **gum.**

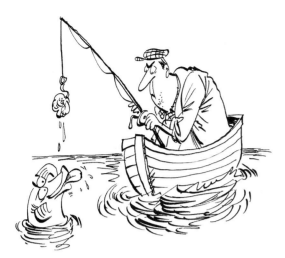

- **Auer rod** in promyelocytic variant

- Immature white blood cells (**blasts**) seen in bone marrow

- **Leukostasis:** high WBC

- **Gum:** gingival hyperplasia seen in monocytic form

- **FISH: F**luorescent **in s**itu **H**ybridization used for cytogenetic testing in leukemias

Figure 12.10 Acute Myelogenous Leukemia

Treatment Options in AML:
- **Chemotherapy**
- **Radiation therapy**
- **Immunotherapy**
- **Stem cell transplantation**

AMIL (AML)
- **A**uer rod
- **M**yeloperoxidase positive in acute promyelocytic leukemia form of AML
- **I**mmature WBC (**blasts**) seen in bone marrow
- **L**ysis syndrome results from rapid destruction of cells during initiation of chemotherapy in patients with AML

- **Down:** associated with Down syndrome in children age <5 (age >5 has higher association with ALL)
- **Stuck:** leukostasis (WBCs) due to high white count makes blood sludge which can lead to complications ie, CVA
- **Gum:** gingival hyperplasia common in the acute monocytic leukemia form of AML

MULTIPLE MYELOMA (PLASMACYTOMA)

Cancer associated with proliferation of a single clone of plasma cells, leads to increased monoclonal Ab (esp IgG, IgA) ±IgM

Etiology/Pathophysiology

- Increased risk: elderly age (>65), African Americans, men, possible exposure to herpes virus and to benzene
- Plasma cells accumulate in bone marrow, interrupting bone marrow's normal cell production

Clinical Manifestations/Physical Exam

- "**BREAK**" your bones in Multiple Myeloma
  - **B**one pain
  - **R**ecurrent infections
  - **E**levated calcium
  - **A**nemia
  - **K**idney failure

Diagnosis

- Serum protein electrophoresis: monoclonal protein spike IgG 60%, IgA (20%)
- Urine protein electrophoresis: Bence-Jones proteins: kappa or lambda light chains
- CBC: Rouleaux formation (RBCs stick together as a result of increased plasma protein and increased ESR)
- Skull x-ray: "punched-out" lytic skull lesions
- Bone marrow: plasmacytosis >10%

Management/Prognosis

- Stem cell transplant (± preceded by chemotherapy eg, thalidomide)
- Chemotherapy usually controls symptoms temporarily; local radiation therapy
- Bisphosphonates for bony involvement

You **"BREAK"** your bones in Multiple Myeloma.

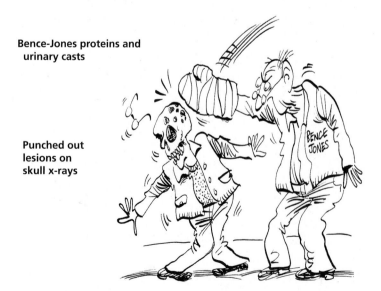

Bence-Jones proteins and urinary casts

Punched out lesions on skull x-rays

Clinical Manifestations:
Bone pain
Recurrent infections
Elevated calcium
Anemia
Kidney failure

Increased incidence (age >65)

Serum and protein electrophoresis

Figure 12.11 Multiple Myeloma

Hematology

Chapter 13

Pharmacology

CYTOCHROME P450 INDUCERS

Increase enzyme activity, thereby decreasing the concentration and effect of a chemical or drug

MOA/Pharmacokinetics

- Medications which induce the cytochrome P450 system may decrease the effectiveness of other drugs (eg, CP450 inducers can reduce serum levels of warfarin, theophylline, phenytoin)

John was **wort**hy when referred and **inducted** into sainthood for giving up **chronic alcohol** use and placing him**self on a real** fast, **fend**ing off **greasy carbs**, leading to **less warfar**e with **theo**logians.

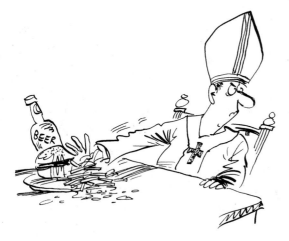

Inducers of the P450:
- **St. Johns wort**
- **Rifampin** (referred)
- **Chronic alcohol use**
- **Sulfonylureas** (self on a real)
- **Phenytoin, phenobarbital** (fend)
- **Griseofulvin** (greasy)
- **Carbamazepine** (carbs)

Figure 13.1 Cytochrome P450 Inducers

Drugs that induce CP450 system can lead to decreased levels of certain drugs, eg, warfarin (less warfare), theophylline (theologians), and phenytoin.

CYTOCHROME P450 INHIBITORS

Decrease enzyme activity, thereby increasing the concentration and effect of a chemical or drug

MOA/Pharmacokinetics

- ○ Medications which inhibit the cytochrome P450 system may increase the effectiveness of other drugs (eg, CP450 inhibitors can increase the serum levels of warfarin, theophylline, and phenytoin)

Despite their **inhibitions**, **Val and Quin** took the **metro** and **met a dean** named **Amio** at bar **Keto** where they sipped on **a cute alcoholic** drink mixed with **grapefruit juice** on **ice** in a wine **flu**te until their **blood levels rose** enough to where they drunk **sexted** a **macro lie** to **sulfonamide.**

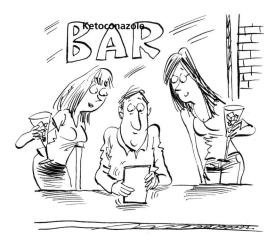

Sodium valproate (Val)
Quinidine
Metronidazole (metro)
Cimetidine (met a dean)
Amiodarone
Ciprofloxacin (sipped)
Acute alcohol intake
Grapefruit juice
Isoniazid (ice)
Fluconazole = flute
Prilo**sec** (omeprazole) = sext
Macrolides = macro lie
Sulfonamides

Figure 13.2 Cytochrome P450 Inhibitors

> Drugs that inhibit the system can lead to increased serum levels of other drugs (eg, warfarin, theophylline, phenytoin).

Pharmacology

CHOLINERGIC DRUGS

Bethanechol, pilocarpine, cevimeline, methacholine, carbachol

MOA/Pharmacokinetics

- Stimulates parasympathetic nervous system (via muscarinic acetylcholine receptors in the peripheral tissues)

Indications

- Acute angle glaucoma (pilocarpine, carbachol), post-operative ileus (bethanechol); post-partum urinary retention (bethanechol); dry mouth (pilocarpine, cevimeline)

Contraindications/Cautions/Side Effects

- Caution with cardiovascular disease, asthma (may cause bronchoconstriction)
- Side effects: bradycardia, diarrhea, nausea, vomiting, incontinence, blurred vision

If you want to Rest on a Pillow and Digest the carbs after eating Carp and Melines you must Chol (call) the waiter first!

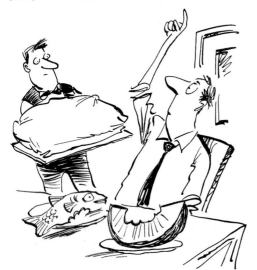

Works on **Parasympathetic** system aka: **Rest and Digest**

Medications Most have -*chol*:
- **Pilocarp**ine
- Cevi**meline**
- **Carbachol**
- Metha**chol**ine
- Bethane**chol**

Figure 13.3 Cholinergic Drugs

ACETYLCHOLINESTERASE INHIBITORS

Neostigmine, pyridostigmine, rivastigmine, edrophonium

MOA/Pharmacokinetics

- MOA: acetylcholinesterase is an enzyme that breaks down acetylcholine in the synapse; inhibition leads to increased acetylcholine (affects both nicotinic and muscarinic receptors)

Indications

Indications: Myasthenia gravis; Alzheimer's disease (donepezil); glaucoma (echothiophate); antidote for atropine poisoning (pyridostigmine)

Contraindications/Cautions/Side Effects

Side effects: dyspnea, muscle fasciculations, prolonged contractions, bradycardia, diarrhea, nausea, vomiting

Stigmine said Ach is **mine** to use if **atropine poisons my organs** but will help **old timers** come to **my graves** faster.

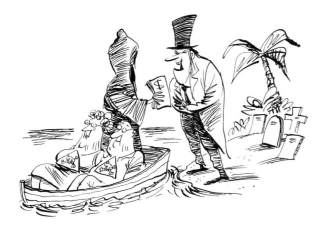

MOA: Increases acetylcholine levels by inhibiting the enzyme that breaks down acetylcholine
Medications: Neo**stigmine**, Pyrido**stigmine**, Riva**stigmine**

Figure 13.4 Acetylcholinesterase Inhibitor

Pharmacology

ANTICHOLINERGICS

Ipratropium bromide; tiotropium, atropine, scopolamine, benztropine, trihexyphenidyl, oxybutynin, tolterodine; propantheline, dicyclomine; ophthalmic: cyclopentolate, homatropine (mydriatic eye drops); GI: hyoscyamine, atropine, scopolamine, phenobarbital

MOA/Pharmacokinetics

Indications

- COPD (ipratropium); bradycardia (atropine); motion sickness (scopolamine); Parkinson's disease (benztropine and trihexyphenidyl); urge incontinence (oxybutynin)

Contraindications/Cautions/Side Effects

- Side effects: dry mouth, blurred vision (dilated pupils), urinary retention, constipation, dry skin, flushing, tachycardia, fever (hyperthermia), HTN, delirium
- Contraindication/caution: acute narrow angle glaucoma, benign prostatic hypertrophy with urinary retention (may worsen both diseases)

During her **flight** to a **trop**ical island, **Donna** used **scope** and suddenly developed **dry mouth**. When she landed, she saw a **panther fighting** a **tall ox** and had **tachycardia** to the point where she was ready to **die.**

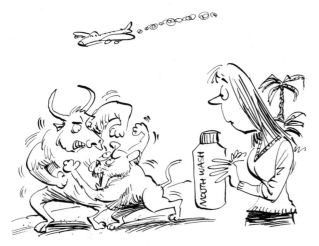

Medications (most have *-trop*):
Ipratropium bromide
Tiotropium
Atropine
Scopolamine
Benztropine
Trihexyphenidyl
Oxybutynin
Tolterodine
Propantheline
Dicyclomine

Ophthalmic:
cyclopentolate
homatropine

Figure 13.5 Anticholinergics

ALPHA-1 RECEPTOR AGONISTS

Phenylephrine, midodrine, epinephrine, oxymetazoline, pseudoephedrine, methylphenidate (ADHD)

MOA/Pharmacokinetics

- α-1 mediated vasoconstriction resulting in increased BP, decreases bleeding, mydriasis during eye examinations, reduces nasal congestion

Indications

- Orthostatic hypotension (midodrine); weight loss (appetite suppressants); phenylephrine (mydriasis), pseudoephedrine (decongestant, stress incontinence); brimonidine (glaucoma)

Contraindications/Cautions/Side Effects

- Syncope, tachycardia (cautious use in patients with HTN)

After eating peanut **M and M's, Alpha** got an allergic reaction and had to use **Epinephrine** so his vessels wouldn't **POP.**

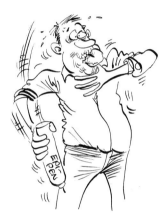

Midodrine and **M**ethylphenidate, **Epinephrine**
Pseudoephedrine, **O**xymetazoline, and **P**henylephrine

Figure 13.6 Alpha-1 Agonists

Pharmacology

ALPHA-2 AGONISTS

Clonidine, methyldopa

MOA/Pharmacokinetics

- Stimulates centrally located α-2 adrenergic receptors; results in decreased sympathetic nervous system activity

Indications

- HTN

Contraindications/Cautions/Side Effects

- Side effects: dry mouth, sedation, fatigue, postural hypotension
- Possible autoimmune hemolytic anemia (methyldopa)

Alpha-2 agonists: another name for 2 is **Di**, so when you activate alpha-2 receptors, you get **Di**lation of the vessels.

When you **Clone Meth,** you will get so **doped** up you will crash your blood pressure and can't say **AHA** due to **dry mouth**!

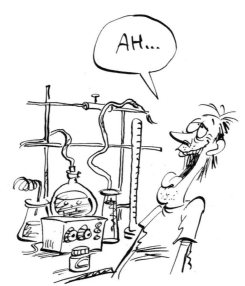

Clonidine and **Meth**yldopa

Figure 13.7 Alpha-2 Agonists

NONSELECTIVE ALPHA-RECEPTOR ANTAGONISTS

Phentolamine, phenoxybenzamine

MOA/Pharmacokinetics

- Blocks both α-1 and α-2 receptors; antihypertensive (vasodilation)

Indications

- Phentolamine (pheochromocytoma preoperative, EpiPen injection reversal), phenoxybenzamine (pheochromocytoma)

Contraindications/Cautions/Side Effects

- Orthostatic hypotension, reflex tachycardia, flushing, nasal congestion, diarrhea, nausea, vomiting, priapism, peptic ulcers, myocardial infarction, stroke, arrhythmias

Non-selective alpha blockers = block alpha-1 and -2 adrenergic receptors

They start with **phen** and end with -*amine*:

Alpha is **Mine! Blocks all alpha receptors.**

- **Phen**tol**amine**
- **Phen**oxybenz**amine**

BETA RECEPTOR ANTAGONISTS (BLOCKERS)

- Cardioselective (β-1 only): metoprolol (most cardioselective), atenolol, esmolol, bisoprolol
- Nonselective (β-1 and β-2): propranolol, nadolol, sotalol, timolol
- Nonselective and Alpha (α-1, β-1 and β-2): labetalol, carvedilol

MOA/Pharmacokinetics

- Beta-receptor blockade decreases cardiac output, heart rate, and contractility; decreases renin secretion, decreases post-myocardial infarction-induced ventricular remodeling

Indications

- HTN, tachyarrhythmia (class II antiarrhythmic), heart failure, angina, acute myocardial infarction, migraine prophylaxis, thyrotoxicosis-associated palpitations, acute angle glaucoma (timolol), benign essential tremor

Contraindications/Cautions/Side Effects

- Caution in those with DM (masks signs of hypoglycemia), asthma/COPD (especially nonselective agents), second-/third-degree heart block, cocaine-induced MI (causes unopposed α1–mediated vasoconstriction), peripheral vascular disease, Raynaud's phenomenon, hypotension, decompensated heart failure
- Side effects: fatigue, depression, impotence

ABCDs of Beta-Blockers: Asthma; heart **B**lock/**b**radycardia; **C**ocaine-induced MI/cardiogenic shock; **D**ecompensated CHF/**d**ecreased systolic BP <90 mm Hg

- **Meto**prolol: cardioselective beta antagonist.
  - When you go on the **METRO** (train), the tracks go one way (selective).
- **Ateno**lol: cardioselective beta antagonist.
  - An **ANTENNA** points up one way (selective).
- **Biso**prolol: isolated to the beta-1 receptor, so it is cardioselective.
- **Es**molol: cardioselective beta antagonist.
  - If you ask esmolol if he is cardioselective, he will say **YES,** I am cardioselective!
- **Nada**lol: noncardioselective beta antagonist.
  - If you ask nadalol if he cardioselective, he will say I am selective to nada (nothing), so not cardioselective.
- **Lab**etalol: noncardioselective beta antagonist.
  - Chemists working in a **LAB** mix all sorts of chemicals (not selective).
- **Pro**pranolol: noncardioselective beta antagonist.
  - When you are a basketball **PRO**, you don't select your opponent because you can compete with anyone (not selective).
- **Car**vedilol: noncardioselective beta antagonist.
  - When you drive your **CAR**, you can go anywhere (not selective).

THIAZIDE AND THIAZIDE-LIKE DIURETICS

- Hydrochlorothiazide, chlorothiazide
- Metolazone, chlorthalidone, and indapamide are "thiazide-like" diuretics with different chemical structures

MOA/Pharmacokinetics

- MOA: decreases BP by decreasing blood volume, prevents kidney sodium/water reabsorption primarily at the distal diluting tubule; lowers urinary calcium excretion

Indications

- HTN (a drug of choice for hypertensive African Americans and patients with no other comorbidities), mild edema (milder natriuretic effect compared to loop diuretics), nephrogenic diabetes insipidus, osteoporosis

Contraindications/Cautions/Side Effects

- Contraindications: allergy to sulfonamides
- Side effects: hyponatremia, hypokalemia, hypomagnesemia, hypercalcemia, mild increase in cholesterol, possible increased digoxin toxicity
- Hyperuricemia and hyperglycemia lead to caution in patients with DM and gout

Diuretics = thiazides deplete all of your electrolytes but can make your **calcium** levels **go up**!

- **Hypercalcemia**/**L**ipidemia/**G**lycemia/**U**ricemia

POTASSIUM-SPARING DIURETICS

Spironolactone, eplerenone (group 1); amiloride, triamterene (group 2)

MOA/Pharmacokinetics

- Group 1: aldosterone antagonist in cortical collecting tubule (inhibits aldosterone-mediated Na/H_2O absorption via reabsorption of K^+ and H^+ ions, thereby "sparing potassium")
- Group 2: inhibits sodium reabsorption at distal convoluted tube, cortical collecting tubule, and collecting duct, specifically at epithelial sodium channel on apical membrane of those cells

Indications

- Group 1: weak diuretic (most useful in combination with loop diuretics to minimize potassium loss), high aldosterone states (eg, ascites, CHF, hyperaldosteronism), HTN, high androgen states (eg, PCOS, female hirsutism, acne) due to spironolactone-induced androgen inhibition
- Group 2: lithium-induced nephrogenic DI, HTN, congestive heart failure

Contraindications/Cautions/Side Effects

- Group 1:
  - Side effects: hyperkalemia, gynecomastia (especially with spironolactone), metabolic acidosis
  - Contraindications: renal failure, hyponatremia
- Group 2:
  - Side effects: hyperkalemia, gynecomastia, metabolic acidosis

Spir**onolact**one: Andrew said, "**O no**, I am **lact**ating."

- Inhibits aldosterone-mediated Na/H_2O absorption
- Inhibits androgens, so leads to **gynecomastia**

ACE INHIBITORS

Captopril, enalapril, ramipril, benazepril, quinapril, lisinopril, trandolapril

MOA/Pharmacokinetics

- MOA: Inhibits ACE; leads to decreased synthesis/production of angiotensin II and aldosterone, causing decreased preload/afterload/BP; potentiates other vasodilators (eg, bradykinin, prostaglandins, nitric oxide)

Indications

- HTN, congestive heart failure, post-myocardial infarction (to prevent ventricular remodeling), diabetic nephropathy (initiate once microalbuminuria is present), proteinuria (causes efferent arteriole dilation, which reduces protein filtration at the glomerulus), hyperaldosteronism

Contraindications/Cautions/Side Effects

- Side effects: 1st dose hypotension; cough and angioedema (due to increased bradykinin), azotemia/renal insufficiency (especially if creatinine >3.0 mg/dL or creatinine clearance <30), hyperkalemia (can be ameliorated with diuretics), neutropenia
- Contraindications: pregnancy (teratogenic), bilateral renal artery stenosis

ACEI work by blocking aldosterone, causing you to develop a **HACK**ing **cough** that can hurt your **RIBS** especially if you are pregnant.

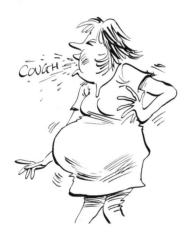

Side Effects: <u>H</u>ypotension <u>A</u>ngioedema <u>C</u>limbing <u>K</u>alemia (hyperK), **Cough**, <u>R</u>enal <u>I</u>nsufficiency, <u>B</u>radykinin <u>S</u>urplus

Contraindications: **Pregnancy**

Figure 13.8 ACE Inhibitors

CALCIUM CHANNEL BLOCKERS

- Dihydropyridines: nifedipine, amlodipine, nicardipine, felodipine
- Non-dihydropyridines: verapamil, diltiazem

MOA/Pharmacokinetics

- Dihydropyridines: potent vasodilators (little to no effect on cardiac contractility or conduction)
- Non-dihydropyridines: affect cardiac contractility and conduction; potent vasodilators; reduce vascular permeability; class IV antiarrhythmics

Indications

- Indications: HTN, angina, achalasia, vasospastic disorders (eg, Prinzmetal's angina, Raynaud's phenomenon, cocaine-induced myocardial infarction), atrial flutter, AFib, migraine prophylaxis

Contraindications/Cautions/Side Effects

- Side effects: vasodilation: headache, dizziness, lightheadedness, flushing, peripheral edema, weakness, bradycardia; constipation with verapamil
- Contraindications/Cautions: patients already on BBs, CHF with ventricular systolic dysfunction (especially nondihydropyridines), second/third heart block
- Dihydropyridines (all end with *-pine*)
  - Potent vaso**Di**lators (little to no effect on cardiac contractility or conduction)
  - All they do is **Di**late and **Drop** your pressure

- Non-dihydropyridines
  - Because they are not only interested in dilating, they affect cardiac contractility and conduction: verapamil and diltiazem

ANTIARRHYTHMIC AGENTS

Medications treating abnormal heart rhythms; 4 classes

Class I: **N**a channel blockers

- Ia: procainamide, quinidine, disopyramide
- Ib: lidocaine, tocainide
- Ic: flecainide, propafenone

Class II: **B**eta-blockers: atenolol, metoprolol

Class III: **K** channel blockers: amiodarone

Class IV: **Ca**lcium channel blockers: verapamil, diltiazem

The **N**ets play in **BK** 4 the **C**hampionships

> These drugs **BANISH** mortality in heart failure
> - **B**eta-blockers
> - **A**CE inhibitors
> - **NI**trates
> - **S**pironolactone
> - **H**ydralazine

CARDIAC AGENTS COMMONLY CONFUSED

- Adeno**S**ine: **S**lows down the AV node
- Amioda**R**one: **R**elaxes the wide QRS and makes it narrow
- Atro**P**ine: **P**icks up rate of heart (anticholinergic)

MOA/Pharmacokinetics

- Adenosine
    - MOA: temporarily decreases SA node automaticity and blocks AV node conduction pathway (by opening K^+ channels); short half-life of approximately 10 seconds (must administer via rapid bolus)
- Amiodarone
    - MOA: Class III anti-arrhythmic (inhibits K^+ efflux leads to increased QT duration); produces vasodilation and slows AV-node conduction via α-1 and β-blockade (Class II properties)
    - Increases QRS duration via inhibition of Na channel (class I properties)
    - Although it is a class III antiarrhythmic, it has properties of class I through IV
    - Prolongs action potential

Indications

- Adenosine
    - Drug of choice for SVT (especially caused by AV node reentry) and narrow, regular, complex tachycardias; can also be used to slow down fast rhythms to differentiate SVT from atrial flutter
- Amiodarone
    - Atrial and ventricular arrhythmias; refractory SVT

Contraindications/Cautions/Side Effects

- Adenosine
    - Side effects: transient flushing, chest pressure/pain; may cause bronchospasm in patients with asthma/COPD
    - Contraindications/Cautions: not used in atrial flutter, AFib, or tachycardia, not caused by AV-nodal reentry
- Amiodarone
    - Side effects: hypotension (most common), bradycardia, vasodilation, heart block or polymorphic VT; long-term use: thyroid disorders (hyperthyroid or hypothyroid), pulmonary fibrosis, corneal deposits (>90% of patients with use >6 months), increased LFTs, blue-green discoloration of the skin
    - Caution: not used together with procainamide

DIGOXIN AND DIGITOXIN

Cardiac glycoside

MOA/Pharmacokinetics

- Positive inotropic agent – Na$^+$/K$^+$ ATPase pump inhibition (decreases intracellular potassium and increases intracellular sodium); the increased intracellular sodium prevents calcium expulsion via the sodium-calcium antiporter leads to increased intracellular calcium contraction
- Increased vagal tone: leads to negative chronotrope (decreases heart rate) and negative dromotrope (slows conduction velocity)

Indications

- Congestive heart failure with left ventricular systolic dysfunction (positive inotrope that decrease hospitalization but has no mortality benefit); possible AFib

Contraindications/Cautions/Side Effects

- Side effects: narrow therapeutic index
  - CNS: seizures, dizziness
  - GI: anorexia, nausea, vomiting, diarrhea (cholinergic effects)
  - Visual: double/blurred vision (objects appear green/yellow), halos around lights
  - Gynecomastia
  - Digitalis effect: T-wave inversion or flattening, shortened QT interval, scooped, down sloping sagging ST segment, junctional rhythms
- Digoxin toxicity
  - ECG may show digitalis effect, premature ventricular contractions (most common) or a wide range of tachy or bradyarrhythmias
  - Electrolyte abnormalities: acute toxicity: may cause hyperkalemia (inhibition of the Na$^+$/K$^+$ ATPase pump increases extracellular potassium); note that in the setting of chronic toxicity, hypokalemia hypomagnesemia, and/or hypercalcemia may worsen toxicity
  - Serum digoxin levels: levels don't always correlate with toxicity
  - Management: antidote digoxin-specific antibody (Fab) fragments

If you take too much digitalis trying to **block** your enemy's **N/k**-47, you will see a **halo around** the **white** light from the gun causing **Kalem to dig up** a grave for you in the **yellow SAND.**

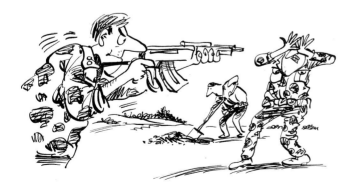

MOA: **Blocks N/K** Pump
Side Effects: **Halos** around lights, yellow green color disturbances, **S**eizures **A**rrhythmias **N**ausea/vomiting **D**ouble vision/**D**izziness.

Figure 13.9 Digoxin Mechanism of Action & Side Effects

Pharmacology

ANTICOAGULANT AGENTS

Unfractionated Heparin

- MOA: potentiates antithrombin III (inhibits conversion of fibrinogen to fibrin) by indirectly inactivating factor Xa and IIa (thrombin); also releases tissue factor pathway inhibitor
- Indications: thrombosis, PE, DVT, PE/DVT prophylaxis, coagulopathies, acute coronary syndrome (UFH does not cross placenta, so safe in pregnancy); usually given as IV bolus and continuous drip
- Side effects: hemorrhage; hyperkalemia; osteoporosis; transaminase elevation; HIT (because heparin is highly negatively charged, may bind to positively-charged platelet factor 4, becoming a hapten); antibodies bind/activates platelets lead to hypercoagulable state with simultaneous thrombocytopenia; occurs most often 5–10 days post-therapy; suspect if platelet <100,000 or >50% from pretreatment
- Cautions: severe thrombocytopenia; safer than low molecular weight heparin in kidney disease
- Must monitor because dosing is unpredictable (heparin can bind to endothelial cells and other plasma proteins and platelet factor 4); half-life 30–60 min depending on binding to other molecules
- Partial thromboplastin time aPTT; titrate to PTT 1.5–2x normal value
- Antifactor Xa levels may be monitored if heparin-resistant
- Antidote: protamine sulfate

> UH: **U**nfractionated **H**eparin must be monitored **U**nder **H**ospital surveillance (used as inpatient).

Low Molecular Weight Heparin (LMWH)

Enoxaparin; dalteparin

- MOA: potentiates antithrombin III (inhibits conversion of fibrinogen to fibrin) causing inactivation of factor Xa (more anti-Xa activity than UFH) but less inhibition of factor IIa (thrombin) 2:1 to 4:1 Xa-IIa ratios; given SQ most commonly
- Indications: thrombosis, PE, coagulopathies, DVT, clot prevention, ACS
- In most cases, better than unfractionated heparin: more predictable, has fewer side effects, has longer half-life, and lacks need for monitoring so better in most cases
- No need to monitor PTT; longer half-life (12 hours); Xa levels can be used to monitor if needed (eg, renal insufficiency, obesity)
- Side Effects: hemorrhage, anemia, thrombocytopenia (all less than UFH), osteoporosis, HIT 5x less likely
- Cautions: renal failure (renally cleared), elderly patients; not as easily reversible as UFH

> LMWH: Patients **Love** LMWH because they can use it at home! **Love**nox

Warfarin

Prevents and treats blood clots

- MOA: inhibits vitamin K-dependent clotting factors II (prothrombin), VII, IX, and X; reduces the functional levels of factor X and prothrombin (which have half-life 24 hrs and 72 hrs, respectively)
- Monitor via PT and INR because common and extrinsic pathway are primarily affected (INR usually 2.0–3.0 [mechanical heart valves 2.5–3.5]); measure every 3–4 wks once therapeutic but more often when initiating
- Side Effects: bleeding (especially when INR above therapeutic range); if INR <10, withhold dose until back in therapeutic range; if >10, try vitamin K (plus FFP); warfarin-induced skin necrosis; vitamin-K dependent anticoagulant proteins C and S have shorter half-life than vitamin K-dependent clotting factors so for first 2–5 days of therapy, patients at increased risk for clots (to prevent clots, bridge patients with heparin for at least 5 days even if INR is within therapeutic range and after 48 hrs of INR being therapeutic; warfarin crosses the placenta
- Interactions: foods containing vitamin K (spinach, kale) may reduce its effectiveness; drugs that inhibit the CP450 system may increase warfarin levels, while drugs that induce the CP450 system may decrease them

Direct Thrombin Inhibitors

- Argatroban, bivalirudin, lepirudin, desirudin
- Dabigatran oral; parenteral
- MOA: bind and inhibit thrombin directly
- Indications: DVT, PE, AFib, prevention of thromboembolism (including CVA); lepirudin and argatroban are treatments of choice for HIT; bivalirudin is an alternative to heparin in patients undergoing PCI, thromboprophylaxis after elective hip arthroplasty
- Side Effects: bleeding, dyspepsia, abdominal pain, increased LFTs
- Contraindications/Cautions: acute bleeding (no reversing agents for most), renal dosing; idarucizumab recently approved as reversal agent for dabigatran
- Monitor lepirudin with aPTT (not ideal test)

Factor X Inhibitors

Fondaparinux (oral), rivaroxaban (oral), apixaban (oral)

- MOA: synthetic selective Factor Xa inhibitor (selectively bind only to antithrombin III); is too short to bridge thrombin so does not significantly inhibit factor IIa formation; does not bind to plasma proteins or platelet factor 4 so its half-life is 17 hrs (usually given 1x/daily) via SC injection
- Indications: DVT/PE/CVA prophylaxis (eg, patients with AFib); DVT/PE treatment similar efficacy to UFH and LMWH; may be used in ACS (however, risk increases for catheter thrombosis); can be used to treat HIT because does not bind to platelet factor 4
- Side Effects: bleeding (no antidote)
- Caution: creatinine clearance <30 mL/min

Factor **Xa** inhibitors all have an **x**:

- Fondaparinu**x**
- Rivaroxaban, apixaban (both ban [inhibit] factor **Xa** (10a)

ANTIPLATELET AGENTS

Adp Inhibitors

Clopidogrel, prasugrel, ticlopidine

- MOA: inhibits ADP-mediated platelet aggregation and activation; irreversibly blocks P2Y12 (the key ADP receptor on platelets)
- Indications: patients with aspirin allergy; in conservative approach or planned PCI due to reduction in death/MI/stroke; may combine with aspirin (eg, stent); prasugrel 10x stronger than clopidogrel
- Prasugrel only indicated in patients undergoing percutaneous coronary intervention
- Side effects: bleeding (especially with prasugrel)—often stopped 5–7 days before major surgery, hematologic
- Caution if coronary artery bypass graft is planned within 7 days; hepatic/renal impairment, bleeding; caution with prasugrel in patients with cerebrovascular disease

Ticagrelor

Administered with aspirin to prevent life-threatening cardiovascular problems

- MOA: oral P2Y12 receptor antagonist (reversible inhibition of ADP); more predictable inhibition compared to clopidogrel, and more effective in reduction of cardiovascular death
- Prevention of thrombotic attacks (eg, CVA, MI), STEMI
- Side effects: bleeding, dyspnea, asymptomatic ventricular pauses of 3 seconds in week 1 of treatment
- Contraindications: history of intracranial bleed or pathological bleeding
- Caution: hepatic impairment; increased plasma levels of ticagrelor when used with inhibitors of the liver enzyme CYP450: 3A4 (ketoconazole, grapefruit juice), CABG surgery; ticagrelor may increase plasma digoxin levels

Glycoprotein IIB/IIIA Inhibitors

- Eptifibatide, tirofiban, abciximab
- MOA: inhibits final pathway for platelet aggregation (GP IIb/IIIa receptor on platelet)
  - Abciximab: antibody that targets the activated receptor
  - Eptifibatide: reversibly binds to receptor
  - Tirofiban: reversibly binds to receptor
- Indications: patients undergoing PTCA (especially if not pretreated with ADP receptor antagonist); tirofiban good for high risk unstable angina
- Contraindications: internal bleeding within 30 days; major trauma/surgery
- Internal bleeding thrombocytopenia (immune-mediated) more likely with abciximab

Salicylate (Acetylsalicylic Acid/Aspirin)

- MOA: non-selectively and irreversibly inhibits cyclooxygenase (COX-1 AND COX-2), decreasing prostaglandin and thromboxane A2 synthesis, producing anti-inflammatory, analgesic, antipyretic effects and reducing platelet aggregation
- Indications: pain, fever, arthritis (anti-inflammatory at high doses); anti-platelet aggregation (eg, ACS, MI/TIA/thromboembolic stroke prevention; rheumatic fever, Kawasaki disease
- Contraindications/Cautions: renal injury (eg, acute renal failure, interstitial nephritis); gastric mucosal injury (eg, gastritis, gastric ulcer, GI bleed) due to loss of the protective effect of prostaglandins; pill-induced esophagitis; decreased uric acid excretion (cautious use in patients with gout)
  - Increased risk of Reye syndrome if used in children with viral infection
  - Asthma exacerbation (arachidonic acid is converted to leukotrienes, leading to bronchoconstriction)
  - Possible hemolytic anemia in patients with G6PD deficiency
  - Contraindicated in hemophiliacs. Increased bleeding with Von Willebrand disease
  - Enhances the effect of lithium warfarin, heparin, digoxin
- Acute toxicity or overdose
  - Tinnitus, hearing loss and vertigo (cranial nerve VIII toxicity)
  - GI symptoms: nausea, vomiting and diarrhea are early symptoms of toxicity
  - Neurologic symptoms: altered mental status changes, lethargy, seizures
  - Noncardiogenic pulmonary edema (acute respiratory distress syndrome)
  - Respiratory alkalosis (early on from respiratory center stimulation, leading to hyperventilation) followed by high anion-gap metabolic acidosis (inhibits oxidative phosphorylation and Krebs cycle, leading to accumulation of lactic acid)
  - Renal insufficiency, hypokalemia, liver injury
- Management of acute toxicity/overdose
  - Supportive care, IV hydration
  - Alkalinization of the urine and serum with IV sodium bicarbonate to increase salicylate excretion and decrease CNS toxicity
  - Activated charcoal to block salicylate absorption in those who ingested salicylate within the past 2 hrs (used in those who are alert with a secured airway)
  - Dialysis (severe cases, eg, salicylate concentration >100 mg/dL)

ASTHMA MEDICATIONS

Beta-2 Receptor Agonists

Albuterol, terbutaline, levalbuterol, metaproterenol (short-acting); salmeterol (long-acting)

- MOA: stimulate β-2 receptor; lead to bronchodilation and uterine relaxation
- Indications: asthma and COPD (short-acting for acute symptoms); delay premature labor (terbutaline); priapism (terbutaline)
- Side effects: β-1 cross reactivity leads to tachycardia, muscle tremor, nervousness, palpitations

Short-acting β-2 agonists: treat the attack before it's too **LATE**:
- **L**evalbuterol
- **A**lbuterol
- **T**erbutaline
- **E**pinephrine

Mast Cell Modifiers

Cromolyn, nedocromil

- MOA: inhibit mast cells and leukotriene-mediated degranulation; improve lung function, decrease airway reactivity (inhibit acute phase response to cold air, exercise, sulfites)
- Minimal side effects (eg, throat irritation)
- Effective prophylaxis may take several weeks

The **mast** of the ship was made of **chrome**, making it **less reactive** in the **cold air**.

Leukotriene Modifiers/Receptor Antagonists

Montelukast. zafirlukast, zileuton

- MOA: inhibit leukotriene-mediated neutrophil migration, capillary permeability, and smooth muscle contraction; montelukast and zafirlukast block leukotriene receptors while zileuton (a 5-lipoxygenase inhibitor) blocks conversion of arachidonic acid into leukotrienes
- Indications: asthmatics with allergic rhinitis/aspirin induced asthma

Luke tried to modify his aspirin allergy by riding a rhino.

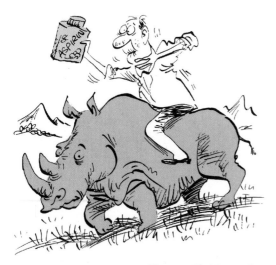

Montelukast, Zafirlukast, Zileuton

MOA: blocks leukotriene-mediated neutrophil migration, capillary permeability, smooth muscle contraction

Indications: asthmatics with aspirin-induced asthma or allergic rhinitis

Figure 13.10 Leukotriene Modifiers/Receptor Antagonist

ANTI-TUBERCULOSIS MEDICATIONS

Drugs used to treat TB, a serious, highly infectious lung disease

Side Effects of Anti-Tuberculosis Medications

Isoniazid (**INH**):

- Inhibitor of the cytochrome P450 system
- Neuropathy (prevented by giving pyridoxine/vitamin B6)
- Hepatotoxicity

Rifampin (**RIF**):

- Red-orange colored secretions
- Inactivity of platelets (thrombocytopenia)
- Flu-like symptoms

Pyrazinamide (**PZA**):

- Photosensitive rashes
- Zaps the liver (hepatitis)
- Arthritis

Ethambutol: **E** = **e**yes (optic neuritis)

Streptomycin (AmiNOglycoside):

- **N**ephrotoxic **O**totoxic
- Covers Gram **N**egatives **O**nly

PEPTIC ULCER DISEASE MEDICATIONS

Proton Pump Inhibitors (PPIs)

Omeprazole, lansoprazole, pantoprazole, rabeprazole, esomeprazole, dexlansoprazole

MOA/Pharmacokinetics

- Irreversibly blocks H^+/K^+ ATP-ase (proton pump) of parietal cell (final step in acid secretion), reducing acid secretion
- More effective than H2 blockers but of little clinical difference after 4 weeks in uncomplicated cases
- Usually given **30 min before meals (especially first meal of the day)** to allow for maximum pump deactivation (number of pumps is greatest after a prolonged fast)

Indications

- PUD, gastritis, persistent GERD, Zollinger-Ellison syndrome, eradication of *H. pylori*
  - May be given in pregnancy (low risk)
- Antisecretory drug of choice (most effective); 90% healing of DU after 4 weeks and GU after 6 weeks

St. Magnum P.I. had a bad omen when he had to defend in the increasing holy war to win the soul of Diaz.

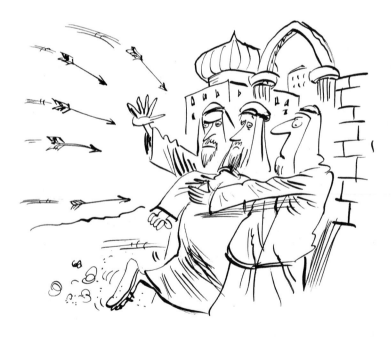

Side Effects:
Diarrhea
Headache
Hypomagnesemia
B12 deficiency
Hypocalcemia

Omeprazole inhibits Cytochrome P450 System: increases Warfarin, phenytoin and Diazepam levels

Magnum: hypomagnesemia, magnum (macrocytic/B12 deficiency)
PI: Proton Pump **I**nhibition, cytochrome **P**450 **I**nhibition
Bad omen: omeprazole interacts with warfarin (war to win) and defends (phenytoin) to increase their levels
Souls: PPIs end in *-zoles*
Dies: diazepam (interacts with diazepam)

Figure 13.11 Proton Pump Inhibitors

Contraindications/Cautions/Side Effects

- Diarrhea
- Headache
- Electrolyte disorders: hypomagnesemia, hypocalcemia
- B12 deficiency (intrinsic factor needs an acidic environment to work), reduction of acidity may also interfere with iron absorption
- Omeprazole and lansoprazole inhibit cytochrome P450 (can cause increased warfarin, phenytoin, theophylline, and diazepam); PPIs may cause methotrexate toxicity
- Omeprazole may decrease clopidogrel and HIV protease inhibitors
- PPIs causing achlorhydria may be associated with decreased absorption of iron, ampicillin, ketoconazole, and digoxin

Histamine-2 Receptor Blockers

Cimetidine, ranitidine, famotidine, nizatidine

- MOA: histamine-2 receptor blocker (indirectly inhibits proton pump) reduces acid/pepsin secretion (especially nocturnal); usually given at night
- Famotidine has few drug interactions; famotidine and nizatidine may cause dyscrasias
- Cimetidine has many drug interactions because it inhibits CP450 (increases serum level of theophylline, warfarin, phenytoin); anti-androgen effects: gynecomastia, impotence
- Caution if renal/hepatic dysfunction
- Side effects: increased LFTs

H2RAs will **block the acid that leads to heart burn** and will allow you **to dine** with your family!

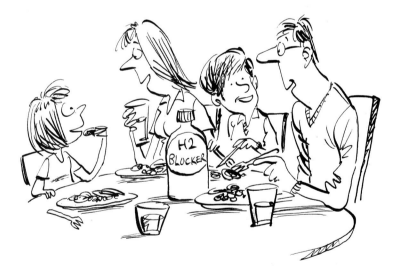

Figure 13.12 H2 Receptor Antagonists

H2 Receptor Antagonists End With -*Tidine*

- Cimetidine
- Ranitidine
- Famotidine
- Nizatadine

Misoprostol

Prevents ulcers and bleeding in the stomach

- MOA: prostaglandin E1 analog that increases bicarbonate and mucous secretions, reduces acid production; good for preventing NSAID-induced ulcers but not for healing already existing ulcers
- Caution with premenopausal women because abortifacient
- Side effects: diarrhea

MISopro**s**tol

- **PRO** at making aspirin-induced ulcers **MISS** their chance of forming
- **PRO** at making mothers **MISS** their babies (most common form of medical abortion)

Sucralfate

Prevents and treats duodenal ulcers

- MOA: forms viscous adhesive ulcer coating; promotes healing; protects stomach mucosa
- Used more as a prophylactic measure than as management of active ulcers
- Cautions: may reduce bioavailability of H2RA, PPIs, and fluoroquinolones when given simultaneously

Sucral**fate** = **S**eals the **fate** of ulcers by applying a coating over them

Serotonin Antagonists

Ondansetron, granisetron, dolasetron

- MOA: blocks serotonin receptors (5-HT3) both peripherally and centrally in the chemoreceptor trigger zone of the medulla, suppressing the vomiting center
- Side effects: headache; GI discomfort: nausea, constipation; fatigue; prolonged QT interval; cardiac arrhythmia

Dopamine Antagonists

Prochlorperazine, promethazine, metoclopramide

- MOA: blocks CNS dopamine receptors (D1, D2) in brain's vomiting center
- Indications: nausea, vomiting, motion sickness
- Side effects:
  - QT prolongation
  - Sedation
  - Constipation
  - Extrapyramidal symptoms: TD, dystonic reactions, parkinsonism
  - Neuroleptic malignant syndrome

Second Generation Antihistamines

- Desloratadine, loratadine, cetirizine, fexofenadine
- Side effects: doesn't cross the blood-brain barrier so much less likely to cause sedation and anticholinergic side effects compared to first generation antihistamines

Des**lora**tadine, **Lora**tadine, **Cetirizine** (city), **Fex**ofenadine (fax)

Lora sent a **fax** to the **Citi** because she **couldn't fall asleep** from all the constant noise.

Doesn't cross the blood-brain barrier so much less likely to cause **sedation (couldn't fall asleep)**.

ANTIEMETIC AGENTS

- Nausea/vomiting are caused by sensory conflict mediated by the neurotransmitters GABA, acetylcholine, histamine, dopamine, and serotonin; antiemetics work primarily by blocking these transmitters
- Antihistamines (often first-line treatment): blocks emetic response via antagonism of central and peripheral H1 receptors; most antihistamines have anticholinergic properties (eg, meclizine, cyclizine, dimenhydrinate, diphenhydramine)
- Dopamine antagonists: metoclopramide, prochlorperazine (IM/rectal); IV promethazine antagonizes dopamine D2 receptors; used to treat severe nausea/vomiting
- Anticholinergics: scopolamine (good for motion sickness and recurrent vertigo); side effects include dry mouth, blurred vision, urinary retention, constipation
- Benzodiazepines: lorazepam, diazepam used in refractory patients (potentiates GABA)

Dopamine

Dopamine Blockers:

- **C**ompazine
- **P**henergan
- **R**eglan

If you **vomit** due to **motion sickness or dope**, you will eventually need **CPR** to help relieve your symptoms.

Serotonin Receptor Antagonists

Ondansetron, **Grani**setron, **Dola**setron **Granny** used up her **Dollas on Dan** the stripper who **held it down** for her by **blocking Tony** from getting into the zone.

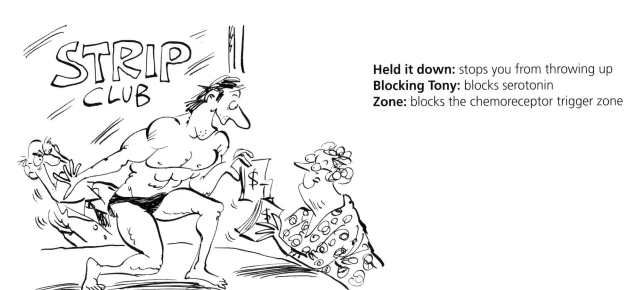

Held it down: stops you from throwing up
Blocking Tony: blocks serotonin
Zone: blocks the chemoreceptor trigger zone

Figure 13.13 Serotonin Receptor Antagonists

Pharmacology

ANTICONVULSANT MEDICATIONS

Ethosuximide

- Blocks calcium channels, leading to motor cortex depression; elevates the stimulation threshold, decreasing neuronal firing
- Indications: absence (petit mal) seizures (drug of choice); can only be used in absence seizures
- Side effects include drowsiness, ataxia, dizziness, headache, rash (SJS), GI upset (nausea/vomiting and diarrhea), weight gain
- Caution: renal or hepatic failure
- Monitor with urinalysis, CBCs, LFTs

Phenytoin

- Stabilizes neuronal membranes by blocking voltage-gates sodium channels
- Indications: seizures (generalized tonic-clonic and focal [simple and complex]); seizure prophylaxis; status epilepticus after benzodiazepines
- Caution: **PHENYTOIN**
  - **P**-450 inducer and induces lupus like syndrome
  - **H**yperplasia of gums and **H**irsutism
  - **E**rythema multiforme
  - **N**eurologic symptoms: vertigo, ataxia, headache
  - **Y**ield: if you don't give it slow it can cause hypotension and arrhythmias
  - **T**eratogenicity (cleft lip and palate, microcephaly)
  - **O**steopenia
  - **I**nhibition of folic acid absorption (megaloblastic anemia)
  - **N**ystagmus

Drug of choice for **Absence** seizures: **Eth**an's **absence** from school kept increasing all because he would **space out** when he would try and put on his **sox** every morning.

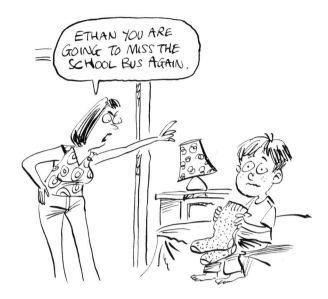

Figure 13.14 Ethosuximide

Pheny put his **toe in**side his mouth, causing his **gingiva** to **enlarge** until he developed **abnormal hair growth** and a **rash** with **multi forms** all over his body.

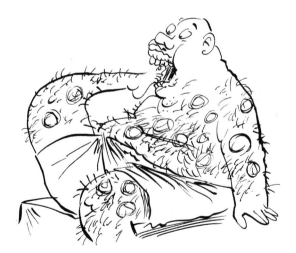

Side Effects:
- Rash, **EM,** Steven-Johnson syndrome
- **Gingival hyperplasia**
- Nystagmus, slurred speech
- Hematologic complications, confusion, dizziness
- Teratogenic, hypotension, arrhythmias
- Increased body hair, alopecia

Figure 13.15 Phenytoin

Progression of Medications for Status Epilepticus:
- Benzodiazepines, then phenytoin loading, then phenobarbital

During her **seizure, Lora Diaz** made **loads** of very large **P**ee **P**ee
- Urinary incontinence may be seen with seizures

Lorazepam and **Diaz**epam are first-line treatment in status epilepticus, followed by **P**henytoin **load**ing; if seizure continues, then give **P**henobarbital

DIABETES MEDICATIONS

Biguanides

Metformin, phenformin

- Metformin MOA: prevents glucose from forming (by decreasing hepatic glucose production) and increases glucose utilization, decreases intestinal glucose absorption, increases insulin sensitivity (has no effect on beta cell, so no hypoglycemia); also decreases triglycerides
- First-line oral therapy for type II DM; not associated with weight gain; also used in some patients with PCOS
- Side effects: GI disturbance very common, macrocytic anemia, lactic acidosis, metallic taste
- Contraindications: renal or hepatic impairment
- Cautions: discontinue metformin 24 hours before iodinated contrast and resume 48 hours later with monitoring of creatinine

Sulfonylureas

- First generation: tolbutamide, chlorpropamide
- Second generation: glipizide, glyburide, glimepiride
- MOA: insulin secretagogue (stimulates pancreatic beta cell insulin release–non-glucose dependent)
- Side effects: hypoglycemia, GI upset (reduced if taken with food), dermatitis, disulfiram reaction, sulfa allergy, weight gain, cardiac dysrhythmias
- Induces CP450 system
- Cautions: chlorpropamide may cause SIADH

Sulfonylureas end with -*m*ide, -*z*ide, and -*ride*

- Cause **Zzz** of glucose (hypoglycemia)
- Must take with **M**eals to decrease GI upset
- **Rides** up levels of insulin (stimulates pancreatic insulin release)

Alpha Glucosidase Inhibitors

Acarbose, miglitol

- MOA: delays intestinal glucose absorption (inhibits pancreatic alpha amylase and intestinal alpha glucosidase hydrolase); does not affect insulin secretion (does not cause hypoglycemia)
- Side effects: GI symptoms (flatulence, diarrhea, abdominal pain)
- Contraindications: hepatitis
- Caution in those with IBD and gastroparesis; delays intestinal glucose absorption

---

You must pay a **toll** to the **car boss** before you can absorb the glucose in your intestine or else you will develop a **flat** tire.

- **F**latulence
- **L**iver inflammation (hepatitis)
- **A**ffects GI tract (both in its MOA and in side effects)
- **T**iming of gastric emptying delayed (gastroparesis)

Thiazolidinediones

- Pioglitazone, Rosiglitazone
- MOA: increases insulin sensitivity at peripheral receptor sites primarily in muscle and adipose tissue; no effect on pancreatic beta cells
- Side effects: hepatotoxicity, weight gain, fluid retention, and edema (CHF)
- Fractures
- Cautions: increased risk of bladder cancer with pioglitazone; cardiovascular toxicity with rosiglitazone

> Thiazolidinediones end with -*ta**zone***
>
> - **T**oxic (to heart and liver)
> - Work in peripheral **zones** (adipose and muscle tissue)

Glucagon-Like Peptide 1 (GLP-1) Agonists

Exenatide, liraglutide

- MOA: lowers blood sugar by mimicking incretin, leading to increased insulin secretion, decreased glucagon secretion
- Side effects: hypoglycemia (less than sulfonylureas because it leads to insulin secretion in a glucose-dependent fashion), pancreatitis
- Contraindications: history of gastroparesis (due to delayed gastric emptying)

> GLP-1 agonists end in -*tide*
>
> Exenatide Liraglutide: drinking too much Tide detergent will lead to Gastroparesis
>
> - **T**itis (inflammation) of the pancreas
> - **I**ncretin mimicker, **I**ncreased Insulin secretion
> - **D**elayed **E**mptying (gastric)
> - **S**erum glucose and glucagon decreased

DPP-4 Inhibitors

Sitagliptin, linagliptin

- MOA: increases GLP-1 by inhibiting dipeptidylpeptidase inhibition
- Side effects: GI upset; pancreatitis; renal failure

> DPP-4 inhibitors: Sitag**liptin**
>
> If you **sit** and **line** your cup with too much sugar in your **Liptin** tea, it can **D**amage your **P**ancreas and affect your **P**ee (kidneys) (DPP).

ANTI-PARKINSONIAN AGENTS

Levodopa/Carbidopa

- MOA: levodopa is converted to dopamine (carbidopa reduces amount of levodopa needed, reducing side effects of the levodopa); most effective treatment for Parkinson's disease
- Side effects: nausea/vomiting, hypotension, somnolence
- Cautions: dyskinesia and "wearing off" associated with long-term use (reduced with amantadine)

Dopamine Agonists

Bromocriptine, pramipexole, ropinirole

- MOA: directly stimulate dopamine receptors; fewer side effects than levodopa
- Indications: used in young patients to delay use of levodopa; if patients are not sensitive to levodopa, they will be insensitive to dopamine agonists
- Side effects: orthostatic hypotension, nausea, headache, dizziness
- Cautions: unpredictable sleepiness

Prami had a **young Bro** named **Mo** who was given **Ropinirole** to help **relieve his resting tremor rolls in bed.** "pill-rolling and resting tremor" associated with Parkinson's

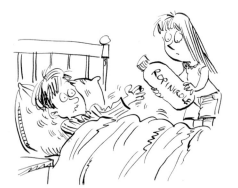

Pramiprexole, **Bromo**criptine, **Ropinirole**

Figure 13.16 Dopamine Agonists

Amanda committed a **sin** when she **met** with her boyfriend by taking **so much dope** for a **long time** that he **swore her off.**

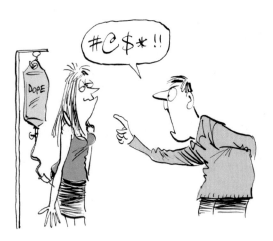

- **Amanta**dine: used synergistically with **Sinemet** to reduce the wearing off of the drug when used long term.

- **Increases dopamine**

Figure 13.17 Amantadine

Al**capone** and Enta**capone** were **good** gangsters straight outta **COMTIN** whose job was to **prevent the breakdown of the dopamine** stores.

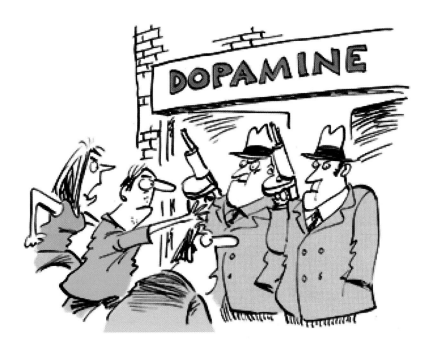

MOA: **prevent dopamine breakdown**

Figure 13.18 COMT Inhibitors

PSYCHOTHERAPEUTIC AGENTS

Selective Serotonin Reuptake Inhibitors

Citalopram, escitalopram, paroxetine, fluoxetine, sertraline, fluvoxamine

- MOA/Pharmacokinetics: selectively inhibit CNS uptake of serotonin, leading to increased serotonin activity in the CNS
- Indications: first-line medical therapy for depression and anxiety disorder: mild side effects and less toxicity than other antidepressants (doesn't affect norepinephrine, acetylcholine, histamine, or dopamine)
- Side effects: GI upset, sexual dysfunction, headache, change in energy level; anxiety, insomnia, change in weight, SIADH, and serotonin syndrome
- Increased suicidality in children and young adults
- Contraindications: citalopram (avoid in those with long QT syndrome)
- On average, antidepressants take 4–6 wks to reach maximum efficacy; if no response, switch to another SSRI

In order to treat your depression, you must be willing to **give up sex** and get a **flu vacc**ine inside your **PECS.**

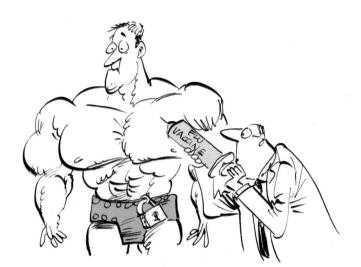

Fluoxetine, **Fluvox**amine
Paroxetine, **E**scitalopram, **C**italopram,
Sertraline

Side Effects:
- **Sexual dysfunction**

- GI upset, headache, change in energy level (fatigue, restlessness); change in weight

  Serotonin syndrome

Figure 13.19 Selective Serotonin Reuptake Inhibitors

Serotonin and Norepinephrine Reuptake Inhibitors

Duloxetine, venlafaxine, desvenlafaxine

- MOA/Pharmacokinetics: inhibit neuronal reuptake of serotonin, norepinephrine, and dopamine
- Indications: extreme fatigue or pain syndromes in association with depression (duloxetine is first-line agent); depression and anxiety disorder (venlafaxine)

Contraindications/Cautions/Side Effects

- Safety, tolerability, and side effect profile similar to those of SSRIs including hyponatremia
- Side effects due to norepinephrine: HTN, dizziness, dry mouth, constipation
- Avoid MAO inhibitor use (renal/hepatic impairment, seizures)
- Avoid abrupt discontinuation
- Caution in those with HTN
- Watch for possible serotonin syndrome if used with St. John's wort

> SNRI: **Venlafax**ine and **Dulox**etine inhibit the reuptake of Dopamine, Norepinephrine, and Serotonin.
>
> **Venla** sent a **fax** to **Dula** that stated he should stop picking up serotonin, norepinephrine, and dopamine along the way.

Tricyclic Antidepressants

Amitriptyline, clomipramine, imipramine, doxepin (tertiary); desipramine, nortriptyline (secondary)

MOA/Pharmacokinetics: inhibit reuptake of serotonin and norepinephrine

- Indications: depression, insomnia, neuropathies (diabetic neuropathic pain, post-herpetic neuralgia), migraine, urge incontinence; used less often because of their side effect profile and severe toxicity with overdose
  - Amitriptyline useful for neuropathy and chronic pain
  - Clomipramine useful for OCD (most serotonin-specific)
  - Imipramine useful for enuresis in children
  - Desipramine least sedating (least antihistaminic) and least anticholinergic
  - Nortriptyline least likely to cause orthostatic hypotension
- Side Effects: anticholinergic effects most common (dry mouth; constipation; urinary retention; tachycardia; orthostatic hypotension; confusion/hallucinations in elderly; sedation, weight gain, prolonged QT interval (best indicator of overdose), lowered seizure threshold, SIADH
- **Overdose** (the 3 Cs)
  - **C**ardiotoxicity: sinus or wide complex tachycardia (due to its Na+ channel blocker effects)
  - **C**onvulsions (seizures) or other neurologic symptoms (eg, respiratory depression)
  - **C**oma
- Caution with use of MAO inhibitors, recent MI, seizure history

> Tricyclic Antidepressants (TCA) mostly end with -*triptyline* or -*ipramine*
> - **T**oxic with overdose
> - **C**ontraindicated with MAO-Inhibitors
> - **A**nticholinergic side effects
>
> **Clom** couldn't go to the prom with **Ami nor Doxe** so she got depressed and developed neuropathic pain and called **Imi and Desi** to come to her aid.

Nonselective MAO Inhibitors

Phenelzine, tranylcypromine, and isocarboxazid

- MOA/Pharmacokinetics: block breakdown of neurotransmitters (dopamine, serotonin, epinephrine, norepinephrine, tyramine) by inhibiting MAO
- Indications: refractory depression or refractory anxiety disorder
- Side Effects: orthostatic hypotension most common; insomnia, anxiety, weight gain, sexual dysfunction
   - Hypertensive crisis after ingesting foods high in tyramine (aged/fermented cheese; some red wine/draft beer/chocolate; and all aged/smoked/pickled/cured meat, poultry, fish)
   - MAO inhibition prevents the breakdown of tyramine, leading to HTN
- Contraindications: increased risk of serotonin syndrome if combined with SSRIs, St. John's wort, MDMA, cocaine, meperidine, tramadol, or dextromethorphan
- Cautions: wait ≥2 wks before switching from MAO inhibitor to SSRI or vice versa; MAO inhibitor + TCA may cause delirium and HT

Parnate the **Nerd** had a **Mar**velous **plan** so he went to **Maui** (MAOI) and ate **cheese and wine** to celebrate but had to cut it short because he was suffering from a hypertensive **crisis.**

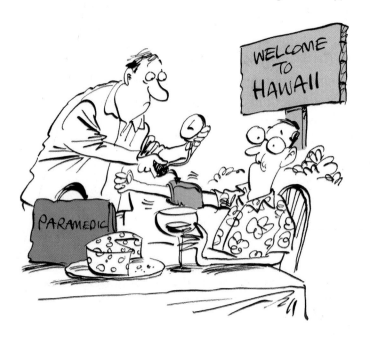

Non-selective A and B
Parnate, Nardil, and **Marplan**

- **HTN crisis if taken with foods that increase tyramine**
  (eg, aged/fermented cheese and wine)

Figure 13.20 Monoamine Oxidase Inhibitors

NEUROLEPTIC AGENTS

First Generation (Typical)

Haloperidol, droperidol, fluphenazine, chlorpromazine, perphenazine, and thioridazine

- MOA/Pharmacokinetics: dopamine-receptor antagonists
- Indications: schizophrenia and acute psychosis
  - Most effective drugs for positive symptoms, minimal effect on negative symptoms but increased risk of extrapyramidal symptoms, TD, neuroleptic malignant syndrome
  - First-line management is a second generation (atypical) antipsychotic: clozapine is never first-line but is the most effective medication for treatment-resistant psychosis (eg, after two medications have been tried); try medications ≥4 wks before evaluating efficacy
- Side Effects: extrapyramidal symptoms e.g., acute dystonia, akathisia, parkinsonism, TD; increased prolactin (more common with first generation)
  - Metabolic: hyperlipidemia, weight gain, hyperglycemia, increased abdominal fat (more common with second generation); aripiprazole and ziprasidone least associated with metabolic changes
  - Neuroleptic malignant syndrome: altered mental status, "lead-pipe" muscle rigidity, autonomic instability (tachycardia, tachypnea, hyperthermia, fever, BP changes, hypersalivation, and diaphoresis), incontinence, leukocytosis, and rhabdomyolysis (increased CPK, LDH, and LFTs)
  - QT prolongation, arrhythmias, and seizures; rash
  - Anti-HAM effects: AntiHistamine, antiAdrenergic, and antiMuscarinic (anticholinergic) effects (more common with first generation)
  - Anticholinergic effects: dry mouth, dry eyes, blurred vision, urinary retention, constipation, and hyperthermia
  - Antihistaminic effects: sedation, weight gain
  - Anti-alpha 1 adrenergic: orthostatic hypotension, sexual dysfunction, cardiac abnormalities

---

PHENOTHI**AZINES** end with "Azine"

- **Chlor**prom**azine**
- Fluphen**azine**
- **Prochlor**per**azine**
- **Promethazine**

MOA: blocks CNS dopamine (D2) receptors (butyrophenones)

The **Pro Chlor**ine cleaner took **meth** and got the **flu,** so she decided to **block dopamine** from her life.

Second Generation (Atypical)

Risperidone, olanzapine, quetiapine, ziprasidone, aripiprazole, and lurasidone

- MOA/Pharmacokinetics: dopamine antagonists (D4 > D2) and serotonin 5-HT2 antagonists
- Indications: first-line agents for schizophrenia and acute psychosis
  - Lower risk of extrapyramidal side effects but increased risk of metabolic side effects
  - Risperidone is one of the most common agents prescribed for schizophrenia; long-acting injectable form
  - Olanzapine is best drug for medication-refractory schizophrenia; decreased incidence of suicide
  - Ziprasidone and aripiprazole less likely to cause weight gain
- Side Effects: extrapyramidal symptoms, increased prolactin, neuroleptic malignant syndrome
  - Metabolic: hyperlipidemia, weight gain and hyperglycemia, increased abdominal fat (more common with second generation); aripiprazole and ziprasidone are least associated with metabolic changes
  - QT prolongation, arrhythmias, and seizures; rash
  - Anti-HAM effects: antiHistamine, antiAdrenergic, and antiMuscarinic (anticholinergic) effects (more common with first generation)
  - Olanzapine: marked weight gain and DM
  - Risperidone: higher incidence of movement disorders
  - Clozapine: agranulocytosis and myositis
  - Ziprasidone: higher incidence of prolonged QT interval

After eating **lox** and **pine**apples for many years, **Olan** realized his **weight gain** and **quit** his **extra** job at the **pyramid** as his **only option** to fit in his **clothes** by eating **low** fat **grains.**

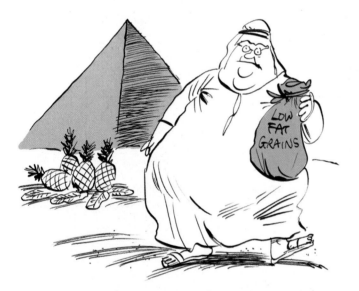

Indications:
- **Clozapine used for those resistant to other antipsychotics**

Side Effects:
- Marked **weight gain with olanzapine**

- **Agran**ulocytosis **(low grain)**

- **Extrapyramidal symptoms**

Figure 13.21 Secondary Generation Atypical Antipsychotics

CHEMOTHERAPEUTIC AGENTS

Cyclophosphamide

- MOA: inhibits DNA replication (by alkylating DNA)
- Indications: leukemias, lymphomas, multiple myeloma, ovarian and breast cancers, retinoblastoma, neuroblastoma, sarcoma
- Side effects: hemorrhagic cystitis (occurrence reduced by increasing water intake), bladder cancer, emesis, myelosuppression, GI mucosal damage (diarrhea), SIADH

> - **Cyclo**phosphamide: **Blocks DNA replication**
> - The **cyclone blocked DNA from replicating** while **damaging the bladder** causing **hemorrhage and bladder cancer.**

Platinum Agents

Cisplatin, carboplatin

- MOA: inhibits DNA replication (by alkylating DNA)
- Indications: leukemias, lymphomas, multiple myeloma, ovarian cancer, breast cancer
- Side effects: neurotoxicity (ototoxicity, neuropathy), renal failure (prevented with IV saline and amifostine), hypomagnesemia, highly emetogenic

> **P**athologic to nerves (neuro**P**athy)
>
> **L**ow magnesium (hypomagnesium)
>
> **A**uditory deficits (ototoxicity); Amifostine prevents renal toxicity associated with cisplatin
>
> **T**hrow up (highly emetogenic)

Anthracyclines

Doxorubicin, daunorubicin

- Cardiotoxicity (dilated cardiomyopathy), bone marrow suppression, alopecia, GI upset

Ruby sat at the docks at dawn because she had dyspnea from dilated cardiomyopathy that could have been disrupted by dexrazoxane.

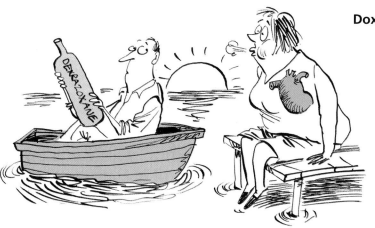

Doxorubicin (docks), Daunorubicin (dawn)

- Dexrazoxane can be used as cardiomyopathy prophylaxis for patients on doxorubicin

- **Dilated cardiomyopathy from use**

Pharmacology

Figure 13.22 Anthracyclines

Bleomycin

- MOA: unknown
- Indications: malignant pleural effusions (also used for pleurodesis), non-Hodgkin lymphoma, Hodgkin lymphoma, squamous cell and testicular cancers
- Side effects: pulmonary fibrosis

> **BL**eomycin: **B**urns the **L**ungs by causing fibrosis

Chapter 14

Procedures

ARTHROCENTESIS

Procedure performed to collect synovial fluid from joint capsule

Indications

- Diagnostic: to rule out septic arthritis, inflammatory arthritis
- Therapeutic: in selected patients to relieve joint pain and promote increased mobility and comfort; in some cases, to remove blood accumulation due to hemarthrosis

Contraindications/Cautions/Complications

- Do not pass through overlying infection (eg, cellulitis) because even if sterile technique is utilized, bacteria may be introduced into the joint
- Caution in patients with bleeding disorders (eg, hemophilia or thrombocytopenia) as they may develop hemarthrosis from the procedure; if the procedure must be performed, factor concentrates in hemophiliacs or correction of the coagulopathy in coagulopaths may reduce complications
- Prosthetic joints are better aspirated by and after evaluation of an orthopedic surgeon or orthopedic surgical team

Equipment/Preparation

- Sterilize the skin, allow sterile solution to dry and then drape the area
- Apply lidocaine to anesthetize the selected area
- Applying a sterile technique, connect a 20-mL syringe to a large gauge needle (eg, 18- or 20-gauge); a larger syringe may be needed if it is a large effusion or be ready to exchange the syringes if more fluid than anticipated is encountered during the procedure
- Make the skin taut over the insertion site by stretching the skin to ensure accurate penetration; joint space entry may be facilitated by slightly flexing the knee 15–20°
  - Insert needle into the joint space (you will often feel it give way) and aspirate until synovial fluid begins to fill the syringe (usually 1–2 cm depth)
  - During aspiration, if fluid stops flowing, reassess your landmarks to make sure you are not in the bone or the tendon; try to apply gentle pressure to the suprapatellar region
- Once aspiration is complete, remove the needle and apply a sterile bandage to insertion site

Procedure

- **Parapatellar approach** (preferred method): find midpoint between the lateral or medial patellar borders; insertion site is 3–4 mm below midpoint with the needle directed toward the intercondylar notch of the femur and perpendicular to the long axis of the femur
- **Suprapatellar approach:** find midpoint of the superolateral or superomedial patellar border; insertion site is at midpoint with the needle directed toward the intercondylar notch of the femur; the suprapatellar approach enters the suprapatellar border
  - In 10–15% of the population, the suprapatellar bursa does not communicate with the knee joint, resulting in a dry tap
- **Infrapatellar approach:** find either side of the inferior border of the patella and patella tendon; insertion site is 5 mm below inferior border of the patellar and lateral to the edge of the patellar tendon; to facilitate the procedure and reduce complications, place patient in an upright position with knee bent at 90° over edge of the bed
  - Caution not to pierce the patellar tendon with insertion of the needle

Procedures

Anatomic Landmarks

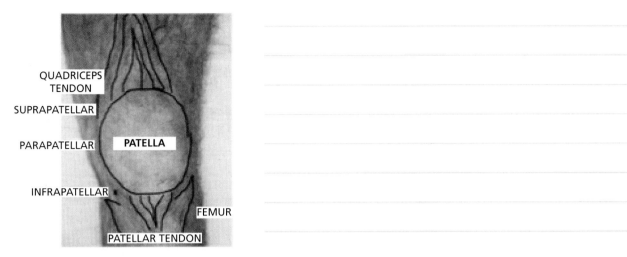

Figure 14.1 Arthrocentesis

Labs

- Synovial fluid
  - Gram stain and culture (aerobic and anaerobic): usually in a sterile culture cup (depending on your institution)
  - Cell count with differential: usually in a purple top blood tube (depending on your institution)
  - Crystals: often in a red top blood tube (depending on your institution)
  - Acid fast bacillus

Arthrocentesis Analysis of Fluid

	WBC/μL	Microscopic	Glucose (mg/dL)
Normal	<150 monocytes/ lymphocytes		Serum levels
Inflammatory Arthritis			
• Gout	<50,000 (<90% PMNs) polymorphonuclear neutrophils = PMNs	• Needle-shaped crystals (negatively birefringent) • Uric acid crystals	<25
• Pseudogout	<50,000 (<90% PMNs)	• Rhomboid-shaped crystals (positively birefringent) • Calcium pyrophosphate crystals	
• Reactive Arthritis and Other Inflammatory Arthritis	<50,000 (<90% PMNs)		
Septic Arthritis	>50,000 ≥ (90% PMNs)	Bacteria, cloudy	<25

THORACENTESIS

Procedure that uses a needle to remove fluid buildup from the pleural space

Indications

- Diagnostic: to remove fluid (or air) from the pleural space to determine if it is transudative, exudative, or empyemic; sometimes done with U/S guidance
- Therapeutic: to relieve dyspnea or pain; to improve lung function (especially in those with large effusions); to remove air (needle decompression) in those with a large pneumothorax or tension pneumothorax; to drain an empyema

Contraindications/Cautions/Complications

- Relative contraindications: coagulation disorders; patients with only one functioning lung; or if there is cellulitis on the chest wall at insertion site
- Complications include hemorrhage; iatrogenic pneumo (or hemo) thorax; hypotension (if a lot of fluid is removed); expansion pulmonary edema (removing <1 L of fluid reduces the incidence)

Equipment/Preparation

- Equipment:
  - Thoracentesis kit includes an 8-French catheter, 7.5-inch (19-cm) needle with a 3-way stopcock
  - Scalpel (11 blade is often used)
  - Drainage bag, drape, sterile towels, tubing set, Luer-lock syringes (5 mL, 10 mL, 60 mL), chlorhexidine solution (or other antiseptic), lidocaine, adhesive dressing, gauze pads
  - 2 vacuum bottles 1 L each
- Preparation:
  - Auscultate the site to determine level of the effusion (penetration is usually best 1–2 intercostal spaces below the fluid level)
  - Place patient in sitting position, leaning forward slightly with head resting on a pillow or table; this allows for access to 7–9th rib along the posterior axillary line

Procedure

- U/S can be used to confirm the size and presence of the effusion and to search for loculations: identify the diaphragm, then pick the optimal insertion site after checking for diaphragm excursion during respiration and assess for the largest collection of fluid
- Optimal puncture site is usually between 7th and 9th rib spaces and between posterior axillary line and the midline; mark the area for puncture site
- Prepare a sterile field by cleaning a large area with antiseptic solution (chlorhexidine is preferred over povidone-iodine); place a sterile drape (with drape opening and adhesive strip) over puncture site
- Place the anesthesia (usually lidocaine 1 or 2%) in the skin, soft tissue, rib periosteum, intercostal muscles, and parietal pleura
- A small skin incision can be made prior to insertion of the needle introducer with a No. 11 scalpel blade; advance the needle introducer over the superior aspect of the rib until pleural fluid is aspirated; in most situations, the catheter should not be advanced >5 cm
- Advance the catheter over the needle introducer (often all the way to the hub)
- Drain the desired amount of pleural fluid with vacuum bottle or syringe pump (depending on if diagnostic or therapeutic) and send for analysis as needed

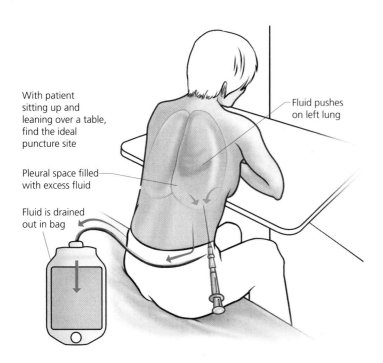

With patient sitting up and leaning over a table, find the ideal puncture site

Fluid pushes on left lung

Pleural space filled with excess fluid

Fluid is drained out in bag

Ideal puncture site should be the **superior aspect of the rib** (usually between 7th and 9th ribs). Make sure to avoid the neurovascular bundle (located at inferior border of the rib).

Figure 14.2 Thoracentesis: Puncture Site

Labs

- Pleural fluid: Gram stain and culture (aerobic/anaerobic) in sterile cup; glucose, protein level, LDH, pH; cell count and differential
- Normal pleural fluid values
  - Clear ultrafiltrate of plasma originating from parietal pleura
  - Glucose content similar to plasma
  - Protein <2% (1–2 g/dL)
  - LDH <50% of plasma
  - pH 7.60–7.64
  - WBCs <1,000
- Cytology (if malignancy suspected); triglycerides (>110 mg/dL indicates a chylous effusion, possibly due to thoracic duct rupture); amylase (if pancreatitis/esophageal perforation suspected); acid fast bacillus

Light Criteria Exclusive to Exudates

- Pleural fluid protein: serum protein >0.5
- Pleural fluid LDH: serum LDH >0.6 or pleural fluid LDH >2/3 upper limit of normal LDH

Pleural Drainage Indications

Drain pleural fluid if empyema present (if **one of the following** is present):

- Pleural fluid pH <7.2
- Glucose <40 mg/dL
- Positive Gram stain of pleural fluid

Procedures

PARACENTESIS

Procedure that uses a needle to obtain peritoneal fluid

Indications

- Diagnostic: to assess the etiology of new-onset ascites (eg, blood due to trauma versus transudate versus exudate), diagnose spontaneous bacterial peritonitis in patients with known ascites, to look for metastatic disease
- Therapeutic: to relieve abdominal pressure in patients with ascites and in patients with respiratory difficulty

Contraindications/Cautions/Complications

- Contraindications:
  - Absolute: acute abdomen
  - Relative: abdominal wall cellulitis; marked thrombocytopenia, eg, platelets <20,000 (may give platelet transfusion prior to procedure); INR >2.0 (may give fresh frozen plasma prior to and even during the paracentesis to reduce bleeding risk); distended urinary bladder; bowel distention
- Complications:
  - Persistent leakage from puncture site (may need suture on skin or temporary ostomy bag)
  - Bleeding or infection
  - Hypotension (if large volumes are removed)

Equipment/Preparation

- Equipment
  - Paracentesis (or thoracentesis kit)
  - Needles: 18-gauge; 22-gauge injection (2); and 25-gauge injection
  - Syringes: 10 or 20 mL; 60 mL; and 5 mL Luer lock
  - 8 French catheter over 18-gauge by 7.5-inch needle with self-sealing valve and 3-way stopcock
  - Tubing set
  - Vacuum container or drainage bag
  - Lidocaine 1%
  - Culture tubes and collection tubes to perform testing
  - Antiseptic swab sticks, adhesive dressing and gauze
- Preparation: have patient urinate beforehand (or assist with Foley catheter) so bladder is empty

Procedure

- Approach either 2 cm below the umbilicus in midline (through linea alba) **or** 5 cm superior and medial to anterior superior iliac spines on either side
- Procedure:
  - Positioning: for mild ascites, left lateral decubitus position ensures better outcome; for severe ascites or large effusion, supine position
  - Create a sterile field by preparing the abdomen with chlorhexidine or other appropriate antiseptic agent; place the fenestrated drape to the area
  - Apply anesthesia to the puncture site using a 25-gauge needle attached to 5-mL syringe by making a small wheal surrounding the ideal puncture site; administer ~5 mL of lidocaine along catheter insertion site (may inject and aspirate intermittently until ascitic fluid is seen in syringe)

- U/S is recommended to determine ideal insertion site and ensure bladder isn't distended
- Make a small nick with the No. 11 blade to facilitate insertion of the catheter
- Insert the catheter slowly, 5 mm each time, until desired depth is reached (to reduce risk of perforation); once a loss of resistance is felt, ascitic fluid should enter the syringe
    - Continue to advance catheter up to 5 mm to avoid displacement (no more than 1 cm past the area ascertained when fluid began to enter the syringe when you anesthetized the area)
    - Use a small gauge needle or make a "Z' shaped track when performing the puncture
- Advance the catheter all the way to the skin and avoid kinking; pull needle out while securing the stopcock
- Attach the 60-mL syringe to the stopcock to remove the ascitic fluid and send for appropriate testing; connect to a vacuum bottle or drainage bag
- After the desired amount of fluid has been removed, remove the catheter, apply pressure to the area and then apply a sterile dressing

Analysis of the Ascitic Fluid

- Gram stain and culture; if SBP is present, common organisms include *E. coli*, *Klebsiella pneumoniae*, enterococcal bacteria, and *S. pneumoniae*
- Cell count
- Total protein level, glucose, lactate dehydrogenase
- Amylase (if pancreatitis suspected), bilirubin (if bowel perforation suspected), cytology (if malignancy suspected)
- Albumin level to calculate SAAG (**SAAG = Serum Albumin − Ascites Albumin**)

Serum Ascites Albumin Gradient

- Must be obtained on same day to be accurate
- Transudative: SAAG $\geq$1.1 g/dL (portal HTN)
    - Hepatic cirrhosis
    - Alcoholic hepatitis
    - Hepatic failure
    - Congestive heart failure
- Exudative SAAG <1.1 g/dL
    - SBP: polymorphonuclear leukocyte count >250/μL (>50% PMN)
    - Inflammation of pancreas or biliary system
    - Peritoneal carcinomatosis
    - Nephrotic syndrome
    - Bowel obstruction or ischemia

PERICARDIOCENTESIS

Procedure that uses a needle and catheter to remove fluid from the pericardium

Indications

- Diagnostic: in certain conditions to determine if the pericardial fluid is inflammatory, malignant, or infectious
- Therapeutic: in patients with pericardial tamponade to prevent or treat obstructive shock or in patients with recurrent malignant pericardial effusions

Contraindications/Cautions/Complications

- Contraindications/Cautions:
  - No absolute contraindications in a hemodynamically unstable patient
  - Relative contraindications in hemodynamically stable patient:
    - Bleeding disorders
    - Some of the traumatic cardiac tamponades you may encounter may be better treated with emergent thoracotomy instead of pericardiocentesis
- Complications
  - Breeching the myocardium: occurs if there are sudden ST elevations on ECG (reflecting a current of injury); if this occurs immediately remove the needle
  - Obtain a follow up chest x-ray to look for complications

Equipment/Preparation

- Pericardiocentesis kit (if available)
- Lidocaine (eg, 1%), syringes (10 mL and 60 mL), antiseptic solution (chlorhexidine or iodine), scalpel with No. 11 blade, sterile drapes, needles (18 gauge 1.5 inches, 25 gauge 5/8 inches, long 18 gauge 7.5–12 cm)
- U/S machine with sterile cover for the probe and sterile gel
- Alligator clip connector to V1 lead of ECG machine

Procedure

- **Subxiphoid approach**: under the xiphoid, process up and leftward through the infrasternal angle (often done with U/S guidance)
  - Place needle at 45° angle and direct it toward left shoulder
  - After sterilizing the entry point, you should be able to access the pericardial space and then aspirate the pericardial fluid
- **Parasternal approach**: through the 5th or 6th intercostal space at left sternal border at the cardiac notch of left lung immediately lateral to the sternum
  - Insert needle perpendicular to the chest (90°) (note that from this view, left anterior descending artery may be lacerated when approaching the pericardium)
  - After sterilizing the entry point, you should be able to access the pericardial space and then aspirate the pericardial fluid

NAIL BED REMOVAL

Procedure performed to remove the nail bed due to injury or infection

Indications

- To repair nail injury, including large subungual hematoma or deformed nail bed

Contraindications/Cautions/Complications

- Nail bed injury
- Nail matrix injury
- Bleeding (reduced with the tourniquet and the hemostat)
- Infection
- Paronychial injury

Equipment/Preparation

- 5-mL syringe
- Lidocaine without epinephrine
- Small gauge needle (eg, 25-gauge)
- Finger tourniquet (eg, finger part of a glove)
- Iris scissors or nail elevator
- 2 straight hemostats
- Nonadherent gauze

Procedure

- Sterilize the finger
- Perform a ring block of the finger
- Use a straight hemostat to firmly secure a finger tourniquet around the base of the finger
- Insert the curved Iris scissors or nail elevator beneath the hyponychium (free edge of the nail); slowly and gently open and close the iris scissors blades or gently put pressure with the nail elevator on the nail bed, advancing slowly and proximally between the nail plate and the nail bed until the nail fold is reached
- Once the nail is separated from the nail bed, it is gently removed by applying steady distal traction with the hemostat

CENTRAL LINE CATHETER

Procedure performed to place a catheter into a large vein, e.g., internal jugular vein, subclavian vein, femoral vein; also called central venous catheter or central venous line

Indications

- To administer potentially caustic medication or fluids to peripheral veins (eg, chemotherapy, calcium chloride, hypertonic saline)
- To assess central venous pressure or oxygenation saturation
- To administer long-term parenteral nutrition or IV antibiotics
- To administer dialysis or plasmapheresis
- To administer IV therapy to those in whom peripheral access cannot be obtained
- To provide rapid administration of fluids/ blood products in emergent situations
- To infuse plasmapheresis or dialysis

Contraindications/Cautions/Complications

Relative Contraindications:

- Internal jugular vein or subclavian vein access in severely coagulopathic individuals; in these patients, femoral access is preferred (because femoral vein can be compressed easier if there are bleeding complications)
- Local infection over the intended site
- Contralateral pneumothorax or hemothorax
- Venous thrombosis
- High-pressure ventilator settings

Equipment/Preparation

- Equipment
  - Central line kit
  - Local anesthetic
  - Scalpel
  - Sterile gel for U/S guidance
  - 18-gauge or similar gauge introducer needle (with saline to detect venous backflow of blood)
  - Tissue dilator
  - Guide wire
  - Indwelling catheter
  - Surgical thread
  - Dressing
  - Sterilizing solution
  - Drape
  - High frequency U/S transducer and U/S machine
  - Sterile gloves
  - Sterile U/S cover and sterile U/S gel
  - Gown, cap, mask, and protective eyewear

- Preparation
  - IJV and stroke volume access: place patient in a slightly Trendelenburg position, with head in a neutral position (maximum head rotation of 30 degrees)
  - Femoral vein access: place patient in a neutral position
  - Position of the practitioner: ipsilateral side of patient is preferred; perform the procedure from the head of the bed and the indicator of the probe should be directed to the operator's left (this corresponds to the left side of patient's body)

Procedure

- Prepare for the procedure by using universal precautions, including sterile gloves, protective eyewear, gown, mask, and cap
- Cleanse patient's skin with povidone iodine solution, chlorhexidine, or other appropriate antiseptic solution
- Vascular cannulation may be accomplished with a catheter-over-needle device or the catheter-over-guidewire technique (Seldinger technique)
- Use the U/S to locate the vessel via the dynamic method (included here) or other methods

Dynamic Method

- Use a sterile sheath and sterile gel/lubricant; place additional sterile transmission gel on the outside of the covered probe
- The vein can be found using the U/S and should be centered on the screen: look for compressibility of the vessel, increased filling (using the Valsalva maneuver), as well as respiratory pulsations
- Anesthetize the selected tract with lidocaine
- Enter the skin with an entry needle, using the U/S to guide the direction of the needle; longitudinal view can make visualization of the needle tip easier and can also be used to visualize the guidewire during that step; once the vein is punctured and the guidewire is placed, remove the entry needle and enlarge the entry site with a No. 11 scalpel blade
- If placed correctly, the vein should be easily flushable and there should be good venous blood return
- Hold the catheter in place with simple interrupted sutures
- Obtain a chest x-ray after the procedure to ensure correct placement and to assess if any complications occurred, such as pneumothorax

LUMBAR PUNCTURE

Procedure performed to obtain CSF by inserting a needle between lumbar vertebrae

Indications

- Diagnostic: to rule out CNS infection, suspected subarachnoid hemorrhage when head CT is negative, and inflammatory CNS disease; can also be used to differentiate between the causes of meningitis
- Therapeutic: to alleviate pain through spinal anesthesia for pregnant women in labor or people with chronic back pain

Contraindications/Cautions/Complications

- Absolute contraindications: infection of skin over incision site; elevated intracranial pressure due to a lesion/mass/abscess; signs of papilledema or focal neurologic deficits, and trauma to the lumbar spine
- Relative contraindications: coagulation disorders
- Complications: hemorrhage; post-procedural headache; infection; herniation in brain

Equipment/Preparation

- Equipment:
  - Lumbar puncture kit (includes 25 gauge × 5/8" needle, Luer-lock syringe, lidocaine, 4 CSF tubes, sponge applicators, gauze pads, fenestrated drape, 20-gauge spinal needle with stylet, and towels)
  - Sterile gloves, cap, gown, drape, sterile towels, Luer-lock syringes (5 mL, 10 mL, 60 mL), chlorhexidine solution (or other antiseptic), lidocaine, adhesive dressing, gauze pads
- Preparation:
  - Palpate patient's spinous processes to identify L3, L4, L5, and the spaces between them; L3–L5 can be found by palpating the posterior iliac crests and moving medially toward midline; once there, palpate to identify L3–L4 and L4–L5; the spaces between L3–L4 or L4–L5 can be used as an entry site for the lumbar puncture
  - Place patient in an upright sitting position or supine in lateral decubitus position with upper back arched and with knees in flexion

Procedure

- Open tray and put on sterile gloves; prepare a sterile field by cleaning a large area with antiseptic solution (chlorhexidine is preferred over povidone-iodine solution); place a sterile drape (with fenestration and adhesive strip) over the puncture site
- Place the anesthesia (usually lidocaine 1 or 2%) in the skin of space between the vertebrae (L3–L4 or L4–L5) and in the deeper soft tissue
- Advance the spinal needle slowly into the space between L3–L4; aim the needle toward the patient's head; make sure the bevel is pointing laterally toward patient's side
  - After advancing the needle approximately 5 cm, you may feel a small popping sensation (but not always felt); when that happens, remove the stylet from the spinal needle and see if there is CSF flow
  - If there is no flow, retract the needle and try again by moving the needle more toward the head of the patient; in most situations, spinal needle should not be advanced >5 cm
- After CSF flow is confirmed, measure the opening pressure by attaching a manometer to the hub of the needle

- Collect approximately 2 mL of CSF fluid in each of 4 tubes provided in kit (or any 4 sterile plastic tubes); if cultures are needed for specific organisms, you may collect >4 tubes
- Remove spinal needle by reattaching stylet to needle first and place pressure over puncture site to reduce changes of CSF leak; apply dressing
- After the desired CSF fluid is collected, the CSF fluid is sent for analysis

Anatomic Landmarks

- Ideal puncture site should be in the arachnoid space between L3–L4 or L4–L5 vertebral bodies
- The spaces between L1–L3 should be avoided

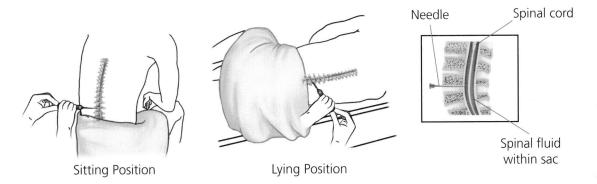

Sitting Position   Lying Position

Figure 14.3 Lumbar Puncture

Labs

- Commonly ordered labs of the CSF
  - Cell count with differential—usually sent in tubes 1 and 4
  - Protein and glucose–usually sent in tube 2
  - Culture and Gram stain—usually sent in tube 3
- Other tests may include immunoglobulins and oligoclonal bands for MS

Table 14.1 Analysis of Cerebrospinal Fluid

	Bacterial	Viral	TB/Fungal
Protein	Increased	Normal to increased	Increased
Glucose	Decreased	Normal	Decreased
Cells	Increased neutrophils	Increased lymphocytes	Increased lymphocytes
Pressure	Increased	Normal	Increased

Procedures

SPLINTING AND CASTING

Procedure performed to immobilize bones and/or joints

Indications

- To set fractures and to stabilize sprains/joints (after reduction of a dislocation)
- To protect deep lacerations across a joint, tendon lacerations

Contraindications/Cautions/Complications

- Complications: ischemia; compartment syndrome; pressure sores (especially if padding is not used); joint stiffness; neurologic injury
- Cautions: while more layers with casting (lower extremities) will provide extra strength, they will also create a bulkier/heavier splint producing more heat to the skin

Equipment/Preparation

- **Equipment:**
  - Plaster or fiberglass casting material; elastic bandages; padding
  - Dipping water and a basin (the warmer the water, the faster the splint will harden)
  - Gloves; adhesive tape or clips; stockinette; pads (to minimize mess from water/plaster)
  - Trauma scissors
- **Preparation:**
  - Assess neurovascular status and document any skin or soft tissue injuries
  - Dress any wounds (to reduce infection)

Procedure

- **Splinting:** Measure the stockinette and cover the area extending ~10 cm past each end of splint site (any excess can be folded over later to pad splint edges); usually stockinette 2–3 inches is used for upper extremities and 4 inches for lower extremities; to ensure proper circulation do not make stockinette too tight
- Estimate the length of the splint and add an additional 1–2 cm at each end (to compensate for shrinking due to the wetting/drying); try to keep splint slightly shorter than the padding
- Thickness of splint depends on patient's size, the extremity involved, and strength desired: upper extremities may require 6–10 layers while lower extremities may require 15
- Submerge splint in water until bubbling from the materials stops; remove and squeeze out excess water
- Place splint on hard surface and smooth out to remove wrinkles
  - Place the extremity in its position of function
  - Place wet splint over the padding and mold it to the contours of the extremity, using only the palm of the hand (using the fingers may cause pressure points)
  - Fold back the stockinette and padding edges, and secure splint with an elastic bandage wrapped in a distal to proximal direction: wrap evenly and overlap each previous layer of the bandage ~50% to avoid potential uneven wrapping
- **Casting** employs a similar technique, although the casting material is wrapped circumferentially with each roll overlapping the previous layer by 50%; the ideal cast isn't too tight or too loose (can be molded while it is still malleable)

INCISION AND DRAINAGE

Procedure performed to drain abscess >4–5 mm

Indications

- To treat paronychia that occurs on medial or lateral aspects of the fingers

Contraindications/Cautions/Complications

- Contraindications
  - Signs of infection without abscess
  - Abscess in certain locations that require consultation should be incised by that specialty; these locations include face, breast, finger pads, palms, rectum, vagina, mouth, and neck
- Complications: deeper infection due to inadequate drainage; fistulas; damage to nerves/vessels; scarring

Equipment/Preparation

- Equipment
  - Face-shield, gown, gloves, iodine solution/chlorhexidine, lidocaine, scalpel (11 blade), iodoform for packing, hemostats (curved), swab for wound culture, saline flushes for irrigation, gauze, sterile water, and tape
- Preparation
  - Palpate the area of the abscess to feel for fluctuance: if difficult to assess or unsure whether abscess exists, use bedside U/S to diagnose; once identified, administer appropriate anesthesia locally and proceed with procedure

Procedure

- Put on protective gear following universal precautions and start by preparing the area with chlorhexidine or iodine; place the anesthesia (usually lidocaine 1% or 2%) in the skin next to the abscess on all sides, creating a field block
- Using the 11 blade scalpel to make a linear incision starting at the area with the most fluctuance and working your way down on both sides
- Once pus is expressed, a wound culture may be taken if necessary; apply pressure on skin surrounding abscess to remove pus from within the cavity and then use the curved hemostat to break apart loculations within the abscess; make sure to break apart the loculations within the entire cavity of the abscess
- Using saline flushes and sterile water, irrigate the abscess cavity to remove excess pus until the fluid is clear
- Packing may then be done using iodoform; apply gauze on the wound; patient should return in 48 hours for removal of the packing and wound should be left to heal by secondary intention

Procedure for Acute Paronychia

- If **paronychia is present without an abscess**, treat with warm soaks for 20 minutes 3 times a day; apply mupirocin to decrease abscess formation
- If **paronychia is present with an abscess**, proceed with incision and drainage
  - Procedure: inject lidocaine to web spaces of involved digit to cause a digit block in that finger
  - Take an 11 blade and make an incision where the cuticle (on affected side of finger) and the skin meet at the side of the nail and extend the incision about 3–5 mm
  - Alternatively, lift up skin on the underside with the blade (so no incision is needed if there is a collection around the edge of the nail and the skin); pus should be seen immediately after incision; packing may be done with iodoform or wound may be left open to heal through secondary intention
  - Antibiotics not needed unless patient is immunocompromised or has high suspicion for infection

Procedures

TRACHEAL INTUBATION

Procedure performed by inserting a flexible tube into the trachea to maintain an open airway

Indications

- Therapeutic: to provide assistance to patients with insufficient ventilation/oxygenation, acute respiratory failure, and an inability to protect their airways (AMS); to assist patients who will undergo surgery receiving general anesthesia

Contraindications/Cautions/Complications

- Contraindications: laryngeal fractures; trauma to oral cavity and/or upper airways
- Caution in patients with burns to upper body and moderate to-severe laryngeal edema
- Complications: trauma to upper airway via laryngoscope; creation of false lumen/intubation in esophagus; damage to vocal cords and/or teeth; hypoxemia if intubation takes too long; aspiration

Equipment/Preparation

- Equipment
  - Endotracheal tube with accompanying stylet; laryngoscope handle with blade (Macintosh or Miller in adults, usually size 3–4); bougie in case unable to intubate with laryngoscope; syringe for inflation of endotracheal tube; tape or ETT holder; end-tidal carbon dioxide monitor; suction; bag with face mask; rescue airway; induction agent (etomidate) and paralyzing agent (rocuronium)
- Preparation
  - Have all equipment prepared beforehand and inflate ETT balloon to look for any leaks; patient should have IV access for medication administration and should be attached to a monitor; preoxygenate patient with a non-rebreather mask or other source; ensure that patient's head is positioned correctly to ensure proper visualization of the epiglottis; stylet should be inside the endotracheal tube
  - Administer induction agent and paralytic agent

Procedure

- Have laryngoscope in hand (with stylet inside) and open patient's mouth
- Move tongue aside to the left with laryngoscope and find the epiglottis (advance slowly and lift up blade to ensure epiglottis hasn't been passed); once found, insert end of the blade into the vallecula
- Lift up laryngoscope toward ceiling (upward) and you should see vocal cords; insert ETT through cords into the trachea (wind pipe)
- Be mindful of placing the tube into trachea; advance tube until 22–23 cm (men)/20–22 (women) from patient's teeth and take out stylet
- Inflate balloon of the ETT; using stethoscope, listen for air movement in lungs bilaterally, and confirm placement using the end-tidal carbon dioxide monitor (look for changes in color when exhaling occurs)
- Secure the ETT with tape or ETT holder; order chest x-ray to confirm placement
- During intubation, make sure to assess patients O_2 saturation; if ≤89, pause intubation and bag mask the patient
- Chest x-ray confirmation of the ETT should be a high priority after intubation
- Patients should be connected to a mechanical ventilator and transferred to the ICU

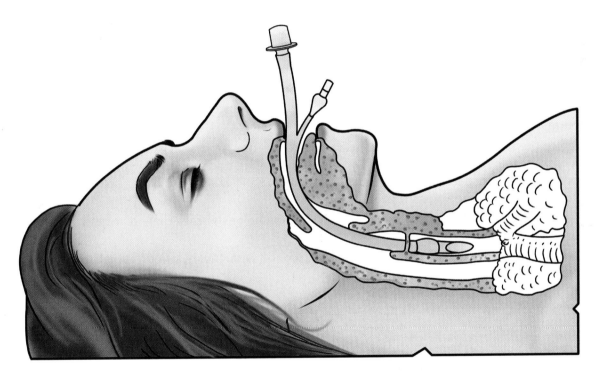

Figure 14.4 Tracheal Intubation

LACERATION REPAIR—SUTURING

Procedure performed to close open wounds

Indications

- To repair wounds that, if left open, would heal with significant scarring; usually on wounds that penetrate through the dermis of the skin
- In most cases skin closure should be done within 24 hours of original laceration to avoid infection within the wound

Contraindications/Cautions/Complications

- Contraindications:
  - Infected wounds; heavily contaminated wounds; suspected foreign bodies in wound; puncture wounds; animal/human bites; superficial abrasions
  - Consults should be called for all open fractures, complicated facial lacerations, heavily contaminated wounds, large wounds that must be sutured under sedation, and lacerations involving nerves and tendons
- Complications: scarring; infections; damage to nerves and vessels

Equipment/Preparation

- Equipment
  - Suture kit (needle driver, hemostat, scissors, forceps, sterile drape and gauze), sterile gloves
  - Iodine solution/chlorhexidine; lidocaine; saline for irrigation, sterile water; non-adhesive gauze; irrigation syringe (60 mL); sutures
- Preparation
  - Before preparing the skin for repair, make sure to perform a physical exam to rule out any nerve damage, tendon malfunctions, and possible foreign bodies in the wound; if radiopaque foreign body is suspected, x-rays should be ordered within the wound edges and make a field block by injecting the lidocaine around the wound
  - Prepare the area surrounding the laceration with iodine or chlorhexidine; place the anesthesia (usually lidocaine 1 or 2%)
  - Using the 60-mL irrigation syringe, irrigate the wound with 100 mL of normal saline or the sterile water per 1 cm of laceration size

Procedure

- Open suture tray and set up sterile field, open suture and drop into sterile field; put on sterile gloves
- **Simple interrupted sutures**
  - Clamp needle onto the driver at its center and use forceps to grab skin and elevate on one side
  - Insert needle at 90° into skin on one side of the laceration and take out of the other side
  - Make sure the distance between the incisions is the same measurement on both sides
  - Needle should penetrate through the skin at the base with same length it penetrates the wound at the surface
  - Make 4–5 knots through an instrument tie
- Clean skin around sutures (peroxide is a good choice); after drying, apply bacitracin ointment to the suture site and cover area with non-stick gauze
- Patient should remove dressing 24 hrs post-procedure and wash wound with soap/water daily (may apply bacitracin as well); patient should return for suture removal in 7–10 days (laceration on extremities) or 5–7 days (laceration on scalp/face)
- Antibiotics are usually unnecessary and should be prescribed on a case-by-case basis

CERVICAL SPINE EVALUATION/CLEARANCE

Assessment performed to rule out the presence of cervical injury

Indications

- To assess the cervical spine in all closed brain/traumatic brain injuries (all patients should first receive C-spine collar)
- Cervical spine "clearance" confirms the absence of cervical spine injury

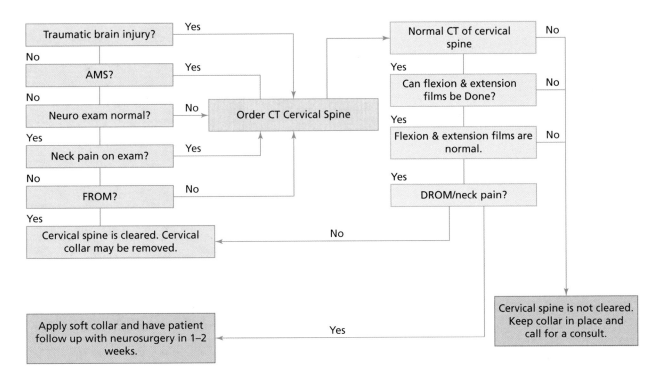

Figure 14.5 Algorithm for C-Spine Clearance

Index

Note: Major treatments are indicated by **bold** page number.

A

Abciximab, 352
Abortion, spontaneous. *See* Spontaneous abortion
Abruptio placentae, **183**
Acarbose, 362
ACE inhibitors, **345**
Acetylcholinesterase inhibitors, **337**
Acetylsalicylic acid/aspirin, 353
Achilles tendon rupture, **121**
Acid-based disorders, 81–82
  metabolic acidosis, 81
  metabolic alkalosis, 81
  mnemonics, 82
  respiratory acidosis, 82
  respiratory alkalosis, 82
  three-step approach to, 82
Acid burns, 148
Acidosis
  metabolic, 81
  respiratory, 82
ACL (anterior cruciate ligament), 117
Acoustic (vestibular) neuroma, **156**
Actinic keratosis, **267**
Acute acalculous cholecystitis, 91
Acute bronchiolitis, **80**
Acute cholecystitis, 91
Acute coronary syndrome, **8–10**
  clinical manifestations/physical exam, 8
  diagnosis, 8
  etiology/pathophysiology, 8
  management/prognosis, 9
  mnemonics, 9
  risk factors, 8
  schema (figure), 10

Acute epiglottitis (supraglottitis), **74**
Acute kidney injury, **212**
Acute lymphocytic leukemia, **324–325**
  clinical manifestations/physical exam, 324
  diagnosis, 324
  etiology/pathophysiology, 324
  management/prognosis, 324
  mnemonic, 325
  risk factors, 324
Acute myeloid leukemia (AML), **330–331**
  clinical manifestations/physical exam, 330
  diagnosis, 330
  etiology/pathophysiology, 330
  management/prognosis, 330
  mnemonics, 331
  risk factors, 330
Acute narrow angle closure glaucoma, **149**
Acute otitis media, **155**
Acute pancreatitis, **94**
Acute pericarditis, 16
Acute respiratory distress syndrome, 77
Adenomyosis, **163**
Adenosine, 348
ADP inhibitors, 352
Adrenocortical insufficiency, chronic, **199**
Adult polycystic kidney disease, **221**
Albuterol, 354

Alkali burns, 148
Alkalosis
  metabolic, 81
  respiratory, 82
Alpha-$_2$ agonists, **340**
Alpha beta receptor antagonists, 342
Alpha glucosidase inhibitors, 362
Alpha-$_1$ receptor agonists, **339**
Alpha thalassemia, 310
Alzheimer's disease, 238
Amantanes, 78
Amenorrhea, **160–161**
  clinical manifestations/physical exam, 160–161
  etiology/pathophysiology, 160
  mnemonic, 161
Amiloride, 344
Aminoglycosides, **283**
Aminopenicillins, 278
Amiodarone, 347, 348
Amitriptyline, 367
Amlodipine, 346
Amphenicol chloramphenicol, **290**
Anemia, **308–309**
  approach to, 308
  clinical manifestations/physical exam, 308
  diagnosis, 308
  etiology/pathophysiology, 308
  iron deficiency, 309
  management/prognosis, 309
  mnemonic, 309
  risk factors, 308
Anemia of chronic disease, **315**

Index

Angina pectoris, **6–7**
  clinical manifestations/physical exam, 6
  diagnosis, 6
  etiology/pathophysiology, 6
  management/prognosis, 6
  mnemonic, 7
  risk factors, 6
Ankle sprains, **120**
Ankylosing spondylitis, 125
Anterior cerebral artery stroke, **246**
Anterior cord syndrome, 254
Anterior cruciate ligament (ACL), 117
Anterior shoulder dislocation, 106
Anthracyclines, 371
Antiarrhythmic agents, **347**
Antibiotics, commonly used. See Commonly used antibiotics for infectious disease
Anticholinergics, **338**
Anticoagulant agents, **350–351**
  direct thrombin inhibitors, 351
  Factor X inhibitors, 351
  low molecular weight heparin, 350
  mnemonic, 351
  unfractionated heparin, 350
  warfarin, 351
Anticonvulsant medications, **360–361**
  ethosuximide, 360
  mnemonics, 360–361
  phenytoin, 360
Antiemetic agents, **359**
Antihistamines, second generation, 358
Anti-Parkinsonian agents, **364–365**
  dopamine agonists, 364
  levodopa/carbidopa, 364
  mnemonics, 364–365
Antiplatelet agents, **352–353**
  ADP inhibitors, 352
  glycoprotein IIB/IIIA inhibitors, 352
  salicylate/acetylsalicylic acid/aspirin, 353
  ticagrelor, 352

Antipseudomonal penicillins, 278
Antistaphylococcal penicillins, 278
Anti-tuberculosis medications, **355**
Aorta, coarctation of the, **27**
Aortic regurgitation/aortic insufficiency, **21**
Aortic stenosis, **20**
Apixaban, 351
Argatroban, 351
Aripiprazole, 370
Arrhythmia
  antiarrhythmic agents, **347**
  sinus, **42**
Arterial disease, peripheral, **37**
Arteries, transposition of the great, **31**
Arteriosus, patent ductus, **28**
Arthritis
  inflammatory, 375
  psoriatic, 261
  septic, 375
Arthrocentesis, **374–375**
  anatomic landmarks, 375
  contraindications/cautions/complications, 374
  equipment/preparation, 374
  indications, 374
  labs, 375
  procedure, 374
Ascitic fluid, analysis of, 378–379
Ascorbic acid (vitamin C) deficiency, 101
Asthma, **56–59**
  clinical manifestations/physical exam, 56
  diagnosis, 56
  management/prognosis, 57
  mnemonics, 58
  risk factors, 56
  stepwise therapy approach, 59
Asthma medications, **354**
Asystole rhythm, 52
Atenolol, 342, 347
Atopic dermatitis (eczema), **258**
Atrial flutter/atrial fibrillation, **45**
Atrial septal defect, **26**
Atrioventricular junctional dysrhythmias, **49**

Atriventricular blocks, **44**
Atropine, 338, 348

B
Babesiosis, **303**
Back pain, **123–126**
  ankylosing spondylitis, 125
  cauda equina syndrome, 123
  emergency back pain, 126
  evaluation, 123
  herniated disk (nucleus pulposus), 123
  lumbrosacral sprain/strain, 124
  mnemonics, 124, 126
  spinal compression fracture, 124
  spinal stenosis (pseudoclaudication), 124
  spondylolisthesis, 125
  spondylolysis, 125
Bacterial meningitis, **252–253**
  clinical manifestations/physical exam, 252
  diagnosis, 252
  etiology/pathophysiology, 252
  management/prognoisis, 252
  mnemonics, 253
Balance, loss of, 157
Basal cell carcinoma, **270**
B_{12} (cobalamin) deficiency, 102–103, **312–313**
  clinical manifestations/physical exam, 312
  diagnosis, 312
  etiology/pathophysiology, 312
  management/prognosis, 312
  mnemonics, 313
Benazepril, 345
Bennett fracture, 112
Benztropine, 338
Berylliosis, 65, 66
Beta-blockers, 347
Beta-2 receptor agonists, 354
Beta receptor antagonists (blockers), **342**
  alpha, 342
  cardioselective, 342
  nonselective, 342
Beta thalassemia, 310

Bethanechol, 336
Biguanides, 362
Bisoprolol, 342
Bivalirudin, 351
Bleomycin, 372
Blepharitis, 140
Blocks, atriventricular, **44**
Bradycardia, sinus, **41**
Broca's area, 243, 244
Bromocriptine, 364
Bronchiectasis, **62**
Bronchogenic carcinoma, **67**
Brown Sequard syndrome, 254
Budd Chiari syndrome, 97
Burn, chemical, **148**

C

Calcium channel blockers, **346**, 347
Calcium levels. *See* Hypercalcemia;
    Hypocalcemia
Campylobacter Jejuni, 104
Cancer
    ovarian, **178**
    papillary thyroid, **191**
    See also Carcinoma
Captopril, 345
Carbachol, 336
Carbidopa, 364
Carboplatin, 371
Carcinoma
    basal cell, **270**
    bronchogenic, **67**
    gastric, **90**
    non-small cell, 67
    small-cell, 67
    squamous cell, **269**
Cardiac agents commonly
    confused, **348**
Cardiac glycoside, 349
Cardiogenic shock, 34
Cardiomyopathy
    dilated, **11**
    hypertrophic, **13**
    restrictive, **12**
Cardioselective beta receptor
    antagonists, 342
Cardiovascular system, **1–52**
    acute coronary syndrome, **8–10**

angina pectoris, **6–7**
aortic regurgitation/aortic
    insufficiency, **21**
aortic stenosis, **20**
atrial flutter/atrial fibrillation, **45**
atrial septal defect, **26**
atrioventricular junctional
    dysrhythmias, **49**
atriventricular blocks, **44**
circulatory shock, **34–35**
coarctation of the aorta, **27**
congenital heart disease, **25**
dilated cardiomyopathy, **11**
ECG cheat sheet, **38**
heart failure, **2–5**
hypertension, **36**
hypertrophic cardiomyopathy, **13**
infective endocarditis, **32–33**
mitral regurgitation, **23**
mitral stenosis (MS), **22**
mitral valve prolapse, **24**
myocarditis, **14**
normal sinus rhythm, **39**
paroxysmal supraventricular
    tachycardia, **47**
patent ductus arteriosus, **28**
pericardial disease, **16–17**
peripheral arterial disease, **37**
restrictive cardiomyopathy, **12**
rheumatic fever, **15**
sick sinus syndrome
    (tachy-brady), **43**
sinus arrhythmia, **42**
sinus bradycardia, **41**
sinus tachycardia, **40**
tetralogy of Fallot, **30**
transposition of the great
    arteries, **31**
valvular disease, **18–19**
ventricular dysrhythmias, **50–52**
ventricular septal defect, **29**
wandering atrial pacemaker and
    multifocal atrial tachycardia, **46**
Wolff-Parkinson-White, **48**
Carvedilol, 342
Cataracts, **153**
Catheter, central line. *See* Central
    line catheter

Cauda equina syndrome, 123
Central cord syndrome, 254
Central line catheter, **382–383**
    contraindications/cautions/
        complications, 382
    dynamic method, 383
    equipment preparation, 382–383
    indications, 382
    procedure, 383
Central retinal artery
    occlusion, **152**
Cephalosporins, **282**
Cerebral artery stroke
    anterior, **246**
    posterior, **247**
Cervical spine evaluation/
    clearance, **391**
Cevimeline, 336
Chalazion, 141
Chemical burn, **148**
Chemoprophylaxis, 78
Chemotherapeutic
    agents, **371–372**
    anthracyclines, 371
    bleomycin, 372
    cyclophosphamide, 371
    mnemonics, 371, 372
    platinum agents, 371
Chlorothiazide, 343
Chlorpromazine, 369
Chlorthalidone, 343
Cholecystitis
    acute, 91
    chronic, 91
Cholesteatoma, **158**
Cholinergic drugs, **336**
Chronic adrenocortical
    insufficiency, **199**
Chronic cholecystitis, 91
Chronic lymphocytic leukemia
    (B cell), **326–327**
    clinical manifestations/physical
        exam, 326
    diagnosis, 326
    etiology/pathophysiology, 326
    management/prognosis, 326
    mnemonic, 327
    risk factors, 326

Chronic myelogenous leukemia (CML), **328–329**
  clinical manifestations/physical exam, 328
  diagnosis, 328
  etiology/pathophysiology, 328
  management/prognosis, 328
  mnemonic, 329
Chronic obstructive pulmonary disease (COPD), **60–61**
  clinical manifestations/physical exam, 60
  diagnosis, 60
  management/prognosis, 60
  mnemonics, 60–61
  risk factors, 60
Cimetidine, 357
Circulatory shock, **34–35**
  etiology/pathophysiology, 34
  management prognosis, 35
  mnemonic, 35
  risk factors, 34
Cirrhosis, **99**
Cisplatin, 371
Citalopram, 366
Clomipramine, 367
Clonidine, 340
Clopidogrel, 352
Cluster headaches, **240–241**
  clinical manifestations/physical exam, 240
  etiology/pathophysiology, 240
  management/prognoisis, 240
  mnemonics, 241
  risk factors, 240
CML. *See* Chronic myelogenous leukemia
Coal worker's lung, 65, 66
Coarctation of the aorta, **27**
Cobalamin deficiency. *See* B$_{12}$ deficiency
Colitis, ulcerative, 95
Collateral ligament injury, **117**
Commonly used antibiotics for infectious disease, **278–279**
  mnemonics, 279
  penicillins, 278
Congenital heart disease, **25**

Congenital hypothyroidism (cretinism), 187
Conjunctivitis (red eyes), **150**
Constrictive pericarditis, 17
COPD. *See* Chronic obstructive pulmonary disease
Corneal abrasion, **147**
Coronary syndrome, acute. *See* Acute coronary syndrome
Corrigan's pulse, 21
Corticosteroids, inhaled, 57
Cretinism (congenital hypothyroidism), 187
Creutzfeldt-Jakob disease, 238
Crigler-Najjar syndrome, 97
Crohn disease, 95
Cromolyn, 354
Cushing's syndrome, **200**
Cyanotic lesions, 25
Cyclopentolate, 338
Cyclophosphamide, 371
Cystic fibrosis, **63**
Cytochrome p$_{450}$ inducers, **334**
Cytochrome p$_{450}$ inhibitors, **335**
Cytomegalovirus (HHV g), **305**

D

Dalteparin, 350
Daunorubicin, 371
Dementia, **238–239**
  Alzheimer's disease, 238
  Creutzfeldt-Jakob disease, 238
  diffuse Lewy body disease, 238
  frontotemporal dementia (Pick's disease), 238
  mnemonics, 239
  vascular disease, 238
De Musset's sign, 21
Dermatology, **257–276**
  actinic keratosis, **267**
  atopic dermatitis (eczema), **258**
  basal cell carcinoma, **270**
  erythema multiforme, **264**
  lichen planus, **259**
  malignant melanoma, **271**
  molluscum contagiosum, **272**
  mumps, **274**
  pityriasis rosea, **260**

  pityriasis (tinea) versicolor, **262**
  psoriasis, **261**
  rosacea, **266**
  roseola (sixth's disease) HHV 6, **273**
  rubella (German measles), **276**
  rubeola (measles), **275**
  seborrheic dermatits, **263**
  seborrheic keratosis, **268**
  squamous cell carcinoma, **269**
  Stevens-Johnson syndrome and toxic epidermal necrolysis, **265**
Desipramine, 367
Desirudin, 351
Desvenlafaxine, 367
Dexlansoprazole, 356
Diabetes insipidus, **204–205**
  clinical manifestations/physical exam, 204
  diagnosis, 204
  etiology/pathophysiology, 204
  management/prognoisis, 204
  mnemonics, 205
Diabetes medications, **362–363**
  alpha glucosidase inhibitors, 362
  biguanides, 362
  DPP-4 inhibitors, 363
  glucagon-like peptide 1 agonists, 363
  mnemonics, 362, 363
  sulfonylureas, 362
  thiazolidinediones, 363
Diabetes mellitus, gestational, **182**
Diabetic ketoacidosis, **203**
Diastolic heart failure, 2, 5
Dicyclomine, 338
Diffuse Lewy body disease, 238
Digoxin/digitoxin, **349**
Dihydropyridines, 346
Dilated cardiomyopathy, **11**
Diltiazem, 346, 347
Direct thrombin inhibitors, 351
Diseases affecting bilirubin, **97–98**
  Budd Chiari syndrome, 97
  Crigler-Najjar syndrome, 97
  Dubin Johnson syndrome, 98
  Gilbert's syndrome, 97
Diseases of gallbladder, **91**

Dislocation
  hip, 113
  shoulder, **106**
Disopyramide, 347
Disseminated intravascular
    coagulation, **322**
Distributive shock, 34
Diuretics
  potassium-sparing, **344**
  thiazide/thiazide-like, **343**
Dizziness, 157
Dopamine, 359
Dopamine agonists, 364
Dopamine antagonists, 358
Doxepin, 367
Doxorubicin, 371
DPP-4 inhibitors, 363
Droperidol, 369
DU (duodenal ulcer), 89
Dubin Johnson syndrome, 98
Duloxetine, 367
Duodenal ulcer (DU), 89
Duroziez's sign, 21
Dysmenorrhea, **162**
Dysrhythmias
  atrioventricular junctional, **49**
  ventricular (See Ventricular
    dysrhythmias)

E
ECG cheat sheet, **38**
Ectopic pregnancy, **176–177**
  clinical manifestations/physical
    exam, 176
  diagnosis, 176
  management/prognoisis, 176
  mnemonics, 177
  risk factors, 176
Eczema, **258**
Edrophonium, 337
EENT, **139–158**
  acoustic (vestibular) neuroma, **156**
  acute narrow angle closure
    glaucoma, **149**
  acute otitis media, **155**
  cataracts, **153**
  central retinal artery occlusion, **152**
  chemical burn, **148**

cholesteatoma, **158**
conjunctivitis (red eyes), 150
eye disorders, **140–141**
foreign body (ocular) and
    corneal abrasion, **147**
globe rupture, **144**
macular degeneration, **145**
ophthalmia neonatorum, **142**
optic neuritis, **151**
orbital floor "blowout"
    fracture, **143**
otitis externa, **154**
retinal detachment, **146**
vertigo, **157**
Ehrlichiosis, **304**
Electrical activity, pulseless, 52
Emergency back pain, 126
Enalapril, 345
Endocarditis, infective. *See*
    Infective endocarditis
Endocrine system, **185–205**
  chronic adrenocortical
    insufficiency, **199**
  Cushing's syndrome, **200**
  diabetes insipidus, **204–205**
  diabetic ketoacidosis, **203**
  hyperaldosteronism, **201**
  hypercalcemia, **194–195**
  hyperthyroidism, **188–189**
  hypocalcemia, **196**
  hypoparathyroidism, **193**
  hypothyroidism, **186–187**
  osteomalacia/rickets, **197**
  papillary thyroid cancer, **191**
  pheochromocytoma, **202**
  prirnary
    hyperparathyroidism, **192**
  renal osteodystrophy, **198**
  subacute granulomatous
    thyroiditis, **190**
Endometrial cancer, **179**
Endometriosis, **164–165**
  clinical manifestations/physical
    exam, 164
  diagnosis, 164
  management/prognoisis, 164
  mnemonic, 165
  risk factors, 164

Endometritis, **170**
Enoxaparin, 350
Enterohemorrhagic *E. Coli*, 104
Epicondylitis, **110–111**
  lateral (tennis elbow), 110
  medial (golfer's
    elbow), 110
  mnemonics, 111
Epidural hematoma, 248
Epinephrine, 339
Eplerenone, 344
Eptifibatide, 352
Erythema multiforme, **264**
Escitalopram, 366
Esmolol, 342
Esomeprazole, 356
Esophageal varices, **86**
Esophagitis, **84**
Essential familial tremor
    (benign), **228**
Ethambutol, 71, 355
Ethosuximide, 360
Ewing's sarcoma, 127
Exenatide, 363
Eye disorders, **140–141**
  blepharitis, 140
  chalazion, 141
  hordeolum (stye), 140
  pinguecula, 141
  pterygium, 141

F
Factor X inhibitors, 351
Famotidine, 357
Felodipine, 346
Fibrillation, atrial, **45**
Fibrillation, ventricular, 50
Flecainide, 347
Fluoroquinolones, **286–287**
  contraindications/cautions/side
    effects, 286
  indications, 286
  mnemonics, 287
  MOA/pharmacokinetics, 286
Fluoxetine, 366
Fluphenazine, 369
Flutter, atrial, **45**
Fluvoxamine, 366

Folate deficiency, **314**

Fondaparinux, 351

Foreign body (ocular), **147**

Fractures, **108–109**
  Galeazzi, 108–109
  hip, 113
  mnemonics, 109
  Monteggia, 108, 109
  orbital floor "blowout," **143**
  proximal humeral, 108
  radial head, 108
  spinal compression, 124
  supracondylar, 108
  thumb, 112

Frontotemporal dementia (Pick's disease), 238

G

Galeazzi fracture, 108–109

Gamekeeper's thumb, 112

Gastric carcinoma, **90**

Gastric ulcer (GU), 89

Gastroesophageal reflux disease, **87**

Gastrointestinal system, **83–104**
  acute pancreatitis, **94**
  cirrhosis, **99**
  diseases affecting bilirubin, **97–98**
  diseases of gallbladder, **91**
  esophageal varices, **86**
  esophagitis, **84**
  gastric carcinoma, **90**
  gastroesophageal reflux disease, **87**
  hepatitis, **92–93**
  inflammatory bowel disease, **95–96**
  invasive diarrhea, **104**
  peptic ulcer disease (PUD), **88–89**
  Plummer-Vinson syndrome, **85**
  vitamin deficiencies, **101–103**
  Wilson's disease, **100**

Genitourinary system, **207–225**
  acute kidney injury, **212**
  adult polycystic kidney disease, **221**
  glomerulonephritis, 210–211
  hyperkalemia, **217**
  hypermagnesemia, **216**
  hypernatremia, **214**
  hypokalemia, **218–219**
  hypomagnesemia, **215**
  hyponatremia, **213**
  incontinence, **224–225**
  nephrolithiasis/urolithiasis, **222–223**
  nephrotic syndrome, **208–209**
  phimosis, **220**

Gestational diabetes mellitus, **182**

Gestational trophoblastic disease, **181**

GI anticholinergics, 338

Gilbert's syndrome, 97

Glaucoma, acute narrow angle closure, **149**

Globe rupture, **144**

Glomerulonephritis, **210–211**
  clinical manifestations/physical exam, 210
  diagnosis, 210
  etiology/pathophysiology, 210
  management/prognoisis, 210
  mnemonics, 210

Glucagon-like peptide 1 (GLP-1) agonists, 363

Glycopeptide vancomycin, **280–281**
  contraindications/cautions/side effects, 280
  indications, 280
  mnemonics, 281
  MOA/pharmacokinetics, 280

Glycoprotein IIB/IIIA inhibitors, 352

Goiter, nontoxic, 187

Golfer's elbow (medial epicondylitis), 110

Gout, **134**, 375

Granulomatosis with polyangiitis, **137**

Graves' disease, 189

Great arteries, transposition of the, **31**

GU (gastric ulcer), 89

Guillain-Barré syndrome, **231**

Guttate psoriasis, 261

H

Haloperidol, 369

Hashimoto's thyroiditis, 187

HAV (hepatitis A virus), 92

HBV (hepatitis B virus), 93

HCV (hepatitis C virus), 92

Headaches, cluster. *See* Cluster headaches

Heart disease, congenital, **25**

Heart failure, **2–5**
  clinical manifestations/physical exam, 2
  diagnosis, 2
  diastolic, 2, 5
  etiology/pathophysiology, 2
  left- vs right-sided, 2, 4
  management/prognosis, 3
  mnemonics, 3
  normal heart circulation vs, 4
  risk factors, 2
  systolic, 2, 5

Helicobacter pylori, 88

Hematology, **307–332**
  acute lymphocytic leukemia, **324–325**
  acute myeloid leukemia (AML), **330–331**
  anemia, **308–309**
  anemia of chronic disease, **315**
  B_{12} (cobalamin) deficiency, **312–313**
  chronic lymphocytic leukemia (B cell), **326–327**
  chronic myelogenous leukemia (CML), **328–329**
  disseminated intravascular coagulation, **322**
  folate deficiency, **314**
  hemolytic uremic syndrome, **321**
  heparin-induced thrombocytopenia (HIT), **320**
  hereditary spherocytosis, **316**
  immune (idiopathic) thrombocytopenic purpura, **318**
  lead poisoning (plumbism), **311**
  multiple myeloma (plasmacytoma), **332**
  sickle cell disease, **317**
  thalassemia, **310**
  thrombotic thrombocytopenic purpura, **319**
  von Willebrand disease, **323**

Hematoma
  epidural, 248
  subdural, 249
Hemolytic uremic syndrome, **321**
Hemorrhage
  intracerebral, 251
  intracranial (See Intracranial
    hemorrhage)
  subarachnoid, 250
Heparin
  low molecular weight, 350
  unfractionated, 350
Heparin-induced
    thrombocytopenia (HIT), **320**
Hepatitis, **92–93**
  hepatitis A virus (HAV), 92
  hepatitis B virus (HBV), 93
  hepatitis C virus (HCV), 92
Hepatitis A virus (HAV), 92
Hepatitis B virus (HBV), 93
Hepatitis C virus (HCV), 92
Hereditary spherocytosis, **316**
Herniated disk (nucleus
    pulposus), 123
Hill's sign, 21
Hip injuries, **113–114**
  hip dislocation, 113
  hip fracture, 113
  mnemonics, 114
Histamine-2 receptor blockers, 357
Homatropine, 338
Hordeolum (stye), 140
Huntington's disease, **230**
Hydrochlorothiazide, 343
Hyoscyamine, 338
Hyperaldosteronism, **201**
Hypercalcemia, **194–195**
  clinical manifestations/physical
    exam, 194
  diagnosis, 194
  etiology/pathophysiology, 194
  management/prognosis, 194
  workup for, 195
Hyperkalemia, **217**
Hypermagnesemia, **216**
Hypernatremia, **214**
Hypertension, **36**
Hyperthyroidism, **188–189**

clinical manifestations/physical
    exam, 188
  diagnosis, 188
  etiology/pathophysiology, 188
  Graves' disease, 189
  management/prognoisis, 188
  mnemonics, 188, 189
  risk factors, 188
Hypertrophic cardiomyopathy, **13**
Hypocalcemia, **196**
Hypokalemia, **218–219**
  clinical manifestations/physical
    exam, 218
  diagnosis, 218
  etiology/pathophysiology, 218
  management/prognoisis, 218
  mnemonic, 219
Hypomagnesemia, **215**
Hyponatremia, **213**
Hypoparathyroidism, **193**
Hypothyroidism, **186–187**
  clinical manifestations/physical
    exam, 186
  cretinism (congenital
    hypothyroidism), 187
  diagnosis, 186
  etiology/pathophysiology, 186
  Hashimoto's thyroiditis, 187
  iatrogenic, 187
  iodine deficiency, 187
  management/prognoisis, 186
  mnemonic, 186
  nontoxic goiter, 187
  risk factors, 186
Hypovolemic shock, 34

I

Iatrogenic hypothyroidism, 187
Imipramine, 367
Immune (idiopathic)
    thrombocytopenic purpura, **318**
Incision/drainage, **387**
Incomplete spinal cord
    injury, **254–256**
  anterior cord syndrome, 254
  Brown Sequard syndrome, 254
  central cord syndrome, 254
  mnemonics, 255–256
  posterior cord syndrome, 254

Incontinence, **224–225**
  mnemonic, 225
  overflow incontinence, 224
  stress incontinence, 224
  urge incontinence, 225
Indapamide, 343
Infant respiratory distress
    syndrome, 77
Infectious disease, **277–306**
  aminoglycosides, **283**
  amphenicol
    chloramphenicol, **290**
  babesiosis, **303**
  cephalosporins, **282**
  commonly used antibiotics for
    infectious disease, **278–279**
  cytomegalovirus (HHV g), **305**
  ehrlichiosis, **304**
  fluoroquinolones, **286–287**
  glycopeptide
    vancomycin, **280–281**
  Lyme disease, **298–299**
  macrolides, **285**
  malaria, **300–301**
  metronidazole, **288**
  osteomyelitis, **294–295**
  rashes that affect palms/soles, **292**
  Rocky Mountain spotted
    fever, **293**
  streptococcal pharyngitis, **291**
  syphilis, **296–297**
  tetracyclines, **284**
  trimethoprim-
    sulfamethoxazole, **289**
  tularemia, **302**
  wound management, **306**
Infective endocarditis, **32–33**
  clinical manifestations/physical
    exam, 32
  diagnosis, 33
  etiology/pathophysiology, 32
  management/prognosis, 33
  mnemonics, 32
Inflammatory arthritis, 375
Inflammatory bowel disease, **95–96**
  Crohn disease, 95
  mnemonic, 96
  ulcerative colitis, 95

Influenza, **78–79**
    clinical manifestations, 78
    diagnosis, 78
    etiology/pathophysiology, 78
    management, 78
    risk factors, 78
    vaccine, 79
Inhaled corticosteroids, 57
Inhibitors
    ACE, 345
    acetylcholinesterase, **337**
    alpha glucosidase, 362
    cytochrome p$_{450}$, **335**
Insufficiency, aortic, **21**
Intracerebral hemorrhage, 251
Intracranial hemorrhage,
    248–251, 250
    epidural hematoma, 248
    intracerebral hemorrhage, 251
    mnemonics, 248–250
    subarachnoid hemorrhage, 250
    subdural hematoma, 249
Intubation, tracheal. *See* Tracheal
    intubation
Invasive diarrhea, **104**
Inverse psoriasis, 261
Iodine deficiency, 187
Ipratropium bromide, 338
Iron deficiency anemia, 309
Isocarboxazid, 368
Isoniazid, 71, 355
IVDA endocarditis, 32

J
Janeway lesions, 292
JNC 8 guidelines, 36
Jones/pseudoJones fracture, **122**

K
Kawasaki syndrome, 292
K channel blockers, 347
Keratosis
    actinic, **267**
    seborrheic, **268**
Kidney disease, adult polycystic, **221**
Kidney injury, acute, **212**

L
LABA (long-lasting beta-2
    agonists), 57

Labetalol, 342
Laceration repair—suturing, **390**
Lansoprazole, 356
Laryngotracheobronchitis
    (croup), **76**
Lateral cruciate ligament (LCL), 117
Lateral epicondylitis (tennis
    elbow), 110
LCL (lateral cruciate ligament), 117
Lead poisoning (plumbism), **311**
Legg-Calvé perthes disease, **115**
Leiomyomata (uterine fibroids),
    166–167
    clinical manifestations/physical
        exam, 166
    diagnosis, 166
    management/prognoisis, 166
    mnemonic, 167
    risk factors, 166
Lepirudin, 351
Leukemia. *See* Acute lymphocytic
    leukemia; Acute myeloid
    leukemia (AML); Chronic
    lymphocytic leukemia (B
    cell); Chronic myelogenous
    leukemia (CML)
Leukotriene modifiers, 354
Leukotriene receptor antagonists,
    57, 354
Levalbuterol, 354
Levodopa, 364
Lichen planus, **259**
Lidocaine, 347
Ligament injury, collateral, **117**
Linagliptin, 363
Liraglutide, 363
Lisinopril, 345
LMWH (low molecular weight
    heparin), 350
Long-lasting beta-2 agonists
    (LABA), 57
Lower motor neuron lesions, **232**
Low molecular weight heparin
    (LMWH), 350
Lumbar puncture, **384–385**
    anatomic landmarks, 385
    contraindications/cautions/
        complications, 384

equipment/preparation, 384
    indications, 384
    labs, 385
    procedure, 384–385
Lumbrosacral sprain/strain, 124
Lung disease, **54–55**
    mnemonics, 54
    obstructive, 54, 55
    restrictive, 54, 55
Lurasidone, 370
Lyme disease, **298–299**
    clinical manifestations/physical
        exam, 298
    diagnosis, 298
    etiology/pathophysiology, 298
    management/prognoisis, 298
    mnemonics, 299
Lymphocytic leukemia
    acute (*See* Acute lymphocytic
        leukemia)
    chronic (*See* Chronic lymphocytic
        leukemia)

M
Macrolides, **285**
Macular degeneration, **145**
Magnesium sulfate, 57
Malaria, **300–301**
    clinical manifestations/physical
        exam, 300
    diagnosis, 300
    etiology/pathophysiology, 300
    management/prognoisis, 300
    mnemonics, 301
Malignant melanoma, **271**
Mast cell modifiers, 57, 354
Medial cruciate ligament
    (MCL), 117
Medial epicondylitis (golfer's
    elbow), 110
Melanoma, malignant, **271**
Meningitis, bacterial. *See* Bacterial
    meningitis
Meniscal tears, **118**
Menopause, **171**
Menstruation
    amenorrhea (*See* Amenorrhea)
    dysmenorrhea, **162**
Metabolic acidosis, 81

Metabolic alkalosis, 81

Metaproterenol, 354

Metformin, 362

Methacholine, 336

Methylphenidate, 339

Metolazone, 343

Metoprolol, 342, 347

Metronidazole, **288**

Middle cerebral artery stroke, **244–245**
  clinical manifestations/physical exam, 244
  mnemonics, 245

Middle cerebral artery syndromes, **243**

Midodrine, 339

Miglitol, 362

Misoprostol, 358

Mitral regurgitation, **23**

Mitral stenosis (MS), **22**

Mitral valve prolapse, **24**

MOA/pharmacokinetics, 356

Molluscum contagiosum, **272**

Monteggia fracture, 108, 109

Montelukast, 354

Motor cortex, 243

Motor neuron lesions
  lower, **232**
  upper, **233**

MS (mitral stenosis), **22**

Müller's sign, 21

Multifocal atrial tachycardia, wandering atrial pacemaker and, **46**

Multiple myeloma (plasmacytoma), **332**

Multiple sclerosis, **236–237**
  clinical manifestations/physical exam, 236
  diagnosis, 236
  etiology/pathophysiology, 236
  management/prognosis, 236
  mnemonics, 237
  risk factors, 236

Mumps, **274**

Musculoskeletal system, **105–137**
  Achilles tendon rupture, **121**
  ankle sprains, **120**

back pain, **123–126**
collateral ligament injury, **117**
epicondylitis, **110–111**
fractures, **108–109**
gout, **134**
granulomatosis with polyangiitis, **137**
hip injuries, **113–114**
Jones/pseudoJones fracture, **122**
Legg-Calvé perthes disease, **115**
meniscal tears, **118**
Osgood-Schlatter disease, **119**
osteoarthritis, **136**
osteochondroma, **128**
polymyalgia rheumatica, **133**
rheumatoid arthritis, **135**
rotator cuff injuries, **107**
sarcoma, **127**
scleroderma (systemic sclerosis), **129**
shoulder dislocation, **106**
Sjögren's syndrome, **132**
slipped capital femoral epiphysis, **116**
systemic lupus erythematosus, **130–131**
thumb injuries, **112**

Myasthenia gravis, **234–235**
  clinical manifestations/physical exam, 234
  diagnosis, 234
  etiology/pathophysiology, 234
  management/prognosis, 234
  mnemonics, 235
  risk factors, 234

Myelogenous leukemia, chronic. *See* Chronic myelogenous leukemia (CML)

Myeloid leukemia, acute. *See* Acute myeloid leukemia (AML)

Myocarditis, **14**

N

Nadolol, 342

Nail bed removal, **381**

Native valve endocarditis (NVE), 32

Nedocromil, 354

Neostigmine, 337

Nephrolithiasis/ urolithiasis, **222–223**
  clinical manifestations/physical exam, 222
  diagnosis, 222
  etiology/pathophysiology, 222
  management/prognosis, 222
  mnemonics, 223

Nephrotic syndrome, **208–209**
  clinical manifestations/physical exam, 208
  diagnosis, 208
  etiology/pathophysiology, 208
  management/prognosis, 208
  mnemonics, 209

Neuramidase inhibitors, 78

Neuroleptic agents, **369–370**
  first generation (typical), 369
  mnemonics, 369, 370
  second generation (atypical), 370

Neurology, **227–256**
  anterior cerebral artery stroke, **246**
  bacterial meningitis, **252–253**
  cluster headaches, **240–241**
  dementia, **238–239**
  essential familial tremor (benign), **228**
  Guillain-Barré syndrome, **231**
  Huntington's disease, **230**
  incomplete spinal cord injury, **254–256**
  intracranial hemorrhage, **248–251**
  lower motor neuron lesions, **232**
  middle cerebral artery stroke, **244–245**
  middle cerebral artery syndromes, **243**
  multiple sclerosis, **236–237**
  myasthenia gravis, **234–235**
  Parkinson's disease, **229**
  posterior cerebral artery stroke, **247**
  Tourette syndrome, **242**
  upper motor neuron lesions, **233**

Niacin/nicotinic acid (B3) deficiency, 103

Nicardipine, 346

Nifedipine, 346
Nizatidine, 357
Non-cyanotic lesions, 25
Non-dihydropyridines, 346
Nonselective alpha-receptor antagonists, **341**
Nonselective beta receptor antagonists, 342
Non-small cell carcinoma, 67
Nonsocomial endocarditis, 32
Nontoxic goiter, 187
Norepinephrine reuptake inhibitors, 367
Normal sinus rhythm, **39**
Nortriptyline, 367
Nucleus pulposus (herniated disk), 123
NVE (native valve endocarditis), 32

O

Obstructive lung disease, 54, 55
Obstructive pulmonary disease, chronic. *See* Chronic obstructive pulmonary disease (COPD)
Obstructive shock, 34
Olanzapine, 370
Omalizumab, 57
Omeprazole, 356
Ophthalmia neonatorum, **142**
Ophthalmic anticholrinergics, 338
Optic neuritis, **151**
Orbital floor "blowout" fracture, **143**
Osgood-Schlatter disease, **119**
Osteoarthritis, **136**
Osteochondroma, **128**
Osteodystrophy, renal, **198**
Osteomalacia/rickets, **197**
Osteomyelitis, **294–295**
    clinical manifestations/physical exam, 294
    diagnosis, 294
    etiology/pathophysiology, 294
    management/prognoisis, 294
    mnemonics, 295
Osteosarcoma, 127
Otitis externa, **154**
Otitis media, acute, **155**

Ovarian cancer, **178**
Overflow incontinence, 224
Oxybutynin, 338
Oxymetazoline, 339

P

Pacemaker, wandering atrial, **46**
Palms, rashes that affect the, **292**
Pantoprazole, 356
Papillary thyroid cancer, **191**
Paracentesis, **378–379**
    analysis of ascitic fluid, 379
    contraindications/cautions/ complications, 378
    equipment/preparation, 378
    indications, 378
    procedure, 378–379
Paraphimosis, 220
Parkinson's disease, **229**
    anti-Parkinsonian agents, **364–365**
Paroxetine, 366
Paroxysmal supraventricular tachycardia, **47**
Patent ductus arteriosus, **28**
PCL (posterior cruciate ligament), 117
PCOS. *See* Polycystic ovarian syndrome
Pelvic organ prolapse (POP), **180**
Penicillins, 278
Peptic ulcer disease (PUD), **88–89**
    clinical manifestations/physical exam, 88
    diagnosis, 88
    duodenal ulcer (DU), 89
    etiology/pathophysiology, 88
    gastric ulcer (GU), 89
    Helicobacter pylori, 88
    management/prognoisis, 88
    risk factors, 88
    See also Peptic ulcer disease medications
Peptic ulcer disease medications, **356–358**
    contraindications/cautions/side effects, 357
    dopamine antagonists, 358

histamine-2 receptor blockers, 357
    indications, 356
    misoprostol, 358
    mnemonics, 356–358
    MOA/pharmacokinetics, 356
    proton pump inhibitors, 356
    second generation antihistamines, 358
    serotonin antagonists, 358
    sucralfate, 358
Pericardial disease, **16–17**
    acute pericarditis, 16
    constrictive pericarditis, 17
    mnemonics, 16, 17
Pericardial effusion, 16–17
Pericardial tamponade, 17
Pericardiocentesis, **380**
Peripheral arterial disease, **37**
Perphanazine, 369
Pertussis (whooping cough), **75**
Pharmacology, **333–372**
    ACE inhibitors, **345**
    acetylcholinesterase inhibitors, **337**
    alpha-$_2$ agonists, **340**
    alpha-$_1$ receptor agonists, **339**
    antiarrhythmic agents, **347**
    anticholinergics, **338**
    anticoagulant agents, **350–351**
    anticonvulsant medications, **360–361**
    antiemetic agents, **359**
    anti-Parkinsonian agents, **364–365**
    antiplatelet agents, **352–353**
    anti-tuberculosis medications, **355**
    asthma medications, **354**
    beta receptor antagonists (blockers), **342**
    calcium channel blockers, **346**
    cardiac agents commonly confused, **348**
    chemotherapeutic agents, **371–372**
    cholinergic drugs, **336**
    cytochrome p$_{450}$ inducers, **334**

cytochrome p$_{450}$ inhibitors, **335**
diabetes medications, **362–363**
digoxin/digitoxin, **349**
neuroleptic agents, **369–370**
nonselective alpha-receptor
    antagonists, **341**
peptic ulcer disease medications,
    356–358
potassium-sparing diuretics, **344**
psychotherapeutic
    agents, **366–368**
thiazide/thiazide-like
    diuretics, **343**
Pharyngitis, streptococcal, **291**
Phenelzine, 368
Phenformin, 362
Phenobarbital, 338
Phenoxybenzamine, 341
Phentolamine, 341
Phenylephrine, 339
Phenytoin, 360
Pheochromocytoma, **202**
Phimosis, **220**
Pick's disease (frontotemporal
    dementia), 238
Pilocarpine, 336
Pinguecula, 141
Pioglitazone, 363
Pistol shot, 21
Pityriasis rosea, **260**
Pityriasis (tinea) versicolor, **262**
Plaque psoriasis, 261
Plasmacytoma, **332**
Platinum agents, 371
Pleural effusion, **69**
Plummer-Vinson syndrome, **85**
Pneumoconiosis, **65–66**
    berylliosis, 65, 66
    coal worker's lung, 65, 66
    mnemonics, 65, 66
    silicosis, 65, 66
Pneumonia, **72–73**
    etiology/pathophysiology, 72
    management/prognosis, 72
    mnemonics, 73
Pneumothorax, **70**
Polycystic kidney disease,
    adult, **221**

Polycystic ovarian syndrome
    (PCOS), **172–173**
    clinical manifestations/physical
        exam, 172
    diagnosis, 172
    etiology/pathophysiology, 172
    management/prognoisis, 172
    mnemonics, 173
Polymyalgia rheumatica, **133**
POP (pelvic organ prolapse), **180**
Posterior cerebral artery stroke, **247**
Posterior cord syndrome, 254
Posterior cruciate ligament
    (PCL), 117
Posterior shoulder dislocation, 106
Postrenal injury, 212
Potassium-sparing diuretics, **344**
PPIs (proton pump inhibitors), 356
Pramiprexole, 364
Prasugrel, 352
Pregnancy, ectopic. *See* Ectopic
    pregnancy
Premature ventricular complex, 50
Premenstrual syndrome, **168–169**
    clinical manifestations/physical
        exam, 168
    diagnosis, 168
    etiology/pathophysiology, 168
    management/prognoisis, 168
    mnemonics, 169
Prerenal injury, 212
Primary hyperparathyroidism, **192**
Procainamide, 347
Procedures, **373–391**
    arthrocentesis, **374–375**
    central line catheter, **382–383**
    cervical spine evaluation/
        clearance, **391**
    incision/drainage, **387**
    laceration repair—suturing, **390**
    lumbar puncture, **384–385**
    nail bed removal, **381**
    paracentesis, **378–379**
    pericardiocentesis, **380**
    splinting/casting, **386**
    thoracentesis, **376–377**
    tracheal intubation, **388–389**
Prolapse, mitral valve, **24**

Propafenone, 347
Propantheline, 338
Propranolol, 342
Prosthetic valve endocarditis
    (PVE), 32
Proton pump inhibitors (PPIs), 356
Proximal humeral fracture, 108
Pseudoclaudication (spinal
    stenosis), 124
Pseudoephedrine, 339
Pseudogout, 375
Psoriasis, **261**
Psoriatic arthritis, 261
Psychotherapeutic agents, **366–368**
    mnemonics, 366–368
    nonselective MAO inhibitors, 368
    selective serotonin reuptake
        inhibitors, 366
    serotonin and norepinephrine
        reuptake inhibitors, 367
    tricyclic antidepressants, 367
Pterygium, 141
PUD. *See* Peptic ulcer disease
Pulmonary embolism, **68**
Pulmonary system, **53–82**
    acid-based disorders, **81–82**
    acute bronchiolitis, **80**
    acute epiglottitis
        (supraglottitis), **74**
    asthma, **56–59**
    bronchiectasis, **62**
    bronchogenic carcinoma, **67**
    chronic obstructive pulmonary
        disease, **60–61**
    cystic fibrosis, **63**
    influenza, **78–79**
    laryngotracheobronchitis
        (croup), **76**
    lung disease, **54–55**
    pertussis (whooping cough), **75**
    pleural effusion, **69**
    pneumoconiosis, **65–66**
    pneumonia, **72–73**
    pneumothorax, **70**
    pulmonary embolism, **68**
    respiratory distress syndrome, **77**
    sarcoidosis, **64**
    tuberculosis, **71**

Pulseless electrical activity, 52
Pustular psoriasis, 261
PVE (prosthetic valve
    endocarditis), 32
Pyrazinamide, 71, 355
Pyridostigmine, 337
Pyridoxine (B6) deficiency, 103

Q

Quetiapine, 370
Quinapril, 345
Quincke's pulse, 21
Quinidine, 347

R

Rabeprazole, 356
Radial head fracture, 108
Ramipril, 345
Ranitidine, 357
Rashes that affect the
    palms/soles, **292**
Red eyes (conjunctivitis), **150**
Red man syndrome, 280
Regurgitation
    aortic, **21**
    mitral, **23**
Renal osteodystrophy, **198**
Reproductive system, **159–183**
    abruptio placentae, **183**
    adenomyosis, **163**
    amenorrhea, **160–161**
    dysmenorrhea, **162**
    ectopic pregnancy, **176–177**
    endometrial cancer, **179**
    endometriosis, **164–165**
    endometritis, **170**
    gestational diabetes
        mellitus, **182**
    gestational trophoblastic
        disease, **181**
    leiomyomata (uterine
        fibroids), **166–167**
    menopause, **171**
    ovarian cancer, **178**
    pelvic organ prolapse (POP), **180**
    polycystic ovarian syndrome
        (PCOS), **172–173**
    premenstrual syndrome, **168–169**
    spontaneous abortion, **174–175**

Respiratory acidosis, 82
Respiratory alkalosis, 82
Respiratory distress syndrome, **77**
Restrictive cardiomyopathy, **12**
Restrictive lung disease, 54, 55
Retinal artery occlusion,
    central, **152**
Retinal detachment, **146**
Rheumatic fever, **15**
Rheumatoid arthritis, **135**
Riboflavin (B2) deficiency, 103
Rickets, **197**
Rifampin, 71, 355
Risperidone, 370
Rivaroxaban, 351
Rivastigmine, 337
Rocky Mountain spotted fever, **293**
Rolando fracture, 112
Ropinirole, 364
Rosacea, **266**
Roseola (Sixth's disease)
    HHV 6, **273**
Rosiglitazone, 363
Rotator cuff injuries, **107**
Rubella (German measles), **276**
Rubeola (measles), **275**

S

SABA (short-acting beta-2
    agonists), 57
Salicylate, 353
Salmeterol, 354
Salmonella, 104
Sarcoidosis, **64**
Sarcoma, **127**
Schwann cells, 156
Scleroderma (systemic
    sclerosis), **129**
Scopolamine, 338
Seborrheic dermatits, **263**
Seborrheic keratosis, **268**
Second generation
    antihistamines, 358
Selective serotonin reuptake
    inhibitors, 366
Sensory cortex, 243
Septal defect
    atrial, **26**
    ventricular, **29**

Septic arthritis, 375
Septic shock, 34
Serotonin antagonists, 358
Serotonin receptor
    antagonists, 359
Serotonin reuptake inhibitors, 367
Sertraline, 366
Shigella dysenteriae, 104
Shock, circulatory. *See*
    Circulatory shock
Short-acting antimuscarinic
    (anticholinergic) agents, 57
Short-acting beta-2 agonists
    (SABA), 57
Shoulder dislocation, **106**
Sickle cell disease, **317**
Sick sinus syndrome
    (tachy-brady), **43**
Silicosis, 65, 66
Sinus arrhythmia, **42**
Sinus bradycardia, **41**
Sinus rhythm, normal, **39**
Sinus syndrome, sick, **43**
Sinus tachycardia, **40**
Sitagliptin, 363
Sixth's disease, **273**
Sjögren's syndrome, **132**
Skier's thumb, 112
Slipped capital femoral
    epiphysis, **116**
Small-cell carcinoma, 67
Soles, rashes that affect the, **292**
Sotalol, 342
Spherocytosis, hereditary, **316**
Spinal compression fracture, 124
Spinal cord injury, incomplete. *See*
    Incomplete spinal cord injury
Spinal stenosis
    (pseudoclaudication), 124
Spironolactone, 344
Splinting/casting, **386**
Spondylitis, ankylosing, 125
Spondylolisthesis, 125
Spondylolysis, 125
Spontaneous abortion, **174–175**
    clinical manifestations/physical
        exam, 174
    diagnosis, 174

etiology/pathophysiology, 174
management/prognoisis, 175
risk factors, 174
Sprains
    ankle, **120**
    lumbrosacral, 124
Squamous cell carcinoma, **269**
Stenosis
    aortic, **20**
    mitral, **22**
Stevens-Johnson syndrome and
    toxic epidermal necrolysis, **265**
Strain, lumbrosacral, 124
Streptococcal pharyngitis, **291**
Streptomycin, 71, 355
Stress incontinence, 224
Stroke
    anterior cerebral artery, **246**
    posterior cerebral artery, **247**
Stye (hordeolum), 140
Subacute granulomatous
    thyroiditis, **190**
Subarachnoid hemorrhage, 250
Subdural hematoma, 249
Sucralfate, 358
Sulfonylureas, 362
Supracondylar fracture, 108
Swimmer's ear, 154
Syphilis, **296–297**
    clinical manifestations/physical
        exam, 296
    diagnosis, 297
    etiology/pathophysiology, 296
    management/prognoisis, 297
Systemic glucocorticoids, 57
Systemic lupus erythematosus,
    130–131
    clinical manifestations/physical
        exam, 130
    diagnosis, 130
    etiology/pathophysiology, 130
    management/prognoisis, 130
    mnemonics, 131
    risk factors, 130
Systolic heart failure, 2, 5

T

Tachycardia
    multifocal atrial, **46**

paroxysmal supraventricular, **47**
    sinus, **40**
    ventricular, 50–51
Tears, meniscal, **118**
Tennis elbow (lateral
    epicondylitis), 110
Terbutaline, 354
Tetracyclines, **284**
Tetralogy of Fallot, **30**
Thalassemia, **310**
Thiamine (B1) deficiency, 102
Thiazide/thiazide-like
    diuretics, **343**
Thiazolidinediones, 363
Thioridazine, 369
Thoracentesis, **376–377**
    contraindications/cautions/
        complications, 376
    equipment/preparation, 376
    indications, 376
    labs, 377
    procedure, 376–377
Thrombocytopenia, heparin-
    induced, **320**
Thrombocytopenic purpura
    immune, **318**
    thrombotic, **319**
Thrombotic thrombocytopenic
    purpura, **319**
Thumb injuries, **112**
Thyroid. *See* Hyperthyroidism;
    Hypothyroidism
Ticagrelor, 352
Ticlopidine, 352
Timolol, 342
Tiotropium, 338
Tirofiban, 352
Tocainide, 347
Tolterodine, 338
Tourette syndrome, **242**
Toxic epidermal necrolysis, **265**
Tracheal intubation, **388–389**
    contraindications/cautions/
        complications, 388
    equipment/preparation, 388
    indications, 388
    procedure, 389
Trandolapril, 345

Transposition of the great
    arteries, **31**
Tranylcypromine, 368
Traube sign, 21
Triamterene, 344
Tricyclic antidepressants, 367
Trihexyphenidyl, 338
Trimethoprim-sulfamethoxazole,
    289
Tuberculosis medications, **355**
Tularemia, **302**

U

Ulcer, peptic, disease medications,
    356–358
Ulcerative colitis, 95
Unfractionated heparin, 350
Upper motor neuron lesions, **233**
Urge incontinence, 225
Urolithiasis. *See* Nephrolithiasis/
    urolithiasis
Uterine fibroids. *See*
    Leiomyomata

V

Valvular disease, **18–19**
    mnemonics, 18, 19
    murmurs, 18
Vascular disease, 238
Venlafaxine, 367
Ventricular dysrhythmias, **50–52**
    asystole rhythm, 52
    fibrillation, ventricular, 50
    premature ventricular
        complex, 50
    pulseless electrical activity, 52
    tachycardia, ventricular, 51
Ventricular septal defect, **29**
Verapamil, 346, 347
Vertigo, **157**
Vestibular neuroma, **156**
Vestibular (acoustic)
    neuroma, **156**
Vitamin A deficiency, 101
Vitamin B deficiency, 102–103
    See also B12 (cobalamin)
        deficiency
Vitamin C (ascorbic acid)
    deficiency, 101

Vitamin D deficiency, 101
Vitamin deficiencies, **101–103**
    mnemonics, 101, 102
    vitamin A deficiency, 101
    vitamin B deficiency, 102–103
    vitamin C (ascorbic acid)
        deficiency, 101
    vitamin D deficiency, 101
Von Willebrand disease, **323**

W
Wandering atrial pacemaker and
    multifocal atrial tachycardia, **46**
Warfarin, 351
Water hammer, 21
Wernicke's area, 243, 244
Wilson's disease, **100**
Wolff-Parkinson-White, **48**
Wound management, **306**

Y
Yersinia Enterocolitica, 104

Z
Zafirlukast, 354
Zileuton, 354
Ziprasidone, 370